SELF AND RELATIONSHIPS

Self and Relationships

CONNECTING INTRAPERSONAL AND INTERPERSONAL PROCESSES

edited by
KATHLEEN D. VOHS
ELI J. FINKEL

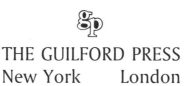

THE GUILFORD PRESS
New York   London

© 2006 The Guilford Press
A Division of Guilford Publications, Inc.
72 Spring Street, New York, NY 10012
www.guilford.com

Printed in the United States of America

This book is printed on acid-free paper.

Last digit is print number: 9   8   7   6   5   4   3   2   1

Library of Congress Cataloging-in-Publication Data

Self and relationships : connecting intrapersonal and interpersonal processes /
edited by Kathleen D. Vohs, Eli J. Finkel.
    p. cm.
  Includes bibliographical references and index.
  ISBN-10 1-59385-271-1 ISBN-13 978-1-59385-271-9 (hardcover)
  1. Self—Social aspects.   2. Self.   3. Interpersonal relations.   I. Vohs,
Kathleen D.   II. Finkel, Eli J.
  BF697.5.S65S45 2006
  158.2—dc22

                           2005028086

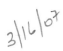
3\16\07

For our families,
who taught us to value both the self
and relationships

About the Editors

Kathleen D. Vohs, PhD, is Assistant Professor in the Carlson School of Management at the University of Minnesota. After receiving her PhD in psychological and brain sciences from Dartmouth College in 2000, Dr. Vohs conducted research at the University of Utah and Case Western Reserve University under a grant from the National Institute of Mental Health. Most recently, she held the Canada Research Chair in Marketing Science and Consumer Psychology at the University of British Columbia. Dr. Vohs has contributed over 60 professional publications, which focus on understanding processes related to self-regulation, self-esteem, interpersonal functioning, impulsive spending, impression management, and bulimia. Her research has been extended to the domains of chronic dieting, sexuality, and personal finances.

Eli J. Finkel, PhD, is Assistant Professor in the Department of Psychology at Northwestern University. After receiving his PhD in social psychology from the University of North Carolina at Chapel Hill in 2001, Dr. Finkel served for 2 years as a postdoctoral fellow at Carnegie Mellon University under a grant from the National Institutes of Health. His research has examined the impact of self-processes (e.g., self-concept, self-regulatory dynamics, narcissistic entitlement) on relationships, and of relationship processes (e.g., interpersonal emotion expression, relationship commitment, social coordination) on the self. Dr. Finkel's most recent research focuses on the interplay between self and relationship dynamics in the first minutes, hours, and days of initial romantic attraction.

Contributors

Christopher R. Agnew, PhD, Department of Psychological Sciences, Purdue University, West Lafayette, Indiana

Arthur Aron, PhD, Department of Psychology, Stony Brook University, Stony Brook, New York

Roy F. Baumeister, PhD, Department of Psychology, Florida State University, Tallahassee, Florida

Ginette C. Blackhart, MS, Department of Psychology, Florida State University, Tallahassee, Florida

Amy B. Brunell, MA, Department of Psychology, University of Georgia, Athens, Georgia

W. Keith Campbell, PhD, Department of Psychology, University of Georgia, Athens, Georgia

Amy Canevello, PhD, Department of Psychology, University of Houston, Houston, Texas

Jennifer Crocker, PhD, Department of Psychology, University of Michigan, Ann Arbor, Michigan

Portia S. Dyrenforth, BA, Department of Psychology, Michigan State University, East Lansing, Michigan

Marie-Joelle Estrada, MA, University of North Carolina, Chapel Hill, North Carolina

Paul E. Etcheverry, PhD, Department of Psychology, University of Texas, Arlington, Texas

Brooke C. Feeney, PhD, Department of Psychology, Carnegie Mellon University, Pittsburgh, Pennsylvania

Eli J. Finkel, PhD, Department of Psychology, Northwestern University, Evanston, Illinois

Catrin Finkenauer, PhD, Department of Social Psychology, Free University, Amsterdam, The Netherlands

Gráinne Fitzsimons, PhD, Department of Psychology, University of Waterloo, Waterloo, Ontario, Canada

Wendi L. Gardner, PhD, Department of Psychology, Northwestern University, Evanston, Illinois

Thomas E. Joiner, Jr., PhD, Department of Psychology, Florida State University, Tallahassee, Florida

Nils B. Jostmann, PhD, Department of Social Psychology, Free University, Amsterdam, The Netherlands

C. Raymond Knee, PhD, Department of Psychology, University of Houston, Houston, Texas

Sander L. Koole, PhD, Department of Social Psychology, Free University, Amsterdam, The Netherlands

Julius Kuhl, DrPhil, Department of Psychology, University of Osnabrück, Osnabrück, Germany

Madoka Kumashiro, PhD, Department of Social Psychology, Free University, Amsterdam, The Netherlands

Mark R. Leary, PhD, Department of Psychology, Wake Forest University, Winston-Salem, North Carolina

Alicia Limke, PhD, Department of Psychology, University of Oklahoma, Norman, Oklahoma

Richard E. Lucas, PhD, Department of Psychology, Michigan State University, East Lansing, Michigan

Lora E. Park, PhD, Department of Psychology, University at Buffalo, State University of New York, Buffalo, New York

Catherine D. Rawn, MA, Department of Psychology, University of British Columbia, Vancouver, British Columbia, Canada

Caryl E. Rusbult, PhD, Department of Social Psychology, Free University, Amsterdam, The Netherlands

Elizabeth A. Seeley, PhD, Department of Management and Organizations, Leonard N. Stern School of Business, New York University, New York, New York

James Shah, PhD, Department of Psychology, Duke University, Durham, North Carolina

Carolin J. Showers, PhD, Department of Psychology, University of Oklahoma, Norman, Oklahoma

Greg Strong, MA, Department of Psychology, Stony Brook University, Stony Brook, New York

Jean M. Twenge, PhD, Department of Psychology, San Diego State University, San Diego, California

Paul A. M. Van Lange, PhD, Department of Social Psychology, Free University, Amsterdam, The Netherlands

Kimberly A. Van Orden, MS, Department of Psychology, Florida State University, Tallahassee, Florida

Kathleen D. Vohs, PhD, Carlson School of Management, University of Minnesota, Minneapolis, Minnesota

Scott T. Wolf, MA, Department of Psychology, University of North Carolina, Chapel Hill, North Carolina

Preface

How does focusing attention on career goals rather than social goals affect Jennifer's perceptions of her friends? How do Jacob's preexisting expectations about relationships influence his interactions with his romantic partner? Can engaging in reassurance-seeking behaviors backfire, causing loved ones to reject you? Why does Betsy experience the urge to work harder after thinking of her mother? Why does Anne feel compelled to eat a pint of ice cream after a bad date? Why do some relationship partners bring out the best in us while others bring out the worst?

Before answering, one might ask: Is there a common thread linking these diverse questions? This book's editors and contributors answer yes. The present volume showcases research on the interrelation between the self and relationships. The questions above illustrate the influence of intrapersonal processes on interpersonal processes, and vice versa. This book proposes a new subfield of social and personality psychology, one that is located at the intersection of the self and relationships.

Psychologists have not arrived at consensual definitions of the terms "self" and "relationship," so we use these terms broadly in the current volume. Self phenomena are defined as those pertaining to the individual that are not dependent upon specific relational contexts. Examples include self-regulation, self-concept, and stable relational schemas. Relationship phenomena are defined as those pertaining to interpersonal dynamics that are more than the sum of the interactants' characteristics. Examples include social acceptance and rejection, interdependence, and the mutual influence of relationship partners' views and expectations regarding the self.

We are grateful for the encouragement we received from Seymour Weingarten, editor-in-chief at The Guilford Press; he provided the optimal balance between freedom and guidance. His professionalism and caring manner have earned him the respect of many in our field, and we join the chorus singing his praises. Carolyn Graham, also at Guilford, was very helpful in smoothing out the bumps along the way and providing us with wisdom and advice at critical points. Finally, we gratefully acknowledge Catherine Rawn for her diligent work preparing the book's index.

We invited authors who are core researchers in either self or relationships and whose work recognizes the importance of merging the two. All authors were given the same task: Tell us about your approach to studying the effect of the self on relationships or of relationships on the self. We wanted a broad collection of state-of-the-art summaries of as many different approaches as we could fit into one book. We emphasized that authors should not simply review their own research for readers of the book, but also examine the mechanisms that account for the interplay between the self and relationships, raise future research questions emerging from their unique perspectives, and theorize about possible bidirectionalities that exist between their self and relationship processes of interest. In doing so, the authors enthusiastically produced creative and innovative ideas that promise to push this new subfield to the forefront of self and relationships research.

KATHERINE D. VOHS, PhD
ELI J. FINKEL, PhD

Contents

PART II

RELATIONSHIPS → SELF

Introduction

Self and Relationships

ELI J. FINKEL
KATHLEEN D. VOHS

The chapters in this volume offer unique perspectives on the interplay between self and relationships. Those in Part I address how the self affects relationships, while those in Part II address how relationships affect the self. They lead the reader on a tour of the latest and most compelling evidence concerning the powerful associations between intrapersonal processes and interpersonal relationships.

The field has not arrived at consensual definitions of the terms "self" and "relationship," so we use these terms broadly in the current volume. *Self* phenomena are defined as those pertaining to the individual that are not dependent upon specific relational contexts. Examples include self-regulation, the self-concept, and stable individual differences in relational schemas. *Relationship* phenomena are defined as those pertaining to interpersonal dynamics that are more than the summation of the interactants' characteristics. Examples include social acceptance and rejection, interdependence, and being influenced by relationship partners' views and expectations regarding the self.

HISTORICAL PERSPECTIVE

"Self" and "relationships" have become hot topics in social and personality psychology over the past several decades. Historically, researchers generally examined psychological processes either within the self or between two individuals. That is, they traditionally engaged in self research or in relationships research, with few scholars linking these two domains (exceptions include Baldwin & Holmes, 1987; Baumeister, 1982; Berkman & Syme, 1979; Bowlby, 1969/1982; Carver, 1975; Dion & Dion, 1973; Markus, Smith, & Moreland, 1985; Reis, Nezlek, & Wheeler, 1980; Shrauger & Schoeneman, 1979; Tesser, 1988; and Wheeler, Reis, & Nezlek, 1983). In the past 15 years, the quantity and quality of research linking these research areas have swelled. Social and personality psychologists are developing exciting new ideas about how self processes influence relationship dynamics and vice versa, and consequently a new subfield of psychology has emerged. Scholars increasingly identify their research interests with phrases such as "self-in-relationships" and "relational self."

One illustration of the transition from viewing self and relationships as separate research areas to seeing their interrelations comes from authors' reactions to the research categories for articles in the *Journal of Personality and Social Psychology* (*JPSP*). *JPSP*, one of the most prestigious Journals in psychology, is divided into three sections: (1) attitudes and social cognition, (2) interpersonal relations and group processes, and (3) personality processes and individual differences. Historically, it seemed that articles fit neatly into one of these three sections. It seems now, however, that articles published in one section frequently could have been published in another. Much of this boundary blurring is emerging at the intersection of self and relationship processes, providing exciting opportunities for social and personality psychologists to produce a more balanced and complete approach to understanding both research domains.

Many psychological scientists are already pursuing research examining the interplay between self and relationships, but we believe that such research is still in the early stages of a steep upswing. The goals of the present volume are (1) to collect in one place discussions of prominent programs of research that examine the interplay between self and relationship processes, and (2) to identify a common *self and relationships* theme connecting these seemingly disparate programs. Moreover, it can serve as a reference guide for researchers interested in perusing research at the intersection of the self and relationships.

Toward these ends, the volume brings together chapters written by influential scholars on research at this intersection. Readers will come away with a new understanding of relevant theoretical perspectives and methodological approaches. We hope to demonstrate to readers (behavioral scientists, students, and professors) the potential of this topic to lead the way in psychological advancements of the 21st century.

OVERVIEW OF THIS VOLUME

Part I (Chapters 2 though 10) examines how intrapersonal processes influence interpersonal relationships; Part II (Chapters 11 through 20) examines how interpersonal relationships influence intrapersonal processes. Each part is further divided into three sections. The Part I sections are "Self-Regulation," "Self-Concept," and "Interpersonal Schemas and Orientations," and the Part II sections are "Interdependence: Overarching Perspectives," "Specific Social Interaction Processes," and "Interpersonal Cognitive Processes."

Part I: Self → Relationships

Chapters 2 and 3 make up the Part I section entitled *Self-Regulation*. In Chapter 2, Rawn and Vohs emphasize the importance of effective self-regulation in promoting successful interpersonal functioning. They review research demonstrating, for example, that the experience of state-level depletion of self-regulatory resources causes people to (1) experience reduced motivation to behave in socially appealing ways, (2) behave narcissistically, (3) be either too intimate or too dismissive in their self-disclosures, and (4) attend closely to attractive alternatives to a current romantic partner. The authors also review compatible evidence demonstrating that poor inhibitory control at a dispositional level has similarly destructive relational consequences.

In Chapter 3, Fitzsimons argues that pursing particular self-regulatory goals (e.g., career goals, social goals, health goals) influences perceptions of and behavior toward close relationship partners who are linked strongly versus weakly to those goals. She asserts that the drive to accomplish a particular goal alters such perceptions and behaviors in a manner that facilitates goal attainment. Relationship partners who are seen by the individual as likely to facilitate goal attainment are evaluated more positively and are behaviorally approached, whereas those who are seen as likely to interfere with goal attainment are evaluated more negatively and are behaviorally avoided. Such evaluative and behavioral processes emerge only when the particular goal is active. Preliminary evidence suggests that these processes indeed facilitate goal achievement.

Chapters 4 through 6 make up the Part I section entitled *Self-Concept*. In Chapter 4, Campbell, Brunell, and Finkel conceptualize narcissism as a positive and inflated self-concept in agentic domains like intelligence, creativity, and physical attractiveness—but not in communal domains like warmth, inti-macy, and closeness. Individuals characterized by narcissistic self-conceptions adopt interpersonal strategies (e.g., dating "trophy partners," engaging in self-serving social comparisons) in which they use others to enhance their percep-tion of themselves. In addition, narcissists frequently employ an impressive arsenal of interpersonal skills (e.g., confidence, charm, charisma) to acquire partners who enhance their narcissistic esteem.

In Chapter 5, Park, Crocker, and Vohs use a new theory based on an old idea first proposed by William James: that people base their self-esteem on performance in certain domains (e.g., academic achievement, moral vir-tue, physical appearance), with their overall feelings of self-worth heavily influenced by positive or negative feedback in those crucial domains. The authors review evidence that people who have self-validation goals—that is, who have a desire to prove that they possess the characteristics on which they base their self-esteem—focus excessively on themselves and conse-quently have less successful relationships with others. In a compelling syn-thesis, they incorporate into their *contingencies of self-worth model* research on rejection sensitivity, insecure attachment styles, and both unstable and low self-esteem.

In Chapter 6, Van Orden and Joiner review research demonstrating that having negative self-views (having low self-esteem or experiencing depres-sion) predicts engaging in excessive reassurance seeking, a maladaptive inter-personal strategy that ultimately leads to social rejection. Although this reassurance-seeking behavior is a self-regulatory strategy oriented toward making individuals feel more secure, it frequently backfires, pushing away the very people they most want close to them.

Chapters 7 through 10 make up the Part I section entitled *Interpersonal Schemas and Orientations*. In Chapter 7, Feeney examines the interpersonal consequences of *attachment working models*, which are relationship schemas that enable individuals to plan their behavior and predict the behavior of oth-ers in response to relationship events. Feeney reviews a stimulating program of research demonstrating that attachment working models influence support-seeking and support-giving behaviors when at least one partner in a romantic relationship experiences distress. Additional evidence indicates that attach-ment working models can systematically bias perceptions of a partner's support-giving behaviors.

In Chapter 8, Knee and Canevello distinguish between two distinct implicit theories of relationships: destiny beliefs and growth beliefs. These theories refer to individuals' implicit assumptions about the stability of their perceptions of partner compatibility (destiny) and the nature and stability of problems in relationships (growth). Implicit theories of relationships influence how partners assign meaning to interpersonal events, and therefore how they respond behaviorally to such events.

In Chapter 9, Showers and Limke build on research examining the structure of self-knowledge by applying a similar analysis to the structure of partner knowledge. They investigate not only whether knowledge of the partner is positive or negative but also whether it is integrated (with positive and negative beliefs about the partner frequently appearing within the same categories of partner knowledge) or compartmentalized (with categories of partner knowledge tending to be purely positive or purely negative). The authors review research demonstrating that when the description of one's partner is generally positive, compartmentalization predicts greater liking and loving toward the partner, but when the description is generally negative, integration is associated with more positive feelings. Follow-up research reveals the intriguing findings that positive compartmentalized individuals have the highest rate of breakup and negative compartmentalized individuals experience especially stable relationships.

In Chapter 10, Van Lange argues that social scientists overestimate the power of self-interest as the dominant orientation with which individuals approach relationships. This overestimation has blinded researchers (including psychologists) from seeing the importance of other interpersonal orientations. Van Lange discusses the relevance of six conceptually distinct orientations (altruism, cooperation, egalitarianism, individualism, competition, and aggression) and suggests that recognizing their impact is essential to understanding topics such as helping, aggression, cooperation, negotiation, and close relationships.

Part II: Relationships → Self

Chapters 11 through 14 make up the Part II section entitled *Interdependence: Overarching Perspectives*. In Chapter 11, Leary observes that the implicit assumption in most self research is that the self is independent of the social world. He takes a different perspective, arguing that "viewing the self as a psychological process without considering its interpersonal functions and origins may lead to an impoverished perspective on self processes" (p. 232). He provides an evolutionary analysis of the origins of selfhood, beginning with the observation that our ancestors depended upon their social groups for survival and reproductive advantages. As a result, humans evolved the ability to monitor other people's thoughts and intentions vis-à-vis the self (e.g., Do they intend to cause me harm?). Although such monitoring was initially performed nonconsciously and automatically, it was eventually accompanied by self-awareness, which allowed individuals to think consciously about other people's reactions toward them. Through the research on "sociometer theory" reviewed in the chapter, Leary argues that the self-esteem system evolved to monitor others' reactions and to alert the individual to possible social exclusion.

In Chapter 12, Blackhart, Baumeister, and Twenge examine the power-ful, adverse effects of social rejection on self-regulation. Experimental evidence reveals that people who have been rejected make poor decisions, engage in unhealthy behaviors, procrastinate, and are unable to delay gratification. In addition, they (1) display aggressive behavior toward others and (2) exhibit reluctance to donate money to an important cause, to volunteer for future studies, and to help after a mishap.

In Chapter 13, Lucas and Dyrenforth examine whether the *existence* of social relationships predicts subjective well-being. Given the overwhelming evidence that having relationships predicts outcomes such as superior physical health and that having high-quality relationships predicts subjective well-being, one might expect that the *existence* of relationships would also predict subjective well-being. Lucas and Dyrenforth's compelling review, however, reveals the surprising finding that the existence of relationships exhibits only weak associations with subjective well-being.

In Chapter 14, Agnew and Etcheverry argue that certain characteristics of social relationships influence self-concept structure. They emphasize the idea that two core features of dyadic interdependence—correspondence of outcomes (the degree to which the two partners have matching behavioral preferences in particular situations) and dependence on the relationship for positive outcomes—influence the degree to which one's self-concept is individuated from (vs. connected to) the partner. They review research demonstrating that relative to participants who experience low dependence on their relationship, those who experience high dependence exhibit greater spontaneous use of plural pronouns (e.g., "we," "us," "our," "ours"), one finding among many to demonstrate the important association of relationship dependence on self-structure.

Chapters 15 through 18 make up the Part II section entitled *Specific Social Interaction Processes*. In Chapter 15, Finkel, Campbell, and Brunell examine the effects of efficient versus inefficient social coordination on the interactants' subsequent self-regulatory success. Although coordination is sometimes efficient and effortless (*low maintenance*), at other times it is inefficient and effortful (*high maintenance*). Findings from a large series of studies reveal that high-maintenance interaction leads to self-regulatory failure, in terms of both diminished achievement motivation and impaired task performance. The chapter concludes by presenting a theoretical model integrating high-maintenance interaction, interpersonal conflict, and self-regulatory failure.

In Chapter 16, Kumashiro, Rusbult, Wolf, and Estrada incorporate concepts from the behavioral confirmation tradition, the self tradition, and the interdependence tradition to identify an interpersonal process they call the *Michelangelo phenomenon*. This phenomenon describes the means by which the self is "sculpted" by a close partner's behavior to approximate the self's ideal. Kumashiro and colleagues review a program of research demonstrating strong associations between partner affirmation (the degree to which a partner's perceptions of and behavior toward the self are congruent with the self's ideal), movement over time toward the ideal self, and, ultimately, personal and couple well-being.

In Chapter 17, Strong and Aron build on *self-expansion theory* to argue that participating in novel and challenging activities with a romantic partner causes individuals to experience excited positive affect, which in turn causes them to experience their relationship as being of higher quality. They suggest that nonexciting positive affect (e.g., calmness, relief) or reduction in any type of negative affect cannot account for the association of shared participation in novel and challenging activities with enhanced relationship quality. The authors review a long and productive line of research examining how relational dynamics can fundamentally alter the composition of the self.

In Chapter 18, Koole, Kuhl, Jostmann, and Finkenauer examine social interaction processes in terms of two types of self-regulatory approaches called "action orientation" and "state orientation". People in an action-oriented frame of mind tend toward change and active self-regulation as they pursue their goals, whereas those in a state-oriented frame of mind tend to be resistant to change and do not engage in active self-regulation. Koole and colleagues argue that differences in action versus state orientation derive from (1) socialization processes that, for example, promote agency (for action-oriented individuals) or inhibit disengagement from undesirable states (for state-oriented individuals) and (2) situation-specific social triggers in which other people serve to bring out action- versus state-oriented coping.

Chapters 19 and 20 make up the Part II section entitled *Interpersonal Cognitive Processes*. In Chapter 19, Shah reviews evidence suggesting that the mental activation of relationship partners who are associated with certain goals influences goal strivings. Additional evidence suggests that these effects are moderated by factors such as number of goals associated with the significant other and the importance of the goal to the significant other. Taken together, evidence suggests that the mere cognitive accessibility of relationship partners can influence self-regulation.

In Chapter 20, Seeley and Gardner argue that social sensitivity and social accountability influence self-regulation. First, they present evidence that efforts aimed at establishing and maintaining harmonious social relationships serve to build self-regulatory capacity. Second, they suggest that the interpersonal accountability that emerges from disclosing goals (e.g., to quit smoking) to close others increases the likelihood of self-regulatory success by removing the burden of choice from the self-control process. Moreover, this effect remains strong over time, even when the discloser is not in the presence of others who know about the goal.

THROWING PERSPECTIVE INTO REVERSE

Although the chapters in Part I emphasize how intrapersonal processes influence interpersonal relationships and those in Part II emphasize how interpersonal relationships influence intrapersonal processes, all chapters also briefly examine the opposite causal pathway. The chapters in Part I also examine how relationship dynamics influence self-regulation, self-concept, or interpersonal schemas and orientations, and those in Part II also examine how intrapersonal processes influence general interdependence processes, specific social interaction processes, and interpersonal cognitive processes. The overarching conclusion is that there is a dynamic and bidirectional interplay between self and relationship processes. Empirical research on such dynamics, however, is sparse. Experimental and longitudinal investigations examining the temporal unfolding of self and relationship processes will provide particularly fertile ground for theory development.

BRIDGING THE PAST TO THE FUTURE

Major ideas linking self and relationships were dominant in the early years of psychological social science. Seminal ideas by scholars such as Cooley (1902), Mead (1934), Erikson (1950), and Sullivan (1953) emphasized the importance of the interplay between processes that take place within persons and those that take place between them. Although such investigations had slowed for decades, they again find themselves at center stage in social and personality psychology. This volume brings together many of the most influential lines of research responsible for this featured location. We recognize that the accelerating pace of research in this domain means that not all of the emerging high-quality work has been captured herein; we eagerly await the wealth of knowledge on the interplay between self and relationships soon to be uncovered.

REFERENCES

Baldwin, M. W., & Holmes, J. G. (1987). Salient private audiences and awareness of the self. *Journal of Personality and Social Psychology, 52,* 1087–1098.

Baumeister, R. F. (1982). A self-presentational view of social phenomena. *Psychological Bulletin, 91,* 3–26.

Berkman, L. F., & Syme, S. L. (1979). Social networks, host resistance, and mortality: A nine year follow-up study of Alameda Country residents. *American Journal of Epidemiology, 100,* 186–204.

Bowlby, J. (1969/1982). *Attachment and loss: Vol. 1. Attachment.* New York: Basic Books.

Carver, C. S. (1975). Physical aggression as a function of objective self-awareness and attitudes toward punishment. *Journal of Experimental Social Psychology, 11,* 510–519.

Cooley, C. H. (1902). *Human nature and the social order.* New York: Scribner's.

Dion, K. L., & Dion, K. K. (1973). Correlates of romantic love. *Journal of Consulting and Clinical Psychology, 41,* 51–56.

Erikson, E. H. (1950). *Childhood and society.* New York: Norton.

Markus, H., Smith, J., & Moreland, R. (1985). Role of the self-concept in the perception of others. *Journal of Personality and Social Psychology, 49,* 1494–1512.

Mead, G. H. (1934). *Mind, self, and society.* Chicago: University of Chicago Press.

Reis, H. T., Nezlek, J., & Wheeler, L. (1980). Physical attractiveness in social interaction. *Journal of Personality and Social Psychology, 38,* 604–617.

Shrauger, J. S., & Schoeneman, T. J. (1979). Symbolic interactionist view of the self-concept: Through the looking glass darkly. *Psychological Bulletin, 86,* 549–573.

Sullivan, H. S. (1953). *The interpersonal theory of psychiatry.* New York: Norton.

Tesser, A. (1988). Toward a self-evaluation maintenance model of social behavior. In L. Berkowitz (Ed.), *Advances in experimental social psychology* (Vol. 21, pp. 181–227). San Diego, CA: Academic Press.

Wheeler, L., Reis, H. T., & Nezlek, J. (1983). Loneliness, social interaction, and sex roles. *Journal of Personality and Social Psychology, 45,* 943–953.

PART I

SELF → RELATIONSHIPS

SECTION I A

SELF-REGULATION

CHAPTER 2

The Importance of Self-Regulation for Interpersonal Functioning

CATHERINE D. RAWN
KATHLEEN D. VOHS

This chapter focuses on the association between self-control and interpersonal relationships. Although these two arenas may on the surface appear to be completely separate—with self-control pertaining to an individual's inner life and interpersonal relationships concerning the behaviors and events that happen between people—we posit that they are intimately tied. The general theme of this chapter is that people's ability to control their unwanted impulses strongly and positively predicts their ability not only to convey the impression that they are good relationship partners but to actually behave as a good relationship partner. We begin with an illustration.

The sport of boxing requires intense daily training schedules that often include daily cardiovascular endurance workouts in the morning, strength and power training in the evening, and sparring with other boxers as often as possible (*How to Train for Boxing*, 2004). Undoubtedly, good self-control is required for such a demanding regimen. Therefore, one might expect that those few individuals who possess the ability to stick to such rigid daily training exercises must also possess good self-control. In addition, one would probably predict that if a person could adhere to a rigid training schedule, then this person could surely behave decently in close relationships. However, this is not always the case.

Consider first Lennox Lewis, a famous heavyweight boxing champion who retired in 2004 (Eisele, 2004a). Lennox Lewis demonstrates intense focus and restraint in many areas of his life, from exercise and eating to sexuality and commitment. Although media interviews with Lewis were rare because he worked to keep his personal life private (perhaps itself a sign of good self-control), sports writers reported that good self-control had become a way of life for Lewis. As one example, although he had a girlfriend whom he loved deeply, Lewis would not have sex with her for several weeks before fights. Lewis explained, "The old-time boxers, they used to refrain from sex for months and it used to get them penned up. I think it's a good sacrifice. It's something you can basically look forward to having afterwards, like a reward. And it [not having sex] clears your mind" (Evans, 2003). Moreover, even with the temptations of newly available attractive women that come with being a heavyweight champion and celebrity, Lewis's monogamous relationship has lasted for years and he has plans to marry his long-term girlfriend (Evans, 2003).

Other successful boxers, however, have failed to show the judicious self-restraint that Lewis has shown. Mike Tyson is famous—and perhaps infamous—for his sensational attacks both inside (he has twice bitten boxers during fights) and outside of the boxing ring. Despite a successful career in boxing (Eisele, 2004b), suggesting that Tyson can exert self-control to achieve his professional goals, Tyson's personal life, which he could not or did not keep out of the media spotlight, was blackened by infidelity, drugs, rape (a charge for which he went to prison for 3 years), numerous assaults, and two failed marriages (Tyson Troubles, 2002). His first marriage, to Robin Givens, in 1988 was reportedly hurried by an unexpected pregnancy, although later that year Givens revealed that Tyson was abusing her and that she had suffered a miscarriage as a result of his abuse (*Mike Tyson*, 2000). In 1989 the couple divorced, with Givens claiming infidelity on Tyson's part, a charge that was repeated 14 years later by his second wife when she too divorced him (Wraga & Abrams, 2002). Despite his controlled physical training, Tyson failed in his interpersonal relationships because of his inability to restrain himself. Not only did Tyson have difficulties controlling himself with others, he admits to being addicted to drugs and has a clinically recognized sexual addiction. Tyson currently struggles to maintain ties to his children and instead cares intimately for 350 pigeons in his Phoenix home (oddly, his penchant for pigeons began as a child when neighborhood bullies forced him to clean their pigeon cages). In a recent interview, Tyson said that he believes that he will die alone and that this would be a just ending to his life (Saracento, 2005).

There is no single answer as to why Lewis and Tyson had similar boxing career trajectories but differed tremendously in their relationships with others. However, we think that the evidence points to a vast difference in their self-control abilities. On the one hand, there is Lewis, who exhibits sexual restraint, strong moral character, and commitment to goals; on the other hand, there is Tyson, who has multiple addictions, a history of violence and sexual deviance, and overall a weak sense of self.

In the remainder of this chapter, we outline the limited resource model of self-regulation, provide evidence that interpersonal relationships are affected by self-regulation, and briefly address how self-regulatory abilities may themselves be influenced by interpersonal relationships. We close with a discussion of future directions for this burgeoning topic.

INTRAPERSONAL PROCESSES OF SELF-CONTROL: THE LIMITED RESOURCE MODEL

The overall framework that we use to understand self-control is the limited resource model initially proposed by Baumeister and Heatherton (1996). In brief, the theory posits that self-control is governed by a limited, global resource. This resource enables all forms of self-regulation, but weakens with each successive exertion. A reduced supply of regulatory resources can, with the right temptations, lead to self-regulation failure. This state of impairment is known as "self-regulatory resource depletion" (also called "ego depletion"). Once a person is depleted, he or she needs time and rest to regain the self-regulatory strength to succeed at another self-control task.

State levels of self-regulatory resources are manipulated in the following experimental paradigm. Participants in the depletion condition exert self-control in an initial task and are then asked to exert self-control a second time in a task associated with an unrelated domain. Compared to control condition participants who do not exert self-control initially, depleted participants are less able to persist on the second task. The results of more than 40 published experiments support this idea (see Baumeister, Schmeichel, & Vohs, in press; Vohs & Baumeister, 2004). Multiple attempts to identify alternative conceptualizations of this mechanism have converged on the limited resource as strength model (Baumeister, Bratslavsky, Muraven, & Tice, 1998).

Trait Self-Control

Chronic self-regulation tendencies influence how susceptible people are to state-level manipulation of self-regulatory resources. *Trait self-control* is conceptualized as the ability to alter internal states and to interrupt undesirable behaviors and urges (Tangney, Baumeister, & Boone, 2004). The degree of self-control exerted in any given situation is a product of this baseline and situational demands, including tests of the limited resource model above.

INTERPERSONAL EFFECTS OF SELF-REGULATION

A great deal of empirical research from the developmental, personality, and clinical subfields of psychology that is consistent with the idea that interpersonal functioning is enhanced by the ability to regulate the self. "Delay of gratification," "ego control," "ego resiliency," and "activity inhibition" are some of the terms that have been used to describe various aspects of the ability to control or regulate one's own behavior. Investigations of self-control have employed a diverse collection of relationship-related dependent measures, including but not limited to having close interpersonal relationships and social support (Gross & John, 2003), socially appropriate behavior (Eisenberg et al., 2003), victimization (Funder, Block, & Block, 1983), abusive tendencies (Mason & Blankenship, 1987), stress management (Shoda, Mischel, & Peake, 1990), and the ability to respond in a relationship-enhancing rather than a destructive manner to transgressions (Finkel & Campbell, 2001). Research on individual differences in self-control also reveals various interpersonal benefits of possessing this trait (Tangney et al., 2004). In this study, having high self-control was related to an absence of problem drinking behaviors; high self-esteem; high conscientiousness, emotional stability, and agreeableness; high family cohesion and low family conflict; secure attachment style but not anxious–ambivalent nor avoidant styles; the ability to take others' perspectives; empathy; low levels of anger and aggression; and taking responsibility for one's transgressions (Tangney et al., 2004).

A Developmental Perspective: Ego Control, Ego Resiliency, and Delay of Gratification

Early research on self-control investigated personality and the ability to delay gratification among children. Two personality constructs, ego control (e.g., Funder et al., 1983) and ego resiliency (e.g., Ayduk et al., 2000; Block & Kremen, 1996; Mischel, Shoda, & Peake, 1988; Shoda et al., 1990) have been linked to others' perceptions of peoples' abilities to engage in social relationships. *Ego control* refers to the ability to control one's emotions, urges, and desires, whereas *ego resiliency* is the ability to alter one's amount of ego control as appropriate for a particular situation (Funder et al., 1983). Low ego resiliency results in levels of ego control inappropriate for a given situation (Block & Kremen, 1996; Funder et al., 1983; Funder & Block, 1989). For example, if one has high ego control, one's desire to sing and dance while walking on the sidewalk can be overridden by one's desire to follow social norms for public behavior. If one has high ego resiliency, behavioral urges are monitored and appeased according to the situation: at a party one sings and dances but in a shopping mall one suppresses this urge.

Ego control in children is positively correlated with interpersonal success among both boys and girls (Funder et al., 1983). Researchers tested the ability to delay gratification as a proxy for ego control in two different situations. In the gift delay situation, the experimenter announced that there was a gift for the child, and that he or she could have it after completing a challenging puzzle. During the puzzle completion task, behaviors directed toward the gift were recorded, including how long it took the child to reach for the gift when told to, and the amount of delay before opening the present. The number of gift-directed behaviors was interpreted as indicative of the degree to which the children could delay gratification, with more of these behaviors indicating less ability to delay gratification. In the second part of this study, a resistance-to-temptation situation was used to measure delay of gratification in the same children. This situation involved instructions for the children to resist playing with attractive toys, and instead to play with the dull and broken toys provided to them. Ability to delay gratification by resisting the attractive toys was assessed through one-way mirrors when the children were left alone. Personality characteristics and the social functioning of each child were rated by schoolteachers at ages 3, 4, 7, and 11. Relative to girls who demonstrated low self-control in the two tasks, girls who were more able to exert self-control in the two tasks were less likely to be victimized by or to take advantage of others, were less emotionally labile, and were more likely to have stable interpersonal relationships. Boys who demonstrated high self-control were described by their teachers as attentive, cooperative, and able to moderate their emotional impulses to a greater extent than boys low in self-control. Both girls and boys who have high self-control are more interpersonally successful than those who have low self-control.

A classic study by Mischel and colleagues (1988) was among the first to demonstrate with longitudinal data that ego resiliency in childhood is related to social success in adolescence. Children participated in a delay-of-gratification task at age 5: they chose between having one marshmallow sooner or two marshmallows later. The experimenter told the children that she was going to leave the room, told them to wait until her return in order to receive the preferred two marshmallows, and then left. They were given the option of ringing a bell to call her back early to receive the less desirable reward of one marshmallow. In this task it is adaptive to exert self-control because the reward is greater when one does not give in to temptation. This is unlike the gift and toy situations of Funder and colleagues (1983) in which the rewards are not contingent on any behavior: whether the puzzle was finished or not, the child still received the gift. Thus delay in the marshmallow task is interpreted as a sign of ego resiliency, whereas delay in the gift and toy situations is viewed as evidence of ego control (Funder & Block, 1989).

The amount of time the preschoolers took before ringing the bell was later correlated with parental ratings of sociability at age 15 (Mischel et al., 1988). Parents of these children were contacted 10 years after the initial experiment to rate their adolescent's social abilities, including their ability to get along with peers and to cope with frustrations. These ratings were predicted by how long the adolescents had been able to wait before calling back the experimenter in the preschool delay-of-gratification task. These results demonstrate that ego resiliency predicts social skills, even with a 10-year time lag between measurements.

The same preschool delay-of-gratification data set used by Mischel and colleagues (1988) was used by Ayduk and colleagues (2000) to investigate the role of ego resiliency in moderating the relationship between rejection sensitivity and interpersonal problems in adulthood. Past research had shown that people who expect that others will reject them (i.e., people who are rejection sensitive) suffer from a host of relational problems including loneliness, social anxiety, unsatisfying relationships, and frequent relationship dissolution. Ayduk and colleagues predicted and then found that the negative effects of rejection sensitivity were avoided among those who were also ego resilient. Among adults sensitive to rejection, the ability to delay gratification in preschool seemed to reduce the negative social outcomes that typically accompany rejection sensitivity. Specifically, among rejection-sensitive adults, ego resiliency in childhood positively predicted self-worth, successful coping strategies, and ego control. Among those with low rejection sensitivity there was no relationship between delay of gratification and these positive functioning variables. These results suggest that the negative interpersonal effects of having high rejection sensitivity are subverted by having high self-control.

In a longitudinal study of young adults, Block and Kremen (1996) found that people with high ego resiliency were more interpersonally adept, even when controlling for IQ scores. Among both women and men, high ego-resilient people were characterized as socially poised, cheerful, and appropriate in their emotional expressions. Conversely, low ego resiliency predicted an inability to trust as well as feelings of inadequacy and vulnerability, especially among women. Men with low ego resiliency were rebellious, hostile, and emotionally labile. The characteristics espoused by those who have low ego resiliency may be destructive to intimate relationships, whereas high ego resiliency is related to qualities that facilitate the initiation and maintenance of interpersonal relationships. The results of these studies show that self-control in general, as well as the ability to regulate self-control in order to meet the demands of a specific situation, are important contributors to interpersonal success across the lifespan.

The Benefits of Self-Control in Close Relationships

Intimate relationships are healthy when each partner can and will sacrifice his or her personal needs for the benefit of the partner and the relationship. What in the short term is a selfless act is often rewarded in the long term with stronger intimate ties. In this way, personal sacrifices lead to better relationships, which in turn benefit the self. This relationship-supporting cycle, however, seems to be hindered by decreased self-regulatory abilities. The ability to prioritize another's needs above one's own requires inhibition of one's selfish impulses. Research shows that responding in a supportive way to a partner's potentially destructive behavior leads to the most positive outcomes for the relationship, but at a cost of psychological resources. Responding in an accommodative fashion to a partner's transgression (e.g., constructively talking about the problem or allowing the incident to pass) has positive outcomes for the longevity of and personal satisfaction in the relationship (Rusbult, Verette, Whitney, Slovik, & Lipkus, 1991), but doing so requires that one exercise self-control in the process (Finkel & Campbell, 2001).

A multimethod investigation led researchers to conclude that both low trait self-control and temporary decrements in self-regulatory ability result in fewer accommodative responses in response to a partner's wrongdoing (Finkel & Campbell, 2001). In one study, participants who recalled responding to partners' transgressions in a destructive fashion were more likely to report experiencing extra self-control demands at that time, compared to those who recalled responding in accommodative ways. These data suggest that self-control is required for accommodative responding in close relationships. Experimental manipulations of the limited resource model of self-regulation also supported this idea. In another study, Finkel and Campbell manipulated self-regulatory resources by having participants either express their emotions naturally or suppress their emotional reactions to an amusing or a sad emotional movie clip. They then were asked to select how they would respond to 12 hypothetical scenarios in which their partners transgressed. Response options represented both accommodative and destructive behaviors. Participants who had suppressed their emotions responded with fewer accommodative responses to the scenarios, relative to those who had responded naturally to the video.

This finding was replicated and extended by Vohs and Baumeister (2005). These researchers also found that self-regulation depletion led people to respond destructively to transgression scenarios similar to those used by Finkel and Campbell (2001). Notably, destructive responses were reported regardless of whether people were thinking of a current, a past, or a hypothetical relationship partner transgressing. These results demonstrate that self-control leads to accommodative responses across many types of interpersonal relationships. Accommodative responses foster positive relationship outcomes (Rusbult et al., 1991), showing once again that self-control contributes to interpersonal success.

Another way relationships can benefit from self-control is by minimizing the *self-serving bias* (SSB), the tendency for people to attribute successes to their internal dispositions and to attribute failures to aspects of the situation, including other people (Sicoly & Ross, 1977). A recent study examined the effects of emotion suppression on the SSB from the perspective of the limited resource model of self-regulation (Vohs & Baumeister, 2005). Dating couples either suppressed their emotional responses to a comedic film or let their emotions flow naturally. The suppression task was presumed to expend self-regulatory resources, leaving fewer resources available for further acts of self-control. Each couple then worked together to build a structure out of blocks. False feedback indicated that the building was either very creative or not creative. Only those who had suppressed their emotions later exhibited the SSB in the joint task: suppressors took credit for creative structures and blamed their partners for uncreative ones. People who had responded freely to the film had retained self-regulatory resources and therefore were able to successfully mitigate self-serving attributions. Because resources remained, selfish impulses were inhibited for the benefit of the relationship.

A third way in which self-control can contribute to the success of intimate relationships is by suppressing attraction to alternative partners. In one study, participants were asked to read drab historical narratives aloud, either with or without the instruction to read these boring narratives emphatically (Vohs & Baumeister, 2005). The additional instruction was again intended to tax self-regulatory resources, since the task required exerting control over facial and emotional expressions. Length of time spent looking through a booklet filled with pictures of scantily clad attractive people was measured. This dependent measure has been used to index consideration of alternative partners (Miller, 1997). The researchers predicted and found that participants who exerted self-control during the reading-aloud task gazed longer at the pictures as compared to participants who read the passage without special emphasis. Of importance, this was particularly true for those in romantic relationships. It is plausible that people in romantic relationships habitually suppress attraction to alternative partners, since giving in to such an impulse could likely lead to the failure of their current relationship. These results show that depletion of self-regulatory resources can make turning away from attractive alternative partners particularly difficult for those in romantic relationships.

Are people who give in to the temptation to gaze at attractive alternatives actually less committed to their current partners? Research suggests that this may be the case. The perceived value of alternative relationship partners negatively predicts peoples' commitment to their current partners (Rusbult, 1980). Moreover, among people already in romantic relationships, the length of time spent gazing at photographs of attractive opposite-sex people predicted whether they would be partnered with the same person 2 months later (Miller, 1997). These findings, taken together, suggest that low self-control can contribute to greater consideration of alternative partners, which may then lead to relationship dissolution.

The Destructive Interpersonal Effects of an Uncontrolled Self

Given the importance of self-control in managing behavioral responses to partner transgressions (Finkel & Campbell, 2001), it seems plausible that lack of self-control may be a contributing factor in domestic abuse. Research confirms such a link. Indeed, physical abuse in intimate relationships was predicted by self-control, commitment to the relationship, and stress (Mason & Blankenship, 1987). Of those who reported high negative stress in the past year, two groups of women were particularly likely to inflict abuse on their male partners: those with high self-control but low commitment to the relationship, and those with low self-control but high commitment to the relationship. Stressful circumstances might facilitate the interaction between commitment and self-control on violence observed by Mason and Blankenship, although the correlational nature of this research makes this type of conclusion a difficult one to draw.

Self-control can also influence interpersonal relationships through its effects on impulse-control disorders. Compulsions and addictions are related to an inability to exert appropriate self-control. These afflictions wreak havoc on interpersonal relationships. For example, compulsive buyers have problems with relationships as a consequence of their inability to control shopping consumption (O'Guinn & Faber, 1989). Self-identified compulsive buyers, some of whom were seeking help for their compulsive purchasing, and members of the general population were surveyed. Reports of envy and nongenerosity were higher among compulsive buyers than in the general population, but there was no difference between groups in the desire to possess items. Compulsive buyers thought of their purchases as ways of improving their self-worth and the quality of their relationships, yet these people reported heavier debt loads, more shame, and more intense marital difficulties. As one compulsive shopper said:

> I didn't have one person in the world I could talk to. I don't drink, I don't smoke, I don't do dope. But I can't stop. I can't control it. I said I can't go on like this. . . . My husband hates me. My kids hate me. I've destroyed everything. I was ashamed and I just wanted to die. . . . My husband said he couldn't deal with this

and he said, "I'm leaving you. We'll get a divorce. That's it. It's your problem. You did it. You fix it up." (in O'Guinn & Faber, p. 9)

These findings are not cause to give up hope. New research has identified a link between positive relationship outcomes and the summed level of self-control for both partners in a romantic relationship (Vohs, Baumeister, & Finkenauer, 2005). Results show that the sum of two partners' self-control scores is a better predictor of relationship satisfaction and longevity than the difference between their scores. Explained another way, being in a relationship in which either partner has high self-control predicts an enduring relationship that is more satisfying. This additive effect can be contrasted with a model in which partner matching is most important, suggesting, for example, that two low self-control partners would be better suited. But this is not the case. Adding to the theme of this chapter, these results show that encouraging good self-control has benefits not only for the self but for relational partners as well.

Conclusion

The interpersonal effects of self-regulation have been demonstrated using a variety of operationalizations, across various developmental time periods, and using both correlational and experimental methods. Research has shown the positive effects of ego control and ego resiliency from preschool age through adulthood. Perhaps most direct is evidence that low self-control results in violent, destructive, and selfish responses in intimate relationships, as well as more consideration of alternative partners—sure signs of poor relationship quality. The message gleaned from this research is clear: low self-control is detrimental to having and maintaining close interpersonal relationships, whereas high self-control brings relational success.

BIDIRECTIONAL LINK: QUALITIES OF INTERPERSONAL RELATIONSHIPS LEADING TO SELF-CONTROL

Thus far we have discussed research evidence showing that the ability to control the self influences how we relate to others and how successful our relationships are. Could it also be that qualities of our relationships influence how much self-control we are able to exert? In terms of the limited resource model of self-regulation, it is conceivable that interpersonal contexts that require one to present the self in a specific way may influence the availability of self-regulatory resources after the interaction. Self-presentational behaviors are important in successfully forming relationships with others, so it follows that they would require considerable effort and possibly drain resources. Across a number of studies, Vohs, Baumeister, and Ciarocco (2005) showed that self-control was related to self-presentation in both directions. Consistent with the thesis of this chapter, decrements in state self-control resulted in impairments in the ability to successfully present a certain image of the self to others. In addition, interpersonally focused self-presentation also influenced intrapersonally focused self-control. Presenting oneself to others in a particularly effortful way impaired self-regulatory strength in the task that followed. These data demonstrate that self-control can be affected by interpersonal processes.

Caregiver–Infant Relationship Influences Later Self-Control

Qualities of the caregiver–infant relationship early in a child's life influence the child's ability to exert self-control years later. The emergence of self-regulation in childhood is facilitated by the coordination of emotional expressions between mothers and infants (Feldman, Greenbaum, & Yirmiya, 1999). Maternal–infant affect synchrony during face-to-face interactions involves mutual regulation of emotion, as mothers reflect the emotions expressed by infants in their facial expressions and verbalizations. Coordination of affect during mother–infant interactions when infants were 3 months old predicted children's ability to delay gratification at age 2.

Other studies have demonstrated that mothers' parenting and disciplining styles predict whether or not preschoolers are able to exert self-control (Mauro & Harris, 2000; Neitzel & Stright, 2003; Putnam, Spritz, & Stifter, 2002). Two-and-a-half-year-old children were instructed not to play with an attractive toy for 1 minute, a period during which mothers and children were left alone and surreptitiously videotaped (Mauro & Harris, 2000). Children who did not delay gratification had mothers who demonstrated a permissive parenting style, in which few demands and limits are set on children's behavior. Mothers of children who successfully delayed gratification used strategies consistent with an authoritative parenting style, a style that balances exertion of control over the child with nurturance for the child, and which involves more rewards than punishments. In another study, techniques mothers used to help their children complete challenging tasks predicted the children's self-regulatory abilities at a second task administered months later (Neitzel & Stright, 2003). Mothers of successfully self-regulating children had provided positive emotional support to their children, and had encouraged their children's autonomy by appropriately relinquishing control of the task to the child.

These studies demonstrate that the quality of the parent–child relationship, from as early as 3 months of age, helps to develop successful self-regulation among children. Recall findings discussed earlier showing that children who successfully self-regulate grow up to be good self-regulators and to have positive interpersonal relationships (Ayduk et al., 2000; Mischel et al., 1988; Shoda et al., 1990). Although such research has yet to explore this linkage directly, the data suggest that qualities of interpersonal relationships very early in a person's development lead to self-regulatory strategies that help him or her achieve interpersonal success well into adulthood.

FUTURE RESEARCH

The links between self-control and interpersonal functioning discussed here lay the foundation for a host of future research endeavors. Future research should test what is known about self-control and relationships to understand risky behavior such as unprotected sex and interpersonal violence, and to inform related policy decisions. According to the limited resource model of self-regulation, people in a resource-depleted state should have fewer self-regulatory resources available for later that day. Resource depletion caused by a stressful work environment during the day, for example, could have severe side effects, such as failing to appreciate the risk involved in having unprotected sex later that evening at a party. Recall research by Mason and Blankenship (1987) indicating a relationship between women's self-control and physical abuse of their partners. Additional work in this area should address male-to-female physical abuse, which typically causes more injuries than the more common female-to-male abuse (Archer, 2000), as well as emotional abuse initiated by both partners.

Another area that self-regulation research has yet to fully address is how the limited resource model of self-regulation applies within other cultures. It is possible that the depletion threshold is influenced by aspects of one's culture. Some research evidence shows that those scoring high on collectivism do not evidence the same degree of depletion from a standard thought suppression task compared to those low on collectivism (Seeley & Gardner, 2003; see also Seeley & Gardner, Chapter 20, this volume). East Asian cultural mores include withholding the expression of emotions and personal opinions lest they interfere with group functioning (Triandis, 1995). Research shows that self-presentation depletes the self-regulatory resources of Western participants (Vohs et al., 2005). Given that East Asians may be more practiced than Westerners at self-presenting, East Asians could have a much greater pool of resources available, and therefore require much more intense and precise self-presentation demands to reach a state of resource depletion than do Westerners. It is important to extend the research of Seeley and Gardner to more fully investigate the impact of culture on self-regulation and self-control by including independent and dependent variables that relate to interpersonal relationships.

Overall, the self-regulation strength model has received much empirical support. Considerable evidence links self-regulatory resources to aspects of the self, although the nature of the resource has yet to be identified precisely. Self-affirmation has been found to act as a buffer against depletion effects: reminding the self of its values seems to counteract the negative consequences of depletion (Schmeichel & Vohs, 2005). In addition, the resource could be neurologically based. It is possible that a certain neurotransmitter in the brain could supply the self with its regulatory abilities, or that a neurological system such as an advanced attentional network facilitates self-regulation (Posner & Rothbart, 2000). These alternatives suggest that there are different levels of examining the nature of self-regulatory resources. We are encouraged by the work being done to identify the resource and await more progress on this front in the years to come.

SELF-REGULATION AFFECTS INTERPERSONAL FUNCTIONING

In the past, self-regulation has been considered an activity *by* the self *for* the self. It may have been obvious to first identify the self as being the greatest source and beneficiary of self-control in early investigations. This notion has not been refuted by the research discussed in this chapter; however, we believe that adding the interpersonal dimension to an understanding of the origins, implications, and development of self-control will serve to promote further theoretical refinement of this construct. Based on the evidence discussed here, it is clear that interpersonal goals are also served through effective self-regulation. The ability to successfully self-regulate predicts more committed, longer lasting, and less abusive relationships and fosters companionship.

Being perceived as likeable, attractive, and intelligent is important in order to become accepted as a group member (Baumeister & Tice, 1990). Being a group member is vital to survival. Conveying the impression to others that one is a worthwhile group member requires successful self-regulation. There is enough evidence that self-regulation is important for interpersonal functioning to suggest that self-regulation may have been adapted in order to glean interpersonal benefits. This hypothesis was put forth by Heatherton and Vohs (1998), who suggested that the ability to self-regulate was an evolutionarily adaptive way to remain a member of the group. If a person was not able to control selfish impulses for the group's benefit, the group would ostracize that person for being uncooperative. The desire to remain a part of the group, thereby reaping the benefits of shared accommodations and additional supports, may have propelled early humans to develop self-control.

Another domain in which self-regulation would have been beneficial to our ancestors is mating (Heatherton & Vohs, 1998). People who could not control the impressions they gave to others might not have been able to attract mating partners. Successful mating partners may have been those who could put forth a positive image of themselves, and who then followed up the positive appearance by suppressing their selfish urges and putting others' needs before their own. The need for companionship may continue to be an important reason for honing one's self-regulatory strength in today's society. As social psychologists, we may have overlooked the role of self-regulation in acquiring group membership (see Seeley & Gardner, Chapter 20, this volume, for more on the interpersonal aspects of self-regulation). Because self-control seems to be such an important component of relationships, furthering research on this topic without considering interpersonal factors may hinder theoretical development.

Self-control is an important aspect of functioning in everyday environments. Many careers in our society require self-control. In the professional world, long hours at work that compete with demands of family and leisure can lead to a constant struggle of the will. Among businesspeople, Donald Trump is one of the richest persons in the world, after having worked diligently to recover from billions of dollars of debt incurred in the early 1990s (Smith, 2004). He has recently begun his third marriage. In an interview, he described why he has been married three times:

> One of my ex-wives once said to me, "You have to work at a marriage." And I said, "That's the most ridiculous thing," because my parents, they didn't work at the marriage. If you have to work at a marriage, it's not going to work. It has to be sort of a natural thing. But my ex-wife would say, "You have to work at this, you have to do this, you have to do that." And I'm saying to myself, "Man, I work all day long, well into the evening. I don't want to come home and work at a marriage. A marriage has to be very easy." (in Smith, 2004, p. 134)

As is demonstrated by the research discussed here, self-control is crucial for interpersonal success. Perhaps if Mr. Trump had listened to his ex-wife and recognized that one's career is not the only domain of life that requires self-control, he would not be a newlywed once again.

REFERENCES

Archer, J. (2000). Sex differences in aggression between heterosexual partners: A meta-analytic review. *Psychological Bulletin, 126*, 651–680.

Ayduk, O., Mendoza-Denton, R., Mischel, W., Downey, G., Peake, P. K., & Rodriguez, M. (2000). Regulating the interpersonal self: Strategic self-regulation for coping with rejection sensitivity. *Journal of Personality and Social Psychology, 79*, 776–792.

Baumeister, R. F., Bratslavsky, E., Muraven, M., & Tice, D. M. (1998). Ego depletion: Is the active self a limited resource? *Journal of Personality and Social Psychology, 74*, 1252–1265.

Baumeister, R. F., & Heatherton, T. F. (1996). Self-regulation failure: An overview. *Psychological Inquiry, 7,* 1–15.

Baumeister, R. F., Schmeichel, B. J., & Vohs, K. D. (in press). Self-regulation and the executive function: The self as controlling agent. In A. W. Kruglanski & E. T. Higgins (Eds.), *Social psychology: Handbook of basic principles* (2nd ed.). New York: Guilford Press.

Baumeister, R. F., & Tice, D. M. (1990). Anxiety and social exclusion. *Journal of Social and Clinical Psychology, 9,* 165–195.

Block, J., & Kremen, A. M. (1996). IQ and ego-resiliency: Conceptual and empirical connections and separateness. *Journal of Personality and Social Psychology, 70,* 349–361.

Eisele, A. (2004a). *Lennox Lewis career record.* Retrieved October 11, 2004, from boxing.about.com/library/bl_lewis.htm.

Eisele, A. (2004b). *Mike Tyson career record.* Retrieved October 11, 2004, from boxing.about.com/library/bl_tyson.htm.

Eisenberg, N., Valiente, C., Fabes, R. A., Smith, C. L., Reiser, M., Shepard, S. A., et al. (2003). The relations of effortful control and ego control to children's resiliency and social functioning. *Developmental Psychology, 39,* 761–776.

Evans, G. (2003). *Heavy hitter.* Retrieved October 11, 2004, from www.obv.org.uk/reports/2003/rpt20030615c.htm.

Feldman, R., Greenbaum, C. W., & Yirmiya, N. (1999). Mother–infant affect synchrony as an antecedent of the emergence of self-control. *Developmental Psychology, 35,* 223–231.

Finkel, E. J., & Campbell, W. K. (2001). Self-control and accommodation in close relationships: An interdependence analysis. *Journal of Personality and Social Psychology, 81,* 263–277.

Funder, D. C., & Block, J. (1989). The role of ego-control, ego-resiliency, and IQ in delay of gratification in adolescence. *Journal of Personality and Social Psychology, 57,* 1041–1050.

Funder, D. C., Block, J. H., & Block, J. (1983). Delay of gratification: Some longitudinal personality correlates. *Journal of Personality and Social Psychology, 44,* 1198–1213.

Gross, J. J., & John, O. P. (2003). Individual differences in two emotion regulation processes: Implications for affect, relationships, and well-being. *Journal of Personality and Social Psychology, 85,* 348–362.

Heatherton, T. F., & Vohs, K. D. (1998). Why is it so difficult to inhibit behavior? *Psychological Inquiry, 9,* 212–217.

How to train for boxing. (2004). Retrieved October 11, 2004, from www.ehow.com/how_16456_train-boxing.html.

Mason, A., & Blankenship, V. (1987). Power and affiliation motivation, stress, and abuse in intimate relationships. *Journal of Personality and Social Psychology, 52,* 203–210.

Mauro, C. F., & Harris, Y. R. (2000). The influence of maternal child-rearing attitudes and teaching behaviors on preschoolers' delay of gratification. *Journal of Genetic Psychology, 161,* 293–317.

Mike Tyson. (2000). Retrieved October 11, 2004, from www.hollywoodauditions.com/Biographies/mike_tyson.htm.

Miller, R. S. (1997). Inattentive and contented: Relationship commitment and attention to alternatives. *Journal of Personality and Social Psychology, 73,* 758–766.

Mischel, W., Shoda, Y., & Peake, P. K. (1988). The nature of adolescent competencies predicted by preschool delay of gratification. *Journal of Personality and Social Psychology, 54,* 687–696.

Neitzel, C., & Stright, A. D. (2003). Mothers' scaffolding of children's problem solving: Establishing a foundation of academic self-regulatory competence. *Journal of Family Psychology, 17,* 147–159.

O'Guinn, T. C., & Faber, R. J. (1989). Compulsive buying: A phenomenological exploration. *Journal of Consumer Research, 16,* 147–158.

Posner, M. I., & Rothbart, M. K. (2000). Developing mechanisms of self-regulation. *Development and Psychopathology, 12,* 427–441.

Putnam, S. P., Spritz, B. L., & Stifter, C. A. (2002). Mother–child coregulation during delay of gratification at 30 months. *Infancy, 3,* 209–225.

Rusbult, C. E. (1980). Commitment and satisfaction in romantic associations: A test of the investment model. *Journal of Experimental Social Psychology, 16,* 172–186.

Rusbult, C. E., Verette, J., Whitney, G. A., Slovik, L. F., & Lipkus, I. (1991). Accommodation processes in close relationships: Theory and preliminary empirical evidence. *Journal of Personality and Social Psychology, 60,* 53–78.

Saracento, J. (2005, June 2). Tyson: "My whole life has been a waste." *USA Today.* Accessed October 8, 2005, at www.usatoday.com/sports/boxing2005-06-02-tyson-saracento_x.htm.

Schmeichel, B. J., & Vohs, K. D. (2005). *Self-affirmation and the executive function of the self.* Manuscript in preparation, Texas A & M University.

Seeley, E. A., & Gardner, W. L. (2003). The "selfless" and self-regulation: The role of chronic other-orientation in averting self-regulatory depletion. *Self and Identity, 2,* 103–118.

Shoda, Y., Mischel, W., & Peake, P. K. (1990). Predicting adolescent cognitive and self-regulatory competencies from preschool delay of gratification: Identifying diagnostic conditions. *Developmental Psychology, 26,* 978–986.

Sicoly, F., & Ross, M. (1977). Facilitation of ego-biased attributions by means of self-serving observer feedback. *Journal of Personality and Social Psychology, 35,* 734–741.

Smith, L. (2004, October 1). At lunch with Liz. *Good Housekeeping,* pp. 130–134.

Tangney, J. P., Baumeister, R. F., & Boone, A. L. (2004). High self-control predicts good adjustment, less pathology, better grades, and interpersonal success. *Journal of Personality, 72,* 271–322.

Triandis, H. C. (1995). *Individualism and collectivism.* Boulder, CO: Westview Press.

Tyson troubles. (2002). Retrieved October 11, 2004, from www.reviewJournal.com/lvrj_home/2002/Jan-27-Sun-2002/sports/17964008.html.

Vohs, K.D., & Baumeister, R.F. (2004). Ego depletion, self-control, and choice. In J. Greenberg, S. L. Koole, & T. Pyszczynski (Eds.), *Handbook of experimental existential psychology* (pp. 398–410). New York: Guilford Press.

Vohs, K. D., & Baumeister, R. F. (2005). *Romantic relationship health is determined by partners' self-control.* Manuscript in preparation, University of Minnesota.

Vohs, K. D., Baumeister, R. F., & Ciarocco, N. J. (2005). Self-regulation and self-presentation: Regulatory resource depletion impairs impression management and effortful self-presentation depletes regulatory resources. *Journal of Personality and Social Psychology, 88,* 632–657.

Vohs, K. D., Baumeister, R. F., & Finkenauer, C. (2005). *Enough for the both of us: Dyadic level of self-control predicts relationship success.* Manuscript in preparation, University of Minnesota.

Wraga, M. P., & Abrams, D. (2002, October 3). Tyson pulls Steele into divorce battle. Gazette.net. Retrieved October 11, 2004, from www.gazette.net/200240/montgomerycty/state/123775-1.html.

CHAPTER 3

Pursuing Goals and Perceiving Others

A Self-Regulatory Perspective
on Interpersonal Relationships

GRÁINNE FITZSIMONS

Via self-regulation, individuals come to realize their dreams and desires—to turn their visions of the future into graspable realities, whether those visions be learning a new language, becoming a better parent, or being the first person in the family to graduate from college. Self-regulation is greatly important because it helps people to create the self and the social world in which they want to live.

Not surprisingly, given its importance, the process of self-regulation is thought to shape many other psychological constructs. Research has uncovered countless routes through which people's needs, goals, and desires can interact with and influence a wide array of psychological mechanisms. For example, New Look theorists demonstrated that needs affect how people perceive objects: Need-relevant objects are perceived to have more value than need-irrelevant objects (see Bruner, 1992). As another example, extensive evidence has illustrated the many ways that self-enhancing or self-protecting motivations can influence perceptions of both the self and others (e.g., Dunning, Leuenberger, & Sherman, 1995; Kay, Jiminez, & Jost, 2002; Kay & Jost, 2003; Kunda, 1990). Similarly, research on prejudice has shown that chronic motivations to avoid prejudice can alter the tendency to use stereotypes when perceiving outgroup members (e.g., Moskowitz, Gollwitzer, Wasel, & Schaal, 1999; Plant & Devine, 1998). Recently, work in social cognition has suggested that goals can even alter automatic attitudes toward everyday objects (Ferguson & Bargh, 2004). These are just a few examples of how goals and motives have been shown to shape psychological processes.

But what of the effects of everyday goals on people's most important social relationships? How do goals, needs, and desires affect the way we see our spouses, our family members, our colleagues, and our friends? Self-regulation likely shapes this important part of our interpersonal lives, but the role that it plays in central social relationships has not received much empirical attention. This chapter focuses on this issue, and emphasizes the idea that the important goals we pursue in everyday life—for example, career goals, social goals, and health goals—profoundly influence our behavior in relationships with family and friends. Integrating work on the intrapersonal processes related to self-regulation with research on interpersonal relationships, this chapter focuses on the hypothesis that evaluations of our most treasured social relationships—and behavior within those relationships—may reflect the connection of those relationships to our self-regulatory success.

Before launching into the integration of the intra- and interpersonal, the chapter first describes each of these processes separately, starting with research on the evaluative effects of self-regulation, and moving on to a brief glance at the subjectively constructed nature of interpersonal evaluations.

SELF-REGULATORY INFLUENCES ON EVALUATIONS

New Look theorists were the first to popularize the integration of motivational and cognitive perspectives (e.g., Bruner & Postman, 1948). They suggested that goals, needs, and desires shape and direct perceptions of the social world, drawing attention to objects and situations that are goal-relevant and simultaneously guiding interpretations of these objects in line with the individual's motivational priorities (Bruner & Goodman, 1947; Bruner & Postman, 1948; Postman, Bruner, & McGinnies, 1948). Chronic values such as religious beliefs, as well as current needs like thirst, were found to influence perceptions of objects and situations (for a review, see Bruner, 1992). In the decades since the New Look, the idea that perception is shaped by motivation has been met with some skepticism (see Nisbett & Ross, 1980), but currently appears to be accepted by mainstream social psychology (e.g., Armor & Taylor, 1998; Dunning et al., 1995; Gollwitzer & Moskowitz, 1996; Kruglanski, 1996; Kunda, 1990). An abundance of theories and empirical findings have supported the role that goals, desires, and needs can play in shaping the way people see themselves, others, and objects (e.g., Dunning et al., 1995; Fein & Spencer, 1997; Kunda, 1990; Taylor & Armor, 1996).

Of particular relevance to the current chapter, and in line with New Look thinking, many theorists have speculated that goals affect evaluations of objects in a particular direction—that is, to enhance self-regulatory success (see Lazarus, 1991). Lewin (1935) theorized that object evaluations depend on the extent to which the objects support versus hinder active goals. Rosenberg (1956) coined the term "instrumentality" to refer to an object's usefulness for goal fulfillment, and proposed that instrumentality was an important feature in object perception and evaluation. Since those early writings on instrumentality, much empirical research has supported the concept that the perceived value of an object varies as people's goals change, depending on the object's relevance to the goal (e.g., Brendl & Higgins, 1996; Brendl, Markman, & Messner, 2003; Shah & Higgins, 2001).

Building on the ideas of Lewin and Rosenberg, appraisal theories of emotion emphasized the idea that affective responses to objects stem from a person's current goals (Lazarus, 1991, 2001). Goal-congruent objects and events (i.e., ones that facilitate goal attainment) are theorized to be evaluated positively, and goal-incongruent objects (i.e., ones that block goal attainment) are theorized to be evaluated negatively (Frijda, 1986; Smith & Ellsworth, 1985). According to appraisal theories, such responses support self-regulation: By avoiding goal-incongruent and approaching goal-congruent objects and situations, individuals can increase their likelihood of achieving their goals and moving toward valued outcomes (Lazarus, 1991). In this fashion, goal-dependent evaluations contribute to individuals' attempts to make progress toward important goals and needs.

Most theorists who have discussed the goal dependency of evaluations have assumed that the effects of goals proceed without conscious awareness (Lazarus, 1991). Indeed, in an everyday situation, given the limited processing capacity of consciousness (Baddeley, 1989; Mandler, 1984), individuals are unlikely to have sufficient resources to evaluate objects as they relate to current and chronic goals in a deliberate and conscious fashion (see Bargh, 1990). Thus the effects of goals on evaluations are likely to occur automatically, with no need for conscious intervention. In the next section, the theories and supportive evidence underlying the potential automaticity of this process are further explicated.

Goals as Cognitive Representations and Automatic Goal Pursuit

The belief that goals may function outside of conscious awareness has resurfaced in social cognition recently, aided by recent research elucidating the cognitive features of goals (Bargh, 1990; Kruglanski, 1996). Such research has suggested that goals are mental representations, just like other constructs such as personality traits and stereotypes (e.g., Bargh, 1990; Kruglanski, 1996), and governed in a joint fashion by both motivational and cognitive principles (see Chartrand & Bargh, 2002; Shah, Kruglanski, & Friedman, 2003). If they are mental representations, then goals should be suitable for studying using the same social-cognitive tools that have been applied to constructs like traits and stereotypes. In addition, if they are mental structures, goals should share some of the features that characterize these other constructs, and should be guided by the same principles of accessibility, activation, and organization (Bargh, 1990; Bargh, Gollwitzer, Lee-Chai, Barndollar, & Troetschel, 2001; Hull, 1931; Kruglanski, 1996; Shah & Kruglanski, 2003).

Applying these basic principles to goals, theorists have hypothesized that the accessibility of goals will vary with the situational context. Contextual cues are thought to have the power to activate or trigger goal constructs directly, without the intervention of consciousness (Bargh, 1990; Higgins, 1996). Contextual cues are thought to gain this power to activate goals via the developing automation of links between goals and features of the situations in which these goals have often been initiated over time (Bargh, 1990; see also Chartrand & Bargh, 2002). With sufficient repetition of the goal–situation association, contextual cues can suffice to directly activate the goal construct and lead to goal pursuit. For example, if Charles always pursues a goal of impression management when he is in his boss's office, with time the office itself will serve as a sufficient cue for that goal to become active, even if Charles does not intentionally or consciously intend to pursue it.

Active goals can operate in two modes that depend on levels of temporary accessibility (e.g., via contextual cue activation) and chronic accessibility (e.g., via individual differences). They can operate *within* conscious awareness or they can become activated and operate *outside* of conscious awareness. Importantly, research suggests that regardless of operating mode, whether conscious or nonconscious, goals shape behavior in much the same fashion (Bargh et al., 2001; Chartrand & Bargh, 1996). Although empirical study of these ideas has begun only recently, strong support for the existence of a nonconscious mode of goal pursuit has already materialized (e.g., Aarts & Dijksterhuis, 2000; Bargh et al., 2001; Chartrand & Bargh, 1996; Ferguson & Bargh, 2004; Fishbach, Friedman, & Kruglanski, 2003; Fitzsimons & Bargh, 2003; Moskowitz et al., 1999; Shah, 2003a, 2003b; Shah, Friedman, & Kruglanski, 2002). In many of these experiments, goals that were activated via priming techniques (and thus outside of conscious awareness or control) were found to guide perception and behavior in an automatic fashion (see Fitzsimons & Bargh, 2004, for a review). Indeed, behaviors triggered by primed goals have now been shown to possess many of the features of goal pursuit that were once defined as requiring consciousness (Bargh et al., 2001; Fitzsimons & Bargh, 2004).

Beyond connections to situational cues, goals are theorized to be part of extensive mental networks, with multiple connections to many other constructs (Shah et al., 2002). Because of these connections, goals have been thought to influence the accessibility of related information and knowledge, possibly facilitating information that is consistent with goal pursuit and inhibiting information that is inconsistent with goal pursuit (Aarts, Dijksterhuis, & DeVries, 2001; Shah et al., 2002). For example, when motivated to lose weight, an individual's knowledge about diets and memories of past workout plans might come to mind more easily.

Especially pertinent for the current chapter, recent research on automatic attitudes (see Bargh, Chaiken, Govender, & Pratto, 1992, and Fazio, 2000, for reviews) has extended this automatic goal research to the evaluative domain, demonstrating that automatic evaluations are also goal-dependent (Ferguson & Bargh, 2004; Moors, De Houwer, & Eelen, 2004). Goal states do not activate all knowledge about goal-related objects in an unbiased fashion; rather, the knowledge they activate has an evaluative tone that depends on the usefulness of the object for goal fulfillment. Further supporting the original New Look theorizing on the nature of evaluations, Ferguson and Bargh (2004) note that as the motivations of a perceiver shift from one context to another, the evaluations of objects change as well, in accordance with the goal "congruence" or "incongruence" of the objects (see Lazarus, 1991). For example, when an individual is motivated to lose weight, he or she generally evaluates alcohol negatively—but if his or her motivation shifts to celebrate a special occasion, a glass of champagne may be seen in a much more positive light. That is, the evaluative criteria depend on the goals that are currently active, a finding that highlights the flexibility with which goals can shape evaluations.

To summarize this research, goals and related motivational constructs such as needs, desires, and wishes can have profound effects on the way that people evaluate themselves and their surroundings. Evaluations appear to depend greatly on the perceiver's goals, needs, and motives; furthermore, the effect of motivations on evaluations can occur completely outside of consciousness. The next section of the chapter examines the factors that are thought to typically underlie evaluations of interpersonal relationships. I then integrate these two areas and examine new evidence that examines how evaluations of important interpersonal relationships may also be goal-dependent.

INTERPERSONAL EVALUATIONS

The maintenance of positive social relationships is at the core of psychological well-being. Thus assessing the quality of these relationships is important for mental health (Leary, 2004; Leary & Downs, 1995). There is no shortage of dimensions on which people can judge the quality of their social relationships; studied dimensions have ranged from the partner's trustworthiness, loyalty, and supportiveness, to the balance of power, equity, and similarity within the relationship (see Berscheid & Reis, 1998). These evaluations are subject to influence from a variety of the perceiver's psychological tendencies as well, including individual differences such as attachment style (Mikulincer

& Horesh, 1999), rejection sensitivity (Downey & Feldman, 1996), trust (Holmes & Rempel, 1989), and naive romantic theories (Franiuk, Cohen, & Pomerantz, 2002; Knee & Canevello, Chapter 8, this volume). Relationship-level motivations have also been shown to influence these evaluations—for example, people with strong intimacy goals have been shown to experience greater relationship satisfaction (Sanderson & Cantor, 2001), and people high in the need to belong tend to have more accurate social perceptions (Pickett, Gardner, & Knowles, 2004). Thus interpersonal evaluations are not necessarily direct reflections of the particular qualities of a given relationship: They also manifest the influence of a number of other psychological variables, and very likely many interactions among these variables.

In sum, interpersonal evaluations are affected by a wide variety of factors, both intrapersonal and interpersonal in nature. These evaluations are subjective and highly malleable, adjusting to reflect the current psychological state of the self and other. The next section of the chapter presents evidence that *personal goals* can also play a role in shaping interpersonal evaluations, in that the link between the self's goal pursuits and the relationship partner can influence the positivity of the self's emotional and motivational response to that partner.

CURRENT RESEARCH: EFFECTS OF SELF-REGULATION ON INTERPERSONAL EVALUATIONS

Integrating the perspectives discussed so far, this next section of the chapter describes recent research suggesting that intrapersonal processes of self-regulation can have powerful effects on interpersonal processes, such as relationship evaluations and relationship behavior (Fitzsimons & Shah, 2005a). At the broadest level, this chapter presents the idea that interpersonal evaluations serve to enhance self-regulatory ability, allowing individuals to more effectively pursue goals and achieve goal fulfillment by selectively engaging in beneficial social relationships and social situations. At a more specific level, this chapter examines the idea that the *instrumentality* of a relationship partner for a given goal—the extent to which this partner promotes self-regulatory progress in this goal domain—is an important underlying factor in how the relationship is evaluated. That is, when a goal is active, relationship partners should be evaluated with respect to how they relate to that goal: People who are "goal-congruent" or "instrumental" should be evaluated more positively, while those who are "goal-incongruent" or "noninstrumental" should be evaluated more negatively, compared to when that particular goal is not active.

The perception that a significant other is instrumental for the self's goal pursuits can arise for a number of different reasons. A significant other can be instrumental by providing direct help with the goal domain (e.g., tutoring you in math), by providing social support for your attempts in that goal domain (e.g., baby-sitting your child so you can take math classes at night, or encouraging you to study), by inspiring you with his or her success in this or another goal domain, or even by serving as a source of competitive energy, causing you to work harder. There are a variety of ways to be instrumental. This chapter focuses simply on the all-inclusive meaning of the word *instrumental* as Rosenberg (1956) first defined it for objects: an instrumental object (or other) is one whose existence makes goal progress more likely.

Perceptions of the instrumentality of a relationship partner for a specific goal may be embedded in mental links connecting the goal construct and the mental representation of the significant other. These links are thought to include knowledge about the other's qualities, intentions, and abilities regarding this goal (see Andersen & Chen, 2002; Baldwin, 1992; Baldwin, Carrell, & Lopez, 1991; Holmes, 2000; Miller & Read, 1991). Empirical support for the existence of direct self–other links comes from findings that activating one of these representations leads automatically to activation of the other. For example, when representations of significant others become activated, either through natural social interactions or via some unobtrusive priming mechanism, they can lead to automatic influences on the self's perception and behavior (see Chen, Andersen, & Fitzsimons, in press, for a review). For example, subliminal exposure to the disapproving face of the Roman Catholic pope caused practicing Catholics to experience lower self-esteem, but did not affect nonpracticing Catholics (Baldwin et al., 1990).

Of particular interest to the current chapter is recent evidence for the inclusion of *goal*-related information in these links between self and other (Andersen, Reznik, & Manzella, 1996; Fitzsimons & Bargh, 2003; Shah, 2003a, 2003b). In a number of studies, significant others have been shown to act as automatic triggers for the self's goals. These findings support the hypothesis that information related to the self's goals, and the other's connection to these goals (such as, perhaps, their instrumentality for this goal), are embedded in these self–other links.

If individuals do use information about instrumentality as a basis for evaluating relationships, this process may help them construct environments that support self-regulatory success. When individuals feel more positively about instrumental significant others, and thus choose to spend more time with them and approach them more readily, they will embed themselves in social situations that enhance their chances of fulfilling their important goals and needs. Similarly, when individuals avoid relationships and social situations that obstruct goal progress, they further contribute to the success of self-regulation attempts.

For example, if Tim desperately wants to make partner in his law firm this year, he may evaluate his friendships accordingly, feeling more positively about a friend (Jason) who offers to "talk him up" to the other partners in the firm, and feeling less positively about a friend (Ryan) who gives him a hard time when he goes home early from a night out at the bars. If Tim's goal to make partner maintains its importance for any length of time, this pattern of goal-dependent evaluations may lead Tim to spend more time with Jason and less time with Ryan. In turn, this should increase the likelihood that Tim will achieve his goal of making partner.

Importantly, like other aspects of self-regulation discussed earlier, this process likely occurs mainly outside of conscious awareness. That is, individuals engaged in goal pursuit should seek goal-congruent others without need for extensive conscious deliberation about the relation of each person to the current goal, or about whether the goal should be used as a basis for evaluation at this time. Furthermore, as people's goals and motivations shift from one context to another, so too should their criteria for evaluation, such that they automatically evaluate and reevaluate other people, objects, and situations with respect to currently active goals (see Ferguson & Bargh, 2004). Automating this process should minimize strain on cognitive capacity and self-regulatory resources, and thereby lead to more successful goal pursuit. Of course, there are limits to the advantages of fully automated processes; ideally, the busy self-regulator would utilize these automated self-regulatory strategies and processes to complement those chosen with fully conscious intent.

Of course, even when goals themselves are fully in consciousness, the effects of those goals on interpersonal evaluations will tend to occur outside of conscious awareness. It is unlikely that people use their beliefs about the instrumentality of others in a conscious fashion to influence their evaluations, even if both the goal and the beliefs about the other person are available to consciousness. It is possible that people might utilize this strategy consciously, but for the average person in an average day it is much more likely that the process will occur outside of conscious awareness.

For example, Tim knows he wants to make partner, and he is aware of pursuing this goal. However, he may not realize how this goal is affecting his evaluations of his friends. He may just find himself enjoying the company of Ryan a little less than usual, without analyzing or understanding that his desire to make partner (and his belief that Ryan does not help this goal) is the underlying reason for his feelings. For evaluations to be affected by goals, very little needs to be consciously thought out or considered. In the fleeting decisions individuals make in an average day, for example, when they decide which friend to call or which colleague to invite to lunch, they are unlikely to recognize the influence of their active goals on their decision.

Empirical support for the general idea that instrumental relationship partners are evaluated more positively is provided by research on social support within close relationships. Perceiving that one is part of a social network that provides support at times of stress is known to provide positive psychological benefits (e.g., Wills, 1991; cf. Bolger, Zuckerman, & Kessler, 2000). Most related to the current hypothesis, Brunstein, Dangelmayer, and Schultheiss (1996) found that partners' support of personal goals was correlated with individuals' perceptions of relationship quality. That is, significant others who were seen as providing opportunities for their partners to work on their goals, being responsive to the importance of these goals, and reliably assisting with goal pursuit were perceived more positively than significant others who did not exhibit this direct goal support.

Providing social support, whether emotional or tangible, is one route through which significant others can be instrumental for goal achievement. As briefly discussed earlier in this section, we propose that there are other routes by which significant others can be instrumental that are not captured within the social support constructs, but may yield the same evaluative effects. For example, others can be instrumental without even intending to be so: a friend may introduce you to people in an industry in which you would like to work; a rival may help you focus and work harder; a colleague may inspire you through her actions. In these cases and many others, the instrumentality of others for the self's goal progress does not depend on the perception that the others intend to help and support the self. And yet, according to the current hypotheses, interpersonal evaluations will be positively affected by all kinds of instrumentality, including that which has this unintended nature.

Turning to data, I now describe a series of empirical tests of the general hypothesis that interpersonal evaluations and relationship behavior are goal-dependent, and address several secondary hypotheses stemming from this overarching idea.

The Effects of Goals on Relationship Evaluations

When a goal is active, relationships with people who facilitate goal progress are theorized to be perceived as closer and more important than relationships with people who do not facilitate goal progress. A series of recent studies has provided evidence for this hypothesis (Fitzsimons & Shah, 2005a). For example, in one study participants nominated good friends who were instrumental or not instrumental for a list of goals, including academic achievement. Later on, participants completed a scrambled sentence task (Srull & Wyer, 1979). For half of the participants, the task was designed to activate achievement goals via the presentation of words related to achievement such as *succeed* and *achieve*. For the other half of the participants, the task presented only neutral, nonmotivational words, matched in length and valence to the achievement goal words. Subsequently, participants evaluated their friendships, and indicated how much time they planned on spending with each of these friends in the upcoming 2 weeks.

As predicted, the currently accessible goal to achieve shaped participants' evaluations of their friendships. Participants primed with a nonconscious achievement goal reported feeling closer to achievement-instrumental friends than friends who were not instrumental for achievement. They also reported relationships with achievement-instrumental friends as more important, and planned to spend more time with them. In contrast, participants in the control condition—who had no primed goal to achieve—did not report feeling any differently about their facilitating and nonfacilitating friends.

Thus our findings suggest that evaluations of good friends are shaped partially by the relationship of these friends to currently active goals. These data further suggest that the goal dependence of interpersonal evaluations is flexible and sensitive to contextual cues. Only when goals are currently active do individuals use their instrumentality as a basis for evaluating their friends; otherwise, they do not use this as a criterion for evaluation. Chronically active goals will of course frequently influence evaluations, and will be active across many contexts, shaping evaluations according to others' instrumentality for these important overarching goals. In a complementary fashion, though, contextual flexibility allows this process to confer self-regulatory benefit: If people always evaluated their friends on the basis of their instrumentality for achievement, they would miss the many other benefits these friendships can provide, the many other goals these friendships nurture and enhance. For example, if Tim's girlfriend breaks up with him and he is feeling despondent, his friend Ryan (who is noninstrumental for his goal of making partner in the law firm) may be very instrumental for the goal of mood repair or stress relief. So in this situation, Tim may benefit from seeing Ryan more positively. That is, the effective self-regulator needs to use this instrumentality-evaluation process in a flexible manner, accommodating to the goals and motives of the moment as well as to more chronically important desires.

The Effects of Goals on the Accessibility of Relationship Partners

A secondary question we set out to examine was whether active goals would also simply "bring to mind" goal-congruent significant others (Fitzsimons & Shah, 2005a). The process of creating links from goals to instrumental others could advance self-regulatory attempts in a very straightforward fashion: If goals are directly linked to representations of instrumental significant others, then when the goal is active, individuals may be more likely to contact that person, spend time with that person, and so on, which could also advance goal progress.

To examine that hypothesis, we conducted a study in which accessibility was the main dependent measure. Participants were asked to provide the name of a good friend who was instrumental for their goal of having a fun social life and the name of a good friend who was not particularly instrumental for this goal. Participants in one condition were exposed to words related to sociability motives in a word task (e.g., *socialize, mingle, party*). All participants completed a "primacy of output" measure (Higgins, King, & Mavin, 1982), in which they listed the first names of all their good friends at college in the order in which they came to mind. The order in which participants received these tasks was counterbalanced, such that half received the goal instrumentality measure first, and half received the priming and accessibility tasks first. As predicted, when a sociability goal was activated, sociability-instrumental friends came more readily to mind, in that their names were generated earlier in participants' list of friends. Similarly, noninstrumental friends were *less* accessible when a sociability goal was activated, compared to a no-goal condition. This suggests that goals can activate, or bring to mind, the mental representations of significant others who are instrumental for goal attainment.

Accessibility versus Evaluations of Goal-Relevant Others

It is of course feasible that both the accessibility and the evaluative effects noted above may reflect the workings of some unrelated third variable—that is, people who are instrumental for a certain goal may also possess some other quality that accounts for their increased accessibility and positive evaluations when the goal becomes active. To further elucidate the nature of these effects, we conducted a follow-up study that examined participants' reactions to three different kinds of friends, who differed in their relation to a goal to achieve at university, and measured both closeness and accessibility to see if the patterns differed.

One type of friend (*instrumental*) was described as being instrumental for the participant's goal but not particularly successful or interested in university; one type of friend (*goal relevant*) was described as being successful and interested in academic achievement but was not particularly facilitative of the individual's goal progress; one final type of friend (*goal irrelevant*) was described as possessing neither quality—this friend was neither accomplished or interested in university, nor was he or she instrumental to the individual's success. For example, one participant nominated the following friends: *instrumental*: "Amanda dropped out last semester, and now she is waitressing at a bar downtown. She is helpful to my studies because she calms me down when I'm stressed and is always excited when I do well."; *goal relevant*: "Becky is great at math, and is doing really well, but she and I don't ever work together and I don't find her helpful in class. I do have fun with her outside of school though!"; *goal irrelevant*: "Lina is not in my department but I do take some classes with her. She doesn't really care about school. She's *a lot* of fun but she doesn't help me do any better here."

By requiring participants to nominate these three kinds of friends, two who are linked to the goal construct—but for different reasons—and one who is not strongly linked to the goal construct, this design disentangled instrumentality from other goal-relevant qualities. To further look at the accessibility versus evaluation question, we also measured both accessibility (via a primacy of output measure) and reported closeness of each friendship to determine if a distinction exists between these two processes.

When participants were primed with an academic achievement goal, we found that *instrumental* friends were more accessible and were also more positively evaluated, replicating earlier findings. Interestingly, *goal-relevant* friends were also found to be more accessible after goal priming, but were not found to be more positively evaluated. That is, active goals did not affect perceptions of closeness for these successful-but-not-helpful friends. *Goal-irrelevant* friends were not made more accessible or closer by the goal priming.

These findings support our self-regulatory interpretation of the earlier studies. To construct a social world that enhances one's ability to achieve important goals, one should evaluate relationships with instrumental others—those who contribute to self-regulatory success—more positively, whether or not they have any other connection to the goal domain. Because of simple semantic spreading-activation processes unrelated to self-regulation, representations of both instrumental and goal-relevant others become more accessible, as evidenced in this study. However, relationships with goal-relevant others who are not instrumental do not contribute to self-regulatory success, and thus they should not receive an evaluative "boost" from their connection to the goal construct. This process causes goal pursuers to draw closer only those friends who can serve the self's higher order goals and motives, providing a functional self-regulatory benefit.

The Effects of Goals on Approach and Avoidance Behavioral Tendencies

For significant self-regulatory benefits to arise, it is likely that instrumentality must go beyond affecting evaluations of relationship partners and shape behavior as well. As a first step toward examining the effects of goals on relationship behavior, we examined approach and avoidance behavioral tendencies, reflections of the most basic human motivations and important drivers of interpersonal relations (Andersen et al., 1996; Baumeister & Leary, 1995; Gable, Reis, & Elliot, 2000; Gray, 1990; Updegraff, Gable, & Taylor, 2004). Approaching others who can help with goal progress—and avoiding others who cannot help with goal progress—should lead to increased self-regulatory success.

Indeed, as predicted, two studies demonstrated that people's approach and avoidance of their relationship partners depended on the partners' instrumentality for an active goal (Fitzsimons & Shah, 2005a). In one study, participants were primed with an achievement goal and then asked about their motivation to approach and to avoid either an instrumental friend or a noninstrumental friend, in a between-subjects design. Participants not primed with any goal reported similar levels of approach and avoidance motivations, whether they were asked about instrumental or noninstrumental friends. In contrast, goal-primed participants reported more approach and less avoidance motivation toward instrumental friends, and less approach and more avoidance motivation toward noninstrumental friends.

In a related study, we found that participants responded faster to approach the names of instrumental friends, and slower to approach the names of noninstrumental friends, when those names were preceded by the subliminal presentation of a goal word. That is, on a trial-by-trial basis, goal primes led to faster approach of friends who were instrumental for the primed goal, and led to slower approach of noninstrumental friends. The complementary pattern of responses was found in trials when participants were instructed to avoid names. In those trials, participants responded faster to avoid noninstrumental friends and slower to avoid instrumental friends. Overall, participants in this study exhibited highly flexible and automatic goal-dependent approach and avoidance tendencies: As goals became active via subliminal exposure to goal-related words, participants responded by automatically altering their behavioral tendencies, and these tendencies responded to moment-by-moment changes in goal-activation levels.

Future research should examine more high-level, more social relationships behaviors in terms of the distinction between instrumental and noninstrumental others. For example, are people more forgiving of the transgressions of goal-instrumental others when the goal is active? Do they raise their standards and become more critical of noninstrumental others when the goal is active? Does their willingness to accommodate the others' wishes depend on the others' instrumentality? These important relationship questions need to be addressed in future research on the behavioral consequences of this process.

Effectiveness of Goal-Dependent Evaluations for Self-Regulation

An explicit assumption of this research is that evaluating relationship partners based on their instrumentality provides the individual with some self-regulatory benefit. Initial data support this assumption, suggesting that individuals who base their evaluations of relationship partners on their instrumentality for important goals make better self-regulatory progress (Shah & Fitzsimons, 2005). In their subjective reports, people who exhibit goal-dependent interpersonal evaluations in the domain of achievement consider themselves to be more effective self-regulators regarding achievement goals. In longitudinal studies, initial data suggest that the stronger the dependence of interpersonal evaluations on goal instrumentality at Time 1, the more perceived goal progress individuals have made at Time 2. Most compellingly, one study demonstrated that individuals who had more goal-dependent interpersonal evaluations at the beginning of the semester (in the domain of academic achievement) went on to receive better grades by the end of that semester. Thus it appears that evaluating relationship partners based on their instrumentality for important goals does lead to more success at goal attainment. Exactly how this occurs is still a question that remains to be answered. For example, does the amount of time individuals spend with their instrumental and noninstrumental friends mediate the relationship between goal-dependent evaluations and subsequent goal progress? Or is it simply that effective self-regulators both engage in this process and make more goal progress? Future research should elucidate the mechanism underlying these evaluative and behavioral effects.

Initial Thoughts on Underlying Mechanisms

This chapter has presented data suggesting that the activation of a personal goal appears to have a strong impact on the evaluations of relationship partners, but without providing any clear answers as to how exactly this process occurs. Although no research has directly examined this mechanism, prior research provides some important clues. When a goal is activated, it is thought to highlight the *relevant aspects* of all associated structures (Shah et al., 2003). For example, people motivated to believe that they possess a certain trait recall more instances in which they behaved in line with this trait (Sanitioso, Kunda, & Fong, 1990); the same has also been shown for people motivated to believe their romantic partner has a particular personality trait (Murray & Holmes, 1997). This motivation-guided biased retrieval of information is one route through which goal effects on interpersonal evaluations could occur. Namely, goals could lead to a biased retrieval of positively valenced information about instrumental significant others, and a biased retrieval of negatively valenced information about noninstrumental significant others, which would thereby alter the overall valence of the active significant other representation. For self-regulatory benefit, this information would not need to be goal-related, but simply valenced in the direction that leads to more approach of the instrumental individual and more avoidance of the noninstrumental individual. For example, Tim's goal to make partner may cause him to remember all the good times he has shared with Jason, such as when Jason bought him lunch and told a hilarious joke. In contrast, he may remember more negative things about Ryan—wholly unrelated to the current goal—like the time he forgot to water Tim's plants when Tim was away or the time he cheated at pool, that may then lead to a more negative overall evaluation of Ryan.

As well as causing the activation of information, motivation may also cause the inhibition or suppression of information (Andersen & Spellman, 1995; Kunda & Sinclair, 1999). That is, goals could lead to an inhibition of valenced information about instrumental and noninstrumental significant others. Unattractive attributes of instrumental significant others could be inhibited in order to maintain positive evaluations and encourage approach of this goal-facilitative person; attractive features of noninstrumental significant others could be temporarily inhibited in order to encourage focus on the active goal. So it may become harder for Tim to remember some of the positive things about Ryan when his "make partner" goal is active. Via either of these routes or through some combination of both of these processes, or by some as yet unconsidered process, personal goals can alter people's evaluations of their interpersonal relationships.

DISCUSSION

The set of findings discussed here suggests that interpersonal evaluations may serve a valuable self-regulatory function, allowing the self-regulator to engage in helpful social relationships and situations, and disengage from less helpful ones, in the name of better progress toward important personal goals. The self-regulator—typically described as an independent agent, whose success or failure is determined by intrapersonal qualities such as strength of will and skill at goal setting—is evidently also an interdependent agent, whose success or failure is shaped by interpersonal processes such as those described in this chapter.

This research highlights the dynamic nature of the interpersonal self, or the links between representations of self and other (Andersen & Chen, 2002). People's perceived closeness to significant others fluctuates depending on the current self-regulatory needs of the individual and the information stored in the goal–significant other links. Because the motivational context is frequently shifting, the self needs to be flexible and responsive to these changes, as well as to any changes in interpersonal contexts (Hardin & Conley, 2001; Hardin & Higgins, 1996). The flexibility of this process contributes to the understanding of the fluid and bidirectional nature of self–other connections that is emerging from work on the relational self (Andersen & Chen, 2002; Baldwin, 1992; Chen et al., in press). Just as the current research suggests that self-regulation influences and shapes interpersonal relationships, so too has much previous research suggested that interpersonal relationships influence and shape self-regulation (Anderson et al., 1996; Fitzsimons & Bargh, 2003; Shah, 2003a, 2003b; see Shah, Chapter 19, this volume).

Interactions of Intra- and Interpersonal Processes

The self-regulatory function of interpersonal relationships has been the main focus of this chapter. Of course, relationships serve many other functions—they do not simply exist to help the self make progress toward personal goals. Evaluations of relationships likely have many other functions and underlying factors that are not related to personal goal progress. Satisfying relationships are the cornerstone of solid mental health and psychological well-being (see Leary, 2004), and relationships may primarily serve to provide the self with a sense of security and belongingness (Baumeister & Leary, 1995). Indeed, the overarching interpersonal motivation to maintain positive relationships is known to shape many aspects of the self, including personal goal pursuit (Hardin & Conley, 2001; Leary, 2004; Leary & Downs, 1995). For example, the self's pursuit of personal goals such as achievement have been shown to serve higher order interpersonal motives such as belonging (Baumeister & Leary, 1995; Deci & Ryan, 1985; Leary, 2004; Leary & Downs, 1995). Thus the dynamic and reciprocal relationship between self-regulatory and interpersonal processes is further highlighted by noting that personal goals can also serve in function of interpersonal relationships, just as relationships can serve in function of personal goals.

These ideas and findings are consistent with many interpersonal theories of the self that propose that people who are interpersonally oriented will be more likely to depend on their significant others for help with goal pursuit (see Markus & Kitayama, 1991; Seeley & Gardner, Chapter 20, this volume). In accordance with these theories, the current research assumes that this is a bidirectional and dynamic process, with interpersonal relationships shaping evaluations of the importance of various personal goals, just as this research has suggested that goals can shape evaluations of the importance of various interpersonal relationships.

In fact, preliminary data suggests that people who are high in relational interdependence are more likely to exhibit goal-dependent interpersonal evaluations (Fitzsimons & Shah, 2005b). Likely because of the close links between self and other, the self's goals have a more profound effect on evaluations of significant others for those who are highly interdependent. In two studies, findings suggest that for participants higher in interdependence, the instrumentality of significant others for currently active goals was more important in determining their feelings and behavior toward these others.

Interestingly, evaluating other people in terms of how useful they are for our own personal goals could be seen as more tied to an *independent* self-construal, where the self's wants and needs take priority over more relational concerns. However, these initial findings are wholly consistent with a relational self perspective: people who have stronger bonds between self and other representations will exhibit stronger effects in either direction, whether it is significant others affecting goal pursuit or goals affecting significant other evaluations.

Concluding Comments

The integration of the studies of self-regulation and interpersonal relationships may yield important insights for both fields. For the study of interpersonal relationships, the inclusion of self-regulatory concepts and processes would serve to broaden the understanding of relationship behavior. Within any social relationship, there are two people with a multitude of personal goals and interpersonal motives, constantly in interaction with each other. The more we understand about the basic and low-level ways in which self-regulation can interact with and influence interpersonal relationships, the more we will understand about real-world relationship behavior. For the study of self-regulation, the inclusion of more interpersonal processes and perspectives would serve to situate the self within the social world in which all goals are pursued and all selves are regulated. Rather than study the self-regulator as a bounded and independent agent, we would immerse the self-regulator into interpersonal contexts, an approach that could shed new light on basic intrapersonal processes. As Berscheid and Reis (1998) noted:

> Further advances in social cognition may depend on gaining an understanding of cognitive processes as they occur in ongoing association with others with whom the individual is interdependent for the achievement of his or her goals and where the actions that result from those processes have potent consequences for the individual's well-being. Without such knowledge, an understanding of social cognition will be incomplete and it also may be inaccurate (see Fiske & Taylor 1991, p. 557).

REFERENCES

Aarts, H., & Dijksterhuis, A. (2000). Habits as knowledge structures: Automaticity in goal-directed behavior. *Journal of Personality and Social Psychology, 78*, 53–63.

Aarts, H., Dijksterhuis, A., & De Vries, P. (2001). The psychology of drinking: Being thirsty and perceptually ready. *British Journal of Psychology, 92*, 631–642.

Andersen, S. M., & Chen, S. (2002). The relational self: An interpersonal social-cognitive theory. *Psychological Review, 109*, 619–645.

Andersen, S. M., Reznik, I., & Manzella, L. M. (1996). Eliciting transient affect, motivation, and expectancies in transference: Significant-other representations in social relations. *Journal of Personality and Social Psychology, 71*, 1108–1129.

Anderson, M. C., & Spellman, B. A. (1995). On the status of inhibitory mechanisms in cognition: Memory retrieval as a model case. *Psychological Review, 102*, 68–100.

Armor, D. A., & Taylor, S. E. (1998). Situated optimism: Specific outcome expectations and self-regulation. In M. P. Zanna (Ed.), *Advances in experimental social psychology* (Vol. 30, pp. 309–379). New York: Academic Press.

Baddeley, A. (1989). The uses of working memory. In P. R. Solomon, G. R. Goethals, C. M. Kelley, & B. R. Stephens (Eds.), *Memory: Interdisciplinary approaches* (pp. 107–123). New York: Springer Verlag.

Baldwin, M. W. (1992). Relational schemas and the processing of social information. *Psychological Bulletin, 112,* 461–484.

Baldwin, M. W., Carrell, S. E., & Lopez, D. F. (1990). Priming relationship schemas: My advisor and the pope are watching me from the back of my mind. *Journal of Experimental Social Psychology, 26,* 435–454.

Bargh, J. A. (1990). Auto-motives: Preconscious determinants of social interaction. In E. T. Higgins & R. M. Sorrentino (Eds.), *Handbook of motivation and cognition: Foundations of social behavior* (Vol. 2, pp. 93–130). New York: Guilford Press.

Bargh, J. A., Chaiken, S., Govender, R., & Pratto, F. (1992). The generality of the automatic attitude activation effect. *Journal of Personality and Social Psychology, 62,* 893–912.

Bargh, J. A., Gollwitzer, P. M., Lee-Chai, A., Barndollar, K., & Troetschel, R. (2001). The automated will: Nonconscious activation and pursuit of behavioral goals. *Journal of Personality and Social Psychology, 81,* 1014–1027.

Baumeister, R. F., & Leary, M. R. (1995). The need to belong: Desire for interpersonal attachments as a fundamental human motivation. *Psychological Bulletin, 117,* 497–529.

Berscheid, E., & Reis, H. T. (1998). Attraction and close relationships. In D. T. Gilbert, S. T. Fiske, & G. Lindzey (Eds.), *The handbook of social psychology* (4th ed., pp. 193–281). New York: McGraw-Hill.

Bolger, N., Zuckerman, A., & Kessler, R. C. (2000). Invisible support and adjustment to stress. *Journal of Personality and Social Psychology, 79,* 953–961.

Brendl, C. M., & Higgins, E. T. (1996). Principles of judging valence: What makes events positive or negative? *Advances in Experimental Social Psychology, 28,* 95–160.

Brendl, C. M., Markman, A., & Messner, C. (2003). The devaluation effect: Activating a need devalues unrelated choice options. *Journal of Consumer Research, 29,* 463–473.

Bruner, J. (1992). Another look at New Look 1. *American Psychologist, 47,* 780–783.

Bruner, J. S., & Goodman, C. C. (1947). Value and need as organizing factors in perception. *Journal of Abnormal and Social Psychology, 42,* 33–44.

Bruner, J. S., & Postman, L. (1948). An approach to social perception. In W. Dennis (Ed.), *Current trends in social psychology* (pp. 71–118). Pittsburgh, PA: University of Pittsburgh Press.

Brunstein, J. C., Dangelmayer, G., & Schultheiss, O. C. (1996). Personal goals and social support in close relationships: Effects on relationship mood and marital satisfaction. *Journal of Personality and Social Psychology, 71,* 1006–1019.

Chartrand, T. L., & Bargh, J. A. (1996). Automatic activation of impression formation and memorization goals: Nonconscious goal priming reproduces effects of explicit task instructions. *Journal of Personality and Social Psychology, 71*(3), 464–478.

Chartrand, T. L., & Bargh, J. A. (2002). Nonconscious motivations: Their activation, operation, and consequences. In A. Tesser, D. A. Stapel, & J. V. Wood (Eds.), *Self and motivation: Emerging psychological perspectives* (pp. 13–41). Washington, DC: American Psychological Association.

Chen, S., Andersen, S. M., & Fitzsimons, G. M. (in press). Automaticity in close relationships. In J. A. Bargh (Ed.), *Automatic processes in social thinking and behavior*. Philadelphia: Psychology Press.

Deci, E. L., & Ryan, R. M. (1985). *Intrinsic motivation and self-determination in human behavior*. New York: Plenum Press.

Downey, G., & Feldman, S. I. (1996). Implications of rejection sensitivity for intimate relationships. *Journal of Personality and Social Psychology, 70,* 1327–1343.

Dunning, D., Leuenberger, A., & Sherman, D. A. (1995). A new look at motivated inference: Are self-serving theories of success a product of motivational forces? *Journal of Personality and Social Psychology, 69,* 58–68.

Fazio, R. H. (2000). On the automatic activation of associated evaluations: An overview. *Cognition and Emotion, 14,* 1–27.

Fein, S., & Spencer, S. J. (1997). Prejudice as self-image maintenance: Affirming the self through derogating others. *Journal of Personality and Social Psychology, 73,* 31–44.

Ferguson, M., & Bargh, J. A. (2004). Liking is for doing: The effect of goal pursuit on automatically activated attitudes. *Journal of Personality and Social Psychology, 87,* 557–572.

Fishbach, A., Friedman, R. S., & Kruglanski, A. W. (2003). Leading us not into temptation: Momentary allurements elicit overriding goal activation. *Journal of Personality and Social Psychology, 84,* 296–309.

Fiske S., & Taylor, S. (1991). *Social cognition*. New York: McGraw-Hill.

Fitzsimons, G. M., & Bargh, J. A. (2003). Thinking of you: Nonconscious pursuit of interpersonal goals associated with relationship partners. *Journal of Personality and Social Psychology, 84,* 148–163.

Fitzsimons, G. M., & Bargh, J. A. (2004). Automatic self-regulation. In R. F. Baumeister & K. Vohs (Eds.), *Handbook of self-regulation* (pp. 151–170). New York: Guilford Press.

Fitzsimons, G. M., & Shah, J. Y. (2005a). *The goal-dependency of interpersonal evaluations and behavioral tendencies*. Manuscript submitted for review.

Fitzsimons, G. M., & Shah, J. Y. (2005b). *Role of self-construal in effects of personal goals on relationship evaluations. Research in progress*. Manuscript in preparation.

Franiuk, R., Cohen, D., & Pomerantz, E. M. (2002). Implicit theories of relationships: Implications for relationship satisfaction and longevity. *Personal Relationships, 9,* 345–367.

Frijda, N. H. (1986). *The emotions*. Cambridge, UK: Cambridge University Press.

Gable, S. L., Reis, H. T., & Elliot, A. J. (2000). Behavioral activation and inhibition in everyday life. *Journal of Personality and Social Psychology, 78,* 1135–1149.

Gollwitzer, P. M., & Moskowitz, G. B. (1996). Goal effects on action and cognition. In E. T. Higgins & A. W. Kruglanski (Eds.), *Social psychology: Handbook of basic principles* (pp. 361–399). New York: Guilford Press.

Gray, J. A. (1990). Brain systems that mediate both emotion and cognition. *Cognition and Emotion, 4*, 269–288.

Hardin, C. D., & Conley, T. D. (2001). A relational approach to cognition: Shared experience and relationship affirmation in social cognition. In G. B. Moskowitz (Ed.), *Cognitive social psychology: The Princeton Symposium on the Legacy and Future of Social Cognition* (pp. 3–21). Mahwah, NJ: Erlbaum.

Hardin, C. D., & Higgins, E. T. (1996). Shared reality: How social verification makes the subjective objective. In R. M. Sorrentino & E. T. Higgins (Eds.), *Handbook of motivation and cognition: Vol. 3. The interpersonal context* (pp. 28–84). New York: Guilford Press.

Higgins, E. T. (1996). Knowledge activation: Accessibility, applicability, and salience. In E. T. Higgins & A. W. Kruglanski (Eds.), *Social psychology: Handbook of basic principles* (pp. 133–168). New York: Guilford Press.

Higgins, E. T., King, G. A., & Mavin, G. H. (1982). Individual construct accessibility and subjective impressions and recall. *Journal of Personality and Social Psychology, 43*, 35–47.

Holmes, J. G. (2000). Social relationships: The nature and function of relational schemas. *European Journal of Social Psychology, 30*, 447–495.

Holmes, J. G., & Rempel, J. (1989). Trust in close relationships. In C. Hendrick (Ed.), *Close relationships* (pp. 187–220). Newbury Park, CA: Sage.

Hull, C. (1931). Goal attraction and directing ideas conceived as habit phenomena. *Psychological Review, 38*, 487–506.

Kay, A. C., Jimenez, M. C., & Jost, J. T. (2002). Sour grapes, sweet lemons, and the anticipatory rationalization of the status quo. *Personality and Social Psychology Bulletin, 28*, 1300–1312.

Kay, A. C., & Jost, J. T. (2003). Complementary justice: Effects of "poor but happy" and "poor but honest" stereotype exemplars on system justification and implicit activation of the justice motive. *Journal of Personality and Social Psychology, 85*, 823–837.

Kruglanski, A. W. (1996). A motivated gatekeeper of our minds: Need-for-closure effects on interpersonal and group processes. In R. M. Sorrentino & E. T. Higgins (Eds.), *Handbook of motivation and cognition: Vol. 3. The interpersonal context* (pp. 465–496). New York: Guilford Press.

Kunda, Z. (1990). The case for motivated reasoning. *Psychological Bulletin, 108*, 480–498.

Kunda, Z., & Sinclair, L. (1999). Motivated reasoning with stereotypes: Activation, application, and inhibition. *Psychological Inquiry, 10*, 12–22.

Lazarus, R. S. (1991). Psychological stress in the workplace. *Journal of Social Behavior and Personality, 6*, 1–13.

Lazarus, R. S. (2001). Relational meaning and discrete emotions. In K. R. Scherer, A. Schorr, & T. Johnstone (Eds.), *Appraisal processes in emotion: Theory, methods, research* (pp. 37–67). New York: Oxford University Press.

Leary, M. R. (2004). The sociometer, self-esteem, and the regulation of interpersonal behavior. In R. F. Baumeister & K. Vohs (Eds.), *Handbook of self-regulation* (pp. 373–391). New York: Guilford Press.

Leary, M. R., & Downs, D. L. (1995). Interpersonal functions of the self-esteem motive: The self-esteem system as a sociometer. In M. Kernis (Ed.), *Efficacy, agency, and self-esteem* (pp. 123–144). New York: Plenum Press.

Lewin, K. (1935.) *A dynamic theory of personality.* New York: McGraw-Hill.

Mandler, G. (1984). The construction and limitation of consciousness. In V. Sarris & A. Parducci (Eds.), *Perspectives in psychological experimentation: Toward the year 2000* (pp. 109–126). Hillsdale, NJ: Erlbaum.

Markus, H., & Kitayama, S. (1991). Culture and the self: Implications for cognition, emotion, and motivation. *Psychological Review, 98,* 224–253.

Mikulincer, M., & Horesh, N. (1999). Adult attachment style and the perception of others" The role of projective mechanisms. *Journal of Personality and Social Psychology, 76,* 1022–1034.

Miller, L. C., & Read, S. J. (1991). On the coherence of mental models of persons and relationships: A knowledge structure approach. In G. J. O. Fletcher & F. D. Fincham (Eds.), *Cognition in close relationships* (pp. 69–100). Hillsdale, NJ: Erlbaum.

Moors, A., De Houwer, J., & Eelen, P. (2004). Automatic stimulus–goal comparisons: Support from motivational affective priming studies. *Cognition and Emotion, 18,* 29–54.

Moskowitz, G. B., Gollwitzer, P. M., Wasel, W., & Schaal, B. (1999). Preconscious control of stereotype activation through chronic egalitarian goals. *Journal of Personality and Social Psychology, 77,* 167–184.

Murray, S. L., & Holmes, J. G. (1997). A leap of faith?: Positive illusions in romantic relationships. *Personality and Social Psychology Bulletin, 23,* 586–604.

Nisbett, R., & Ross, L. (1980). *Human inference: Strategies and shortcomings of social judgment.* Englewood Cliffs, NJ: Prentice-Hall.

Pickett, C. L., Gardner, W. L., & Knowles, M. (2004). Getting a cue: The need to belong and enhanced sensitivity to social cues. *Personality and Social Psychology Bulletin, 30,* 1095–1107.

Plant, E. A., & Devine, P. G. (1998). Internal and external motivation to respond without prejudice. *Journal of Personality and Social Psychology, 75,* 811–832.

Postman, L., Bruner, J. S., & McGinnies, E. (1948). Personal values as selective factors in perception. *Journal of Abnormal and Social Psychology, 43,* 142–154.

Rosenberg, M. J. (1956). Cognitive structure and attitudinal affect. *Journal of Abnormal and Social Psychology, 53,* 367–372.

Sanderson, C. A., & Cantor, N. (2001). The association of intimacy goals and marital satisfaction: A test of four mediational hypotheses. *Personality and Social Psychology Bulletin, 27,* 1567–1577.

Sanitioso, R., Kunda, Z., & Fong, G. T. (1990). Motivated recall of autobiographical memories. *Journal of Personality and Social Psychology, 59,* 229–241.

Seeley, E. A., & Gardner, W. L. (2003). The "selfless" and self-regulation: The role of chronic other-orientation in averting self-regulatory depletion. *Self and Identity, 2,* 103–117.

Shah, J. Y. (2003a). Automatic for the people: How representations of significant others implicitly affect goal pursuit. *Journal of Personality and Social Psychology, 84*(4), 661–681.

Shah, J. Y. (2003b). The motivational looking glass: How significant others implicitly affect goal appraisals. *Journal of Personality and Social Psychology, 85,* 424–439.

Shah, J. Y., & Fitzsimons, G. M. (2005). *Interpersonal strategies for personal goal progress*. Manuscript in preparation.

Shah, J. Y., Friedman, R., & Kruglanski, A. W. (2002). Forgetting all else: On the antecedents and consequences of goal shielding. *Journal of Personality and Social Psychology, 83*, 1261–1280.

Shah, J. Y., & Higgins, E. T. (2001). Regulatory concerns and appraisal efficiency: The general impact of promotion and prevention. *Journal of Personality and Social Psychology, 80*, 693–705.

Shah, J. Y., & Kruglanski, A. W. (2003). When opportunity knocks: Bottom-up priming of goals by means and its effects on self-regulation. *Journal of Personality and Social Psychology, 84*(6), 1109–1122.

Shah, J. Y., Kruglanski, A. W., & Friedman, R. (2003). Goal systems theory: Integrating the cognitive and motivational aspects of self-regulation. In S. J. Spencer, S. Fein, M. Zanna, & J. Olson (Eds.), *The Ontario Symposium: Vol. 8. Motivated social perception* (pp. 134–145). Mahwah, NJ: Erlbaum.

Smith, C. A., & Ellsworth, P. C. (1985). Patterns of cognitive appraisal in emotion. *Journal of Personality and Social Psychology, 48*, 813–838.

Srull, T. K., & Wyer, R. S. (1979). The role of category accessibility in the interpretation of information about persons: Some determinants and implications. *Journal of Personality and Social Psychology, 37*, 1660–1672.

Taylor, S. E., & Armor, D. A. (1996). Positive illusions and coping with adversity. *Journal of Personality, 64*, 873–898.

Updegraff, J. A., Gable, S. L., & Taylor, S. E. (2004). What makes experiences satisfying? The interaction of approach–avoidance motivations and emotions in well-being. *Journal of Personality and Social Psychology, 86*, 496–504.

Wills, T. A. (1991). Social support and interpersonal relationships. In M. S. Clark (Ed.), *Prosocial behavior* (pp. 265–289). Newbury Park, CA: Sage.

SELF-CONCEPT

Narcissism, Interpersonal Self-Regulation, and Romantic Relationships

An Agency Model Approach

W. KEITH CAMPBELL
AMY B. BRUNELL
ELI J. FINKEL

Narcissism is at the center of the human condition, resting at the place where the desires of the self intersect with relationships with others. Are you better than others, more deserving, more special? Or are you on the same plane as others, connected and part of a larger whole? From this intersection of self and other, narcissism is manifested in inflated self-conceptions, interpersonal self-regulation, and relationships at all levels of human behavior, from cultural independence to private fantasies of power.

In this chapter, we focus on narcissists' interpersonal self-regulatory efforts with a focus on narcissists' romantic life. We do so in an effort to narrow our discussion and also as a nod to the myth of Narcissus, which pitted the romantic love of self against the love of another. However, we also bring into the discussion findings from a range of interpersonal settings. The manifestations of narcissism in romantic relationships differ little from those in friendships, work relationships, or stranger relationships.

We begin by offering an abbreviated history of narcissism. We next focus on the construct itself, with particular attention directed at narcissistic self-regulation. We present an *agency model* of narcissism that we find useful for thinking about many of its effects. We then turn our attention directly to narcissism in the context of romantic relationships.

HISTORY OF NARCISSISM

Freud

The application of the myth of Narcissus to psychological phenomena was first made by Havelock Ellis (1898). However, it was with Freud's famous monograph *On Narcissism: An Introduction* (Freud, 1914/1957) that interest in narcissism took off. Freud's approach to narcissism had two important outcomes. First, he presented narcissism in such a way that its importance in normal human development, in psychopathology, and in normal adult psychology and behavior was clear. Second, he made his presentation in such a confusing manner that researchers and clinicians would be forced to spend years simply trying to untangle his ideas (Baranger, 1991). The study of narcissism has thus been one of broad interest, from clinical and developmental psychology to sociology, management, and political science. This breadth, however, has barely concealed rampant confusion about the construct itself.

For our purposes, it is important to extract just a few key ideas from Freud's monograph. Freud distinguished between two types of individual experiences of love. "Anaclitic," or attachment-type, individuals focus their love outward, preferring love objects reminiscent of past attachment figures. In contrast, narcissistic-type individuals focus their love inward toward the self. The narcissistic object of affection represents: "(a) what he himself is (i.e., himself), (b) what he himself was, (c) what he himself would like to be, (d) someone who was once part of himself" (Freud, 1914/1957, p. 90). In a sense, Freud was arguing that love could be about connection (anaclitic type) or about the self (narcissistic type). As we will see, in this regard he was not that far off the mark.

Freud returned again to narcissism as a personality variable in a later work, *Libidinal Types* (Freud, 1931/1950). In this essay, he notes that those of the narcissistic type are independent, energetic, confident, and aggressive. This same pattern was suggested in Reich's phallic–narcissistic character (Reich, 1949). This personality approach appeared to be linked primarily to extraversion/surgency and low agreeableness. Indeed, this is relatively consistent with the empirically demonstrated Big Five correlates of narcissism that include extraversion/surgency and openness to experience, along with low agreeableness (e.g., Paulhus & Williams, 2002).

Kernberg and Kohut

In terms of the modern psychodynamic understanding of narcissism, the two most influential thinkers have been Kernberg (1974, 1975) and Kohut (1977) (for reviews, see Akhtar & Thompson, 1982; Greenberg & Mitchell, 1983). Both of these individuals took more of a deficit approach to narcissism: either narcissism was a defense against feelings of abandonment and its associated rage (Kernberg, 1975), or it was a response to not getting enough mirroring and idealization in childhood (Kohut, 1977). These approaches resulted in the notion that narcissistic personality is a defensive structure.

Murray

Henry Murray must be noted as the first researcher to our knowledge to empirically assess and examine correlates of "narcism" (his term; his alternate term was "egophilia.") Murray's work on narcissism grounded it in the empirical, personality tradition. Although his narcism scale differs from what we use today, it remains important historically (Murray, 1938).

Narcissistic Personality Disorder

The inclusion of narcissistic personality disorder (NPD) in the *Diagnostic and Statistical Manual of Mental Disorders* (DSM-III) dramatically increased interest in narcissism. Unfortunately, the creation of NPD also changed the image of narcissism from a normal personality trait (e.g., Freud, 1931/1950; Murray, 1938) to a disorder that afflicts less than 1% of the population (American Psychiatric Association, 1994). Furthermore, because normal individuals with high narcissism scores do not typically seek therapy—Why would they? They view themselves as winners—the clinical impression of narcissism was arguably subject to a sample bias. The narcissists seen in clinical settings may have been overly represented by "failed" narcissists, that is, those narcissists who could not function smoothly in normal life. This sample bias, we argue, skewed the clinical picture of narcissists in the direction of individuals with fragile self-esteem covering up inner depression and self-loathing (Campbell, 2001; Campbell & Baumeister, in press).

The Narcissistic Personality Inventory

Fortunately, Raskin and Hall (1979) brought narcissism back into the territory of social and personality psychologists with the creation of the Narcissistic Personality Inventory (NPI). This measure is based on the DSM description of narcissism but is designed for use in normal samples. It is typically a 40-

item (Raskin & Terry, 1988) scale in a forced-choice format, although there are several other versions in circulation that provide similar results (e.g., Emmons, 1984). The vast majority of empirical research on narcissism uses the NPI.

Summary

Narcissism has worn many guises throughout the years, from a developmental stage to a clinical disorder. There are two ways to approach this history. One is to try and think deeply about it and try to find some resolution; the other is to ground our ideas in empirical research and use the past simply as a source of inspiration. We are of the mind that a critical mass of empirical research in social and personality psychology has been reached; the focus should be on theory development that reconciles empirical findings, not historical theoretical approaches.

WHY STUDY NARCISSISM?

Whenever you study an individual difference variable such as narcissism, the first question to ask yourself is: Why? (or, as reviewers like to put it, "Who cares about narcissism?"). The individual differences space can be divided up in infinite ways. The Big Five and its variants were initially derived from natural language. These are ways that individuals naturally describe others. Many other personality models share similar empirical heft. In contrast, narcissism is originally derived from psychoanalytic theory. It is not alone: Attachment research, for example, is in part an outgrowth of object relations theory, also a psychoanalytic theory. Neither of these models, however, is the result of the empirical grind that led to the Big Five. Thus it is particularly important to state why it is useful to study narcissism. We can think of at least five benefits.

     First, as noted, we would argue that narcissism stands at the potential point of conflict between a focus on the self and a focus on others. This tension between egotism and affiliation has been a key element in human interaction throughout human existence (e.g., Boehm, 1999). At a social level, this tension is one between dominance and egalitarianism: Am I different from and better than others, or am I the same as and equal to others? This tension has been noted by a range of psychologists who have given the concept various names, from getting along versus getting ahead (Hogan, 1983), to moving against others versus moving toward others (Horney, 1937), to power versus tenderness (Sullivan, 1953). This is a basic theme in human relations and narcissism is at its heart.

     Second, narcissism can be thought of as a bridge variable. By that, we mean that it can be used to bridge multiple approaches to a single issue. Narcissism sits at the nexus of personality, the self, self-regulation, and relationships. In the case of romantic relationships, for example, we can link a personality variable (narcissism) to a self-concept (I am a winner!), to a self-regulation strategy (I want others to see that I am a winner), to a relationship behavior (I will date a supermodel) (Campbell, 1999). This linkage is thus directly related to the topic of this volume. Narcissism can bridge different levels of analysis as well. For example, narcissism is relevant to understanding physiological responding to stress (Kelsey, Ornduff, McCann, & Reiff, 2001), fantasy life (Raskin & Novacek, 1991), decision making (Campbell, Goodie, & Foster, 2004), attribution (Campbell, Reeder, Sedikides, & Elliot, 2000), self-conceptions (Gabriel, Critelli, & Ee, 1994), self-esteem (Raskin, Novacek, & Hogan, 1991), interdependent relationships (e.g., Campbell & Foster, 2002), group-level processes (Hogan & Hogan, 2002), societal processes (Campbell, Bush, Brunell, & Shelton, 2005), and cultural processes (Foster, Campbell, & Twenge, 2003).

Third, and also directly relevant to the present chapter, narcissism provides a window to self-enhancement processes that would not normally be open. For example, if you ask psychologically close individuals to engage in a dyadic, interdependent task (e.g., a creativity task), give them false negative feedback, and then ask them to attribute responsibility for the failure, you will not find a self-serving bias. That is, close individuals tend to share responsibility for failure rather than blame each other (Sedikides, Campbell, Reeder, & Elliot, 1998). The reasonable conclusion is that close relationships reliably mitigate the self-serving bias. However, if you assess narcissism and run the same study, a somewhat different picture emerges: Yes, close relationships attenuate the self-serving bias, on average. But the underlying pattern is that narcissists still show the self-serving bias and nonnarcissists actually show an other-serving bias (Campbell et al., 2000).

Fourth, narcissism has the potential for several important applications. This is because narcissism is linked to a range of behaviors that have a negative effect on both individual performance and social outcomes. Narcissism, for example, is linked to diminishing academic performance (Robins & Beer, 2001) and poor decision making (Campbell, Goodie, & Foster, 2004). On a more social level, narcissism is linked to corrupt leadership (Hogan & Hogan, 2002), counterproductive workplace behaviors (Penney & Spector, 2002), aggression and violence (Bushman & Baumeister, 1998; Twenge & Campbell, 2003), rape (Bushman, Bonacci, van Dijk, & Baumeister, 2003), incarceration (Bushman & Baumeister, 2002), and exacerbation of the tragedy of the commons (Campbell et al., 2005).

Fifth, narcissism is interesting to study in part to find out how life would be without it. If the self-regulatory impulse that drives narcissism were not part of the human psyche, what would the experience of life be like? It is arguable that narcissism is a roadblock to a perception of the world that is unmediated or unhindered by the ego (or, at least, by egotism). Narcissism is a very effective roadblock because narcissists feel good about themselves, are happy, and function reasonably well (Rose & Campbell, 2004). In dynamic systems terminology, narcissism may be a "local minimum": It is a moderately positive and self-reinforcing self-regulatory strategy that makes it difficult to enter a less distorted, more reality-consistent level of awareness.

NARCISSISM AS A SOCIAL PERSONALITY CONSTRUCT

Narcissism has three fundamental characteristics. The first is a positive and inflated self-concept. The inflation is evident in comparisons made between self-reports and objective criteria (e.g., Gabriel et al., 1994; John & Robins, 1994). Narcissists have positive opinions about themselves on several agentic domains (e.g., intelligence and creativity), as well as on physical attractiveness (Gabriel et al., 1994). This is largely because narcissists care primarily about agentic issues. This is evident both in self-reports (e.g., Bradlee & Emmons, 1992; Campbell, Rudich, & Sedikides, 2002) and in projective tests such as the Thematic Apperception Test (TAT; Carroll, 1987). The narcissistic self also includes a fundamental sense of specialness. This is reflected in a heightened sense of uniqueness (Emmons, 1984) and psychological entitlement (Campbell, Bonacci, Shelton, Exline, & Bushman, 2004). There may even be a deeply held sense that others exist to serve the narcissist (Sedikides, Campbell, Reeder, Elliot, & Gregg, 2002).

The second characteristic is a relative lack of interest in close, warm, or intimate relationships. For example, narcissists place less importance on communal traits (Campbell, Rudich, & Sedikides, 2002). Narcissists also express a relatively weak intimacy motive on the TAT (Carroll, 1987). Indeed, it is this relative lack of interest in communal traits that separates narcissists from those with high self-esteem. Narcissism is not simply "very high" self-esteem. Narcissists limit their overly positive self-views to agentic domains; individuals with high self-esteem have positive self-views in both the agentic and the communal domains (Campbell, Rudich, & Sedikides, 2002).

The third characteristic of narcissism, and the one most directly related to the topic of the present chapter, is self-regulation. The trouble with inflated self-beliefs is that their inconsistency with reality needs to be bolstered and supported. This makes self-enhancement, both intrapsychically and interpersonally, central to narcissists. Because narcissists are temperamentally extraverted, sensation seeking, and approach-oriented (e.g., Bradlee & Emmons, 1992; Emmons, 1991; Rose & Campbell, 2004), these self-enhancement processes are largely (although not exclusively) "offensive" rather than "defensive." That is, narcissists spend time looking for opportunities to augment the self; they do not simply remain at status quo reacting defensively to threats.

The intrapsychic efforts to self-enhance include fantasizing about power and status (Raskin & Novacek, 1991), maintaining beliefs that one is better than others (i.e., the better-than-average effect) (Campbell, Rudich, & Sedikides, 2002), and taking credit for successes and blaming situational forces for failure (Farwell & Wohlwend-Lloyd, 1998; Rhodewalt & Morf, 1995).

Perhaps the more interesting aspect of narcissistic self-regulation in regards to this chapter is interpersonal self-regulation. Narcissists are masters at using the social environment to maintain their sense of status and esteem. This skill reflects in large part narcissists' social extraversion and high energy level (Bradlee & Emmons, 1992), as well as their relative lack of interest in close, warm social relationships (and the lower levels of guilt and social anxiety that go with that; see Gramzow & Tangney, 1992). Some examples of this self-regulation are as follows: Narcissists adopt "colorful" personae to draw attention to themselves and establish specialness (Hogan & Hogan, 2002). General Douglas MacArthur, for example, deliberately used dramatic props such as his corncob pipe and large aviator glasses to set himself apart from other generals. In conversation, narcissists will direct the topic toward themselves (Raskin & Shaw, 1988; Vangelisti, Knapp, & Daly, 1990). They will brag, show off, and seek attention (Buss & Chiodo, 1991). Narcissists will also be energetic and entertaining (Paulhus, 1998). Narcissists are highly competitive, constantly on the lookout for opportunities to best or dominate others (Bradlee & Emmons, 1992; Emmons, 1984). They will jump at the opportunity to win for public glory (Wallace & Baumeister, 2002), and steal credit from or place blame on coworkers (Campbell et al., 2000; Gosling, John, Craik, & Robins, 1998; John & Robins, 1994). Narcissists also punish those who threaten their self-conceptions. This can be seen in aggression following ego threat (Bushman & Baumeister, 1998) and social rejection (Twenge & Campbell, 2003). This aggression is part of a basic externalizing response among narcissists to threatening information and is linked to externalizing attributions (Stucke, 2003).

It is worth noting two additional aspects regarding narcissistic self-regulation. First, narcissists' internal and external self-enhancement strategies are not necessarily independent. Their fantasies, for example, involve an imagined audience, and their predilection to talk about themselves may be as much for themselves as it is for the public. Second, narcissism is not a socially unappealing trait. Indeed, for narcissistic self-regulation to be effective, narcissists need to be popular, admired, and respected by other powerful and important people. One outcome of this is that narcissists are liked in the short term (e.g., Paulhus, 1998). Recent research on NPD has even found that narcissists were viewed as likeable by others after seeing 30-second "thin slices" of narcissists' behavior (Oltmanns, Friedman, Fiedler, & Turkheimer, 2004), although narcissism seems to fall apart (at least in the eyes of others) in the longer term. Narcissists' general lack of interest in others' welfare and overinterest in the self eventually leads others to dislike them (Paulhus, 1998).

THE AGENCY MODEL

The central goal of this chapter is to describe narcissistic self-regulation within the context of romantic relationships. Before jumping into the research findings, however, we would like to present a model of narcissism that we find useful for thinking about the issue of self-regulation in relationships. For lack of a better name, we call this the *agency model of narcissism*. The model itself is an outgrowth of several other models of narcissism. It borrows esteem regulation, agency seeking, and interpersonal self-regulation from the self-orientation model (Campbell, 1999); it borrows a dynamic self-regulatory approach from the dynamic self-regulatory processing model (Morf & Rhodewalt, 2001); it starts with the assumption that narcissism is grounded in a basic agentic–communal asymmetry as does the minimalist model (Paulhus, 2001); it uses self-esteem as an important regulatory goal from the self-esteem management model (Raskin et al., 1991); it includes a broader view of esteem, however, based on the addiction model of narcissism (Baumeister & Vohs, 2001) and the model of self-conscious emotions (Tracy & Robins, 2004); and it assumes that narcissism is largely offensive/approach-oriented rather than defensive (e.g., Rose & Campbell, 2004).

Central to the agency model, narcissism has certain fundamental elements or qualities:

1. Narcissists focus on agentic rather than communal concerns (e.g., Campbell, 1999; Campbell, Foster, & Finkel, 2002) and this is linked to their basic personality structure (Bradlee & Emmons, 1992; Paulhus, 2004).
2. Narcissists are approach-oriented (Campbell & Rose, 2004).
3. Narcissists' self-regulation is focused on acquiring self-esteem (Campbell, 1999; Raskin et al., 1991).
4. Narcissism is linked to entitlement in interpersonal self-regulation (Campbell, Bonacci, et al., 2004).
5. Narcissists have an inflated view of themselves on many dimensions.

See Figure 4.1 for an illustration of the agency model as applied to interpersonal self-regulation.

The agency model is presented as a system. Narcissism is linked to two basic processes: interpersonal skills and interpersonal strategies (again, there are other processes, such as intrapsychic self-regulation, but we are focusing more on interpersonal self-regulation). To take one path, narcissists' interper-

The Agency Model: An Esteem-Generating System

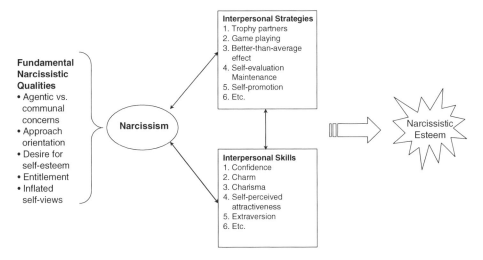

FIGURE 4.1. Visual representation of the agency model.

sonal skills (e.g., confidence, charm, resilience) make their self-regulatory strategies (e.g., game playing, acquiring "trophy" [i.e., high self-presentational value] romantic partners) possible. All elements of the system feed back into each other. For example, confidence and extraversion leads the narcissist to date a highly attractive partner. This, in turn, further strengthens the narcissist's self-views, which then leads to greater confidence, and so on.

One important outcome of this system in action is what we call "narcissistic esteem." We see this as more than simple self-esteem. Rather, it is a dominance-related self-esteem (Brown & Zeigler-Hill, 2004; Campbell, 1999) with a hint of pride (Tracy & Robins, 2004) and a rush of possibly addictive excitement (Baumeister & Vohs, 2001). We do not argue that self-esteem is the "ultimate goal" of narcissistic self-regulation—in fact, narcissistic esteem is likely to feed back into the system and increase the workings of the other components. The question of the "ultimate goal" of narcissism is a tricky one. Some have argued for self-image defense or aggrandizement (e.g., Morf & Rhodewalt, 2001); others have argued for self-esteem (e.g., Raskin et al., 1991). The agency model makes clear that the various outcomes (esteem, inflated self-views, excitement) are associated, but does not theoretically identify a single "ultimate goal" of narcissism. The inflated self-image and the desire for narcissistic esteem are both important to the system.

Finally, we should also note that we find it useful to think about narcissism visually by using the interpersonal circumplex (e.g., Leary, 1957; Wiggins, 1991). We are not arguing for a strict circumplex form, nor for the

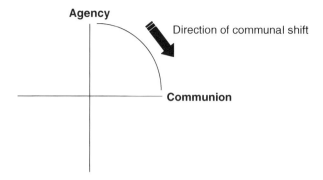

FIGURE 4.2. Visual representation of agency and communion in circumplex. We find this to be a useful visual heuristic for conceptualizing change in narcissism.

exact elements on the circumplex. These are topics for a different discussion. Rather, we find it useful to think about two basic sets of traits, values, and approaches to interpersonal relationships. These have been referred to as agency and communion (e.g., Bakan, 1966), alpha and beta (e.g., Digman, 1997), dominance and friendliness (e.g., Leary, 1957), and egoistic and moralistic (Paulhus & John, 1998). We use the terms "agency" and "communion" because they are broad and they convey more meaning than the terms "alpha" and "beta." Furthermore, we find it useful to think of these two traits as being represented in circumplex form (see Figure 4.2). This makes it easy to conceptualize individuals as being high in agency and high in communion; high in agency, low in communion; and so on. Also, it makes it easy to visualize individuals shifting along the circumference of the circumplex. For example, a narcissist who is high in agency but slightly low or middling in communion would conceivably become a better partner by shifting toward the communion end of the circumplex. We have more to say on this topic later; for now, we turn to narcissists' romantic relationships.

APPLYING THE AGENCY MODEL TO ROMANTIC RELATIONSHIPS

The agency model is useful for understanding narcissism in romantic relationships. Narcissists' approach to relationships is a self-reinforcing, self-regulatory system that generates narcissistic esteem. This is especially evident in the relative desire for agentic goals (status, dominance, autonomy) versus communal goals (warmth, caring, emotional intimacy). Narcissists' self-regulation will be coupled with a generally confident and extraverted interpersonal style. This self-regulatory agenda will infuse all aspects of narcissists' romantic life. This includes narcissists' desired partners, relationship initiation strategies, behavior in relationships, experience of love, and sexuality. Similarly, the agency model can be used to explain not just narcissists' behaviors, but also the reason why others are attracted to narcissists (i.e., agentic traits and confidence). Finally, the agency model suggests approaches for mitigating the negative outcomes of narcissism for romantic relationships.

Our discussion is arranged in three parts. First, we tackle narcissists' approach to relationships. Second, we look at the partners of narcissists and their experiences in these relationships. Third, we speculate about ways in which narcissism can be a positive for romantic relationships.

Before we begin, however, we should briefly note that almost none of these findings is qualified by gender. Narcissistic males and females generally act the same way in romantic relationships. There are three important caveats: First, there are gender main effects for many of these relationship findings. Men, for example, reliably report greater levels of unrestricted sociosexuality than women. Second, men are on average more narcissistic than women (Foster et al., 2003). Third, there is some evidence that males and females experience narcissism differently (e.g., Tschanz, Morf, & Turner, 1998), so the possibility of gender interactions certainly should not be ruled out.

Narcissists' Approach to Relationships

Attraction

The principles underlying narcissists' romantic attraction are consistent with the agency model. Narcissists are looking for partners who can provide them with self-esteem and status. How can a romantic partner provide status and esteem? First, he or she can do so directly: a romantic partner who admires me and thinks that I am wonderful elevates my esteem. Second, he or she can do so indirectly through a basic association: my partner is beautiful and popular, therefore I am too. This indirect esteem generation is clear from a range of social psychological research, from the self-evaluation maintenance (SEM) model (Tesser, 1988) to Basking in Reflected Glory (BIRGing; Cialdini et al., 1976). This indirect esteem provisioning is évident in the term "trophy" partner.

There is good empirical evidence that narcissists like targets who provide esteem and status both directly and indirectly (Campbell, 1999). There is also an important interaction effect. Namely, narcissists like popular and attractive partners, especially when those others admire them. Narcissists, however, are not particularly interested in admiration from just anybody. This finding is inconsistent with the "doormat hypothesis." Narcissists are not looking for someone they can walk on and who worships them; rather, narcissists are looking for someone ideal who also admires them.

The next question, of course, is what characteristics of a potential partner make them able to provide narcissists with narcissistic esteem? Not surprisingly, what narcissists particularly look for in a partner are physical attractiveness and agentic traits (e.g., status and success). A narcissist's ideal partner is like a narcissist's ideal self (recall Freud's comments): attractive, successful, and admiring of the narcissist. Indeed, in our research, narcissists report that part of the reason that they are drawn to attractive and successful partners is that these people are similar to them (Campbell, 1999).

Initiation: Confidence and Mate Poaching

In a recent conversation with a hairstylist, one of us (WKC) heard the following description of how she (the hairstylist) was approached by a gentleman at a bar:

> HIM: Hey, I know you from the store.
>
> HER: Yes, I've seen you there.
>
> HIM: Well, I'm hot, you're hot, what do you say we get out of here and go back to my place?
>
> HER: Are you kidding me?
>
> HIM: (*pointing*) Look, I could have her or her or her, but I'm talking to you.

One of us asked from the barber chair, "Did this approach work?" She responded that she did give him her number because he "really was hot."

This is a classic example of a narcissistic approach to relationship initiation. It relies on extreme extraversion and confidence, as well as on resilience in the face of rejection. (These approaches have very low base rates for success when employed by men, unless the invitation is for a date; see Clark & Hatfield, 1989.) Also, note that this approach relies on traits narcissists care about. It is not about caring or feelings, but about physical attractiveness.

We have conducted several studies looking at reports of relationships initiated by narcissists and nonnarcissists (more on these later; Brunell, Campbell, Smith, & Krusemark, 2004). What we find is that the relationships with narcissists are initiated more rapidly, and that the narcissists are described as confident and charming. They are also described by their relationship partners as physically attractive, which contradicts the data that narcissists are no more attractive than nonnarcissists (Gabriel et al., 1994). There are a couple of possible explanations for this. It could be that in still photos narcissists are not more attractive, but they are in interpersonal settings because of the way that they carry themselves and/or attire themselves. It also could be that attractive narcissists are the ones out there using these confident dating strategies. Our hunch is that it is the former, but more data are needed.

Research on "mate poaching" (Schmitt & Buss, 2001) also is consistent with the idea that narcissists use high-confidence initiation strategies. Narcissists are more likely to lure dating partners away from preexisting relationships (i.e., to mate poach) (Foster, Shrira, & Campbell, 2004).

Finally, an additional line of research has found that narcissists are prone to distort their memories of romantic rejection in such a way that narcissists' egos remain unbruised (e.g., "I never liked him anyway") (Rhodewalt & Eddings, 2002). In short, it is apparent that narcissists are confident in their interactions.

If the agency model holds, narcissists should also use their relationship initiation strategies in order to directly gain esteem. There is no research evidence for this prediction. However, there is certainly anecdotal evidence of individuals collecting "phone numbers" in an effort to gain status among their friends and esteem. Thus we suspect that there is a direct enhancement agenda present, but will withhold judgment on this issue until data are collected.

Self-Serving Biases

Although narcissists look for attractive, high-status partners, they tend to maintain positive self-views by favorably comparing themselves to their partners. This can be seen in work on the better-then-average effect, where narcissists are asked to rate themselves on a series of traits relative to their dating partner. Narcissists rate themselves more highly than they rate their partners. Consistent with the agency model, the more inflated ratings are on agentic traits (Campbell, Rudich, & Sedikides, 2002).

To the best of our knowledge, no experimental research has been done on romantic partners using a classic self-serving bias or self-evaluation maintenance paradigm. However, research with other close relationships has found evidence that narcissists are more self-serving (e.g., Campbell et al., 2000). Given that self-enhancing responses are typically attenuated in close relationships (Alicke, Klotz, Breitenbecher, Yurak, & Vredenberg, 1995; Beach, Tesser, Mendolia, & Page, 1996; Sedikides et al., 1998), narcissists' self-enhancing self-regulatory strategies do not bode well for relationship longevity.

Attachment

Narcissism arguably has important parallels with attachment theory. In a sense, both can be modeled with a basic interpersonal circumplex. Narcissists have positive views of themselves and report relatively little interest in warm relationships with others. The parallel to this in attachment theory terminology would be dismissive attachment (Bartholomew & Horowitz, 1991). At first blush, the clear prediction would be that narcissists would report dismissive attachment styles. Indeed, there is some reported evidence for a positive correlation between dismissive attachment and narcissism (Campbell & Foster, 2002; Neumann & Bierhoff, 2004), as well as psychological entitlement (Campbell, Bonacci, et al., 2004).

We view this conclusion with caution, however, because we have several data sets that do not show this effect. It is possible that there may be important differences between narcissism and dismissive attachment. Dismissive attachment may include more emotional constriction than narcissism (Carlson, 2002). Narcissists, in contrast, tend to be outgoing and engaging. Narcissists may shun emotional closeness, but they need interpersonal contact to effectively regulate narcissistic esteem. This is not necessarily the case with individuals with a dismissive attachment style, which may be linked to a general dislike of relationships altogether. In personality disorder terminology, it is arguable that dismissive attachment contains some elements of both Cluster A (e.g., schizoid) and Cluster B traits (e.g., narcissistic). Thus, it does not strongly correlate with a Cluster B trait like narcissism.

It is also arguable that the developmental roots of dismissive attachment and narcissism differ. Dismissive attachment is based on social rejection. Narcissism, in contrast, may be derived from a combination of warm parental involvement that is contingent upon performance coupled with parental permissiveness consisting of loose social restraints in childhood and adolescence (Horton, Bleau, & Drwecki, in press). Future research is clearly needed in this area.

Materialism

When one thinks about romantic relationships, materialism is not the first thing that comes to mind. We have found, however, that this is a major complaint among those who date narcissists. The problem from the perspective of those dating narcissists is that the narcissists spend too much energy and attention on possessing material goods. This is arguably detrimental to the relationship because it takes away from energy that could be directed toward deepening intimacy (material relationships are basically "shallow" in that there is no reciprocal and deepening self-disclosure with an object—unless it is a volleyball named Wilson).

Why would narcissists be materialistic? Based on the agency model, narcissists' materialism would be in the pursuit of agentic goals that are used to regulate self-views, social success, and narcissistic esteem. Fortunately, there is some evidence for narcissistic materialism as an interpersonal, self-regulatory process (Vohs & Campbell, 2004). Narcissists self-report being more materialistic, and the stated reason is largely to meet their esteem needs. In other words, narcissists like high-status "stuff" because it makes them look and feel good (e.g., narcissistic esteem). Indeed, when initiating interpersonal interactions with strangers, narcissists prefer to discuss their material goods rather than more emotional topics. This is especially true when they want to impress high-status others of the opposite sex.

Probably the most interesting implication of narcissistic materialism is the potential substitutability of things for people. In order to meet intimacy needs, you need to interact with a person (or, rarely, an object imbued with a lot of human qualities). This is because intimate relationships involve reciprocal communication and self-disclosure (Reis & Shaver, 1988). In order to meet narcissistic esteem needs, however, an object may serve equally to a person. Chas, the narcissist, can gain narcissistic esteem by showing up at a party with his attractive girlfriend or in his new Porsche. From the perspective of esteem regulation, the experience of the two events may even be the same.

Commitment and Interdependence

One approach to investigating narcissism in romantic relationships is to apply interdependence theory (Thibaut & Kelley, 1959). According to this approach, relationship outcomes can be considered emergent properties of the relationship. Commitment, for example, is seen as a motive that emerges from the interaction of the two partners in the relationship (i.e., a macromotive).

The most influential model in the interdependence tradition for examining commitment is the investment model (Rusbult, 1980, 1983). According to the investment model, commitment in a relationship is the result of three predictors: satisfaction, investments, and alternatives. Satisfaction is the reward supplied by the relationship minus the costs. Investments include things such as time, shared friends, or children that would be potentially lost if the relationship were to end. Alternatives are other possible dating partners or being alone.

When placed within the context of the investment model, narcissists report lower commitment. Importantly, this lower commitment is driven primarily by increased alternatives. Put another way, narcissists perceive greater alternatives to their relationships and this leads to lesser commitment (Campbell & Foster, 2002).

Why the greater alternatives? The agency model would suggest that this is linked to self-regulation, approach orientation, and extraversion. There is some evidence of approach orientation in narcissists' alternatives. In particular, narcissists score particularly high on what is known as "attention to alternatives" (Miller, 1997). This is a measure of how much effort one applies to identifying and spending time with alternative partners. It is not that the alternatives come to the narcissist; rather, narcissists are actively seeking out potential alternatives. As for narcissistic esteem regulation, there is no direct evidence linking alternatives to esteem. We think it is plausible to assume that narcissists are "looking for a better deal" or "looking to trade up." If they can find the partner who will bring them more status and esteem, they will go for it.

Sexuality

Sexuality is not just a physical act. It is also a social process that is suffused with meaning (Baumeister & Tice, 2000). Based on the agency model, one would predict that, for narcissists, sex can be a self-regulatory act that invokes positive feelings of agency rather than communion. This is indeed the case. Narcissists are more likely to use agentic words to describe sex, such as daring, power, and domination (Foster, Shrira, & Campbell, in press). This agentic view of sex has positive self-regulatory benefits for narcissists, but has social costs for them as well. First, it is linked to lesser relational commitment (Foster et al., in press). Second, it is associated with greater unrestricted sociosexuality. Narcissists are more likely to perceive sex as divorced from emotional warmth and closeness, and also to desire greater sexual diversity. This same research also found that narcissists conceived of sex more in terms of personal pleasure than in terms of emotional intimacy. Basically, it is a selfish and self-serving activity (Foster et al., in press). (Of course, there is also the possibility that narcissists could strive to be "dynamos" in bed in order to gain narcissistic esteem. This would be an example of a behavior where the interests of narcissistic selfishness and partner needs may be aligned.) Finally, one line of research directly examined predicted infidelity in newly married couples (Buss & Shackelford, 1997). These researchers found that narcissistic wives were more likely than nonnarcissistic wives to predict being unfaithful (although actual infidelity was not assessed) to their husband.

Love

There is a Western cliché that you have to love yourself before you can love others. Using narcissism as a model for self-love, this statement is far from accurate. Narcissists' approach to love is consistent with the tenets of the agency model. Narcissists are extraverted, socially confident, and approach-oriented. They are interested in their own agentic goals and not interested in communal goals. Their style of loving reflects this state of affairs.

In terms of the typology of love styles operationalized by Hendrick and Hendrick (1986), narcissists report being selfish (low agape) and pragmatic (high pragma). What really separates narcissists from nonnarcissists, however, is a game-playing (ludic) approach to love (Campbell, Foster, & Finkel, 2002; Le, in press). Narcissists see love as a game and enjoy keeping their partner uncertain about their commitment to the relationship. This approach not only plays on narcissists' social strengths, but is also an excellent self-regulatory strategy for narcissists. By keeping the partner uncertain of commitment, increased power and autonomy (agentic traits) accrue to the narcissist (Campbell, Finkel, Kumashiro, & Rusbult, 2004).

This process relies on a social psychological process known as "the principle of least interest" (Waller, 1938). Simply put, the individual with the least interest in the relationship has the most power. Imagine that you are dating someone to whom you are very attracted, but who is really not very interested in you. Saturday night rolls around, and she says that she would like to go "clubbing." You have no desire to go clubbing because you don't really like crowds, dancing, or dressing in black. But because you have more to lose in the relationship by saying no, you put on your black attire and head out the door.

In sum, narcissists' approach to love is a clear example of social self-regulation in action. Importantly, it demonstrates how certain groups of individuals (narcissists) can increase agentic self-views (power and autonomy) by employing a specific love style (game playing) that, in turn, activates a basic social psychological process (principle of least interest.)

Aggression

On occasion, the self-regulatory agenda of narcissists will lead to physical violence. Although no research has looked directly at narcissism and aggression in the context of ongoing romantic relationships, a wealth of data suggests a link between narcissism and aggression under conditions of ego threat (Baumeister, Smart, & Boden, 1996). The seminal research on the topic placed narcissists in a condition of ego threat (i.e., negative performance feedback). Aggression against the person who provided the critique using a white noise blast was then assessed. Narcissism was linked to increased aggression following threat (Bushman & Baumeister, 1998). Additional research has replicated this same pattern in the context of relational rejection. Individuals were brought to a lab and asked to choose two other people who they "liked and respected" to be in a group. Each individual was then given false rejection feedback (nobody chose them) and then offered the opportunity to set the level of white noise blasts directed toward the rejecting group. Under conditions of rejection, narcissists were more aggressive (Twenge & Campbell, 2003).

Recent research has also linked narcissistic aggression following threat directly to external attributions (Stucke, 2003). Basically, narcissists blame others for the negative feedback and disrespect that they receive. They then reassert dominance and punish those who provided the negative feedback. This tendency on the part of narcissists is especially troubling given that narcissists are more likely to perceive hostile intent in the eyes of others (McCullough, Emmons, Kilpatrick, & Mooney, 2003).

An additional and particularly harmful self-regulatory behavior that may be displayed by narcissists is rape (Baumeister, Catanese, & Wallace, 2002; Bushman et al., 2003). The model guiding this research is consistent with agentic self-regulation. Narcissists are told they cannot have something (sexual access to a woman) and they react by taking it anyway. Narcissists do not have the usual constraint of empathy to restrict this behavior. Narcissists' sense of power and entitlement is preserved, but with tragic consequences for the victim.

The Partners of Narcissists

Given the above, it is reasonable to conclude that narcissists would make lousy dating partners. They are game playing, unfaithful, low in commitment, and selfish. Yet narcissists are strangely adept—maybe more adept than nonnarcissists—at starting romantic relationships. Why do narcissists find it so easy to find romantic partners?

The truth is that narcissists are not all bad. If they were, they would be avoided. Instead, narcissists have many positive qualities. These are located in agentic domains: Narcissists are confident, extraverted, and energetic. They are exciting and, at least in the reports of their dating partners (although not in ratings of photographs [Gabriel et al., 1994]), good looking. These are all attractive qualities. Even Charles Manson—or Scott Peterson for that matter—still has women interested in him, despite his murderous past. Unfortunately for their relationship partners, narcissists' agentic traits are not balanced by communal concerns. Narcissists are not all that interested in caring or intimacy. Finally, add to this mix our speculation that in relationships agentic traits are good for attraction and communal traits are good for relational durability. The result is that narcissists can be very appealing at the early stages of romantic relationships, but not so appealing in the longer term. In a sense, the course of romantic relationships is similar to that found by Paulhus in group interactions (Paulhus, 1998). Namely, narcissists are well liked in initial interactions, but disliked after repeated interactions.

In line with these ideas, we gathered narrative accounts of those who have dated narcissists and nonnarcissists (Brunell et al., 2004; Foster, Shrira, & Campbell, 2003). The main pattern of findings is that narcissists are more confident, outgoing, exciting, and attractive (but not necessarily nice) at the initial stages of relationships. Indeed, relationships with narcissistic partners were reported to be more satisfying during the early stages, but satisfaction level dropped dramatically until it was well below that in relationships with nonnarcissists. Part of this drop was accounted for by the lack of emotional intimacy in relationships with narcissists, as well as by the narcissists' alleged game playing, infidelity, and overcontrolling behavior. Relationships with nonnarcissists started more slowly, and they were initially less satisfying and consistently less exciting than relationships with narcissists. Relationships with nonnarcissists ultimately became more satisfying than those with narcissists, however, and even at the end of the relationship those relationships with nonnarcissists were more satisfying.

In a sense, relationships with narcissists reflect poor self-regulation on the partners' part, somewhat equivalent to eating a chocolate donut. Relationships with narcissists have the sugary rush consistent with high agency, but lack the nutritious sustenance supplied by communal traits. Hence, dating narcissists results in the satisfaction equivalent of a sugar crash. The difference between donuts and narcissists, of course, is that nobody really believes donuts are healthy. Narcissists, however, can arguably feign communal traits to some extent, these communal traits can reasonably be inferred by the partner, or partners can hope to increase the communal qualities of their partner. This combination of positive agentic qualities and misrepresented, unknown, or potential communal qualities make narcissists hard to avoid.

One additional question involves the personalities of those who date narcissists. A commonly held belief is that people with low self-esteem are attracted to narcissists because they want the abuse. This "doormat model," however, does not hold, on average. When we collect data on past relationships, the far more common finding is that most individuals have dated both narcissists and nonnarcissists. When we examine ongoing relationships that are committed enough that one partner can get the other partner to come to a psychology study, we find that narcissists tend to date other narcissists (Campbell, Foster, & Finkel, 2002). This same pattern is found with sociopathy (Krueger, Moffitt, Caspi, Bleske, & Silva, 1998). In marriage, however, we have not found evidence that narcissism correlates across partners.

In sum, narcissists' agentic traits make them satisfying partners in the short term, but they are also associated with more rapid relationship deterioration. The result for narcissists is a churning of relationships—engaging in a series of shallow short-term relationships rather than fewer emotionally deep relationships. This pattern of self-regulation may well work for narcissists. The partners of narcissists, to the extent that they want emotional intimacy, are likely to suffer in the longer term from dating narcissists.

Can Narcissism Ever Be Positive for Relationships?

We conclude our discussion of narcissists' relationships by describing some instances where narcissism can be positive for relationships (beyond, of course, the exciting initial stage). Given the tenets of the agency model, one possible avenue for improving narcissists' relationships is not to diminish narcissists' agentic self-regulation, but instead to enhance narcissists' communal self-regulation. If narcissists are able to become more communal in their approach to relationships, they would become desirable partners. Indeed, this is a plot in many Hollywood movies, where the narcissistic partner becomes more communal after an intense event. These communal elicitation events include electric shock (Mel Gibson in What Women Want), falling from riches to rags (Hugh Grant in Two Weeks Notice), and being shot in the head (Harrison Ford in Regarding Henry). Plot devices are wonderful things, but they are not appropriate in the lab and have little utility outside of it. Nevertheless, they are consistent with the theoretical possibility that this communal change or shift can happen.

One way that this communal shift could happen is in the context of an ongoing relationship. In a relationship, communal traits could conceivably be elicited by the partner. This is consistent with a range of research on self-concept change in relationships (e.g., Aron, Aron, Tudor, & Nelson, 1991; Drigotas, Rusbult, Wieselquist, & Whitton, 1999; Murray, Holmes, & Griffin, 1996; see also Strong & Aron, Chapter 17, and Kumashiro, Rusbult, Wolf, & Estrada, Chapter 16, this volume). We found evidence for such a communal shift in a longitudinal study of marriage partners. The narcissists who felt that their partner made them more communal actually became more committed and less interested in alternatives across a period of several months(Campbell, Finkel, Kumashiro, & Rusbult, 2004). This study strongly suggests a direction for improving the relational functioning of narcissists.

Another line of research looked at narcissism and resilience to relational threat. Relationship partners can at times be exposed to doubts about the other's commitment. If these doubts are not successfully resisted, relational problems can ensue (Murray, Holmes, Griffin, Bellavia, & Rose, 2001). Consistent with the agency model, it was predicted that narcissists would be more resilient to such doubts. In one study, for example, individuals were asked to list 10 reasons why their partner was committed or was not committed to the relationship. After this threat manipulation, relational commitment and fidelity were assessed. Narcissists were resistant to this threatening information. They found it harder to list reasons why their partner was not committed. Importantly, after this threat, narcissists actually reported being more committed to their relationship than did nonnarcissists. In short, narcissists were particularly adept at resisting information threatening to the relationship. Of course, when narcissists listed reasons why their partners were highly committed to the relationship, narcissists reported less relational commitment and a greater interest in alternative partners. Nevertheless, although there are possibly some circumstances in which narcissists will actually be better partners than nonnarcissists, it is more reasonable to expect that they will be lousy partners than to wait for their positive relationship qualities to emerge.

CONCLUDING THOUGHTS

We have spent a good deal of time discussing the link between narcissism, self-concept, self-regulation, and interpersonal relationships. We hope that we have presented a theoretical model of narcissistic self-regulation that is useful for explaining past findings and generating future research. We also hope that we have conveyed some of the complexities of narcissists' approach to relationships. Narcissism is neither uniformly good nor uniformly bad. Rather, narcissism is associated with a series of trade-offs. It is well suited for providing the narcissist with a positive self-concept and narcissistic esteem in the short term. In the long term, however, the narcissist will have trouble maintaining relationships. Likewise, the partner of the narcissist may get a short-term jolt of satisfaction and excitement from the relationship, but he or she is likely to suffer in the long term from the narcissist's lack of communal qualities. Finally, we hope that we have sketched out a possible strategy for making narcissists better partners—namely, the communal shift.

ACKNOWLEDGMENT

We thank Josh Foster for feedback and suggestions.

REFERENCES

Akhtar, S., & Thompson, J. A. (1982). Overview: Narcissistic personality disorder. *American Journal of Psychiatry, 139,* 12–20.

Alicke, M. D., Klotz, M. L., Breitenbecher, D. L., Yurak, T. J., & Vredenberg, D. S. (1995). Personal contact, individuation, and the better-than-average effect. *Journal of Personality and Social Psychology, 68,* 804–825.

American Psychiatric Association. (1994). *Diagnostic and statistical manual of mental disorders* (4th ed., rev.). Washington, DC: Author.

Aron, A., Aron, E. N., Tudor, M., & Nelson, G. (1991). Close relationships as including other in the self. *Journal of Personality and Social Psychology, 60,* 241–253.

Bakan, D. (1966). *The duality of human existence: Isolation and communion in Western man.* Boston: Beacon Press.

Baranger, W. (1991). Narcissism in Freud. In J. Sandler, E. S. Person, & P. Fogany (Eds.), *Freud's "On narcissism: An introduction"* (pp. 108–130). New Haven, CT: Yale University Press.

Bartholomew, K., & Horowitz, L. (1991). Attachment styles among young adults: A test of a four-category model. *Journal of Personality and Social Psychology, 61,* 226–244.

Baumeister, R. F., Catanese, K. R., & Wallace, H. M. (2002). Conquest by force: A narcissistic reactance theory of rape and sexual coercion. *Review of General Psychology, 6,* 92–135.

Baumeister, R. F., Smart, L., & Boden, J. M. (1996). Relation of threatened egotism to violence and aggression: The dark side of high self-esteem. *Psychological Review, 103*, 5–33.

Baumeister, R. F., & Tice, D. M. (2000). *The social dimension of sex*. New York: Allyn & Bacon.

Baumeister, R. F., & Vohs, K. D. (2001). Narcissism as addiction to esteem. *Psychological Inquiry, 12*, 206–210.

Beach, S. R. H., Tesser, A., Mendolia, M., & Page, A. (1996). Self-evaluation maintenance in marriage: Toward a performance ecology of the marital relationship. *Journal of Family Psychology, 10*, 379–396.

Boehm, C. (1999). *Hierarchy in the forest*. Cambridge, MA: Harvard University Press.

Bradlee, P. M., & Emmons, R. A. (1992). Locating narcissism within the interpersonal circumplex and the five-factor model. *Personality and Individual Differences, 13*, 821–830.

Brown, R. P., & Zeigler-Hill, V. (2004). Narcissism and the non-equivalence of self-esteem measures: A matter of dominance? *Journal of Research in Personality, 38*, 585–592.

Brunell, A. B., Campbell, W. K., Smith, L., & Krusemark, E. A. (2004, February). *Why do people date narcissists?: A narrative study*. Poster presented at the annual meeting of the Society for Personality and Social Psychology, Austin, TX.

Bushman, B. J., & Baumeister, R. F. (1998). Threatened egotism, narcissism, self-esteem, and direct and displaced aggression: Does self-love or self-hate lead to violence? *Journal of Personality and Social Psychology, 75*, 219–229.

Bushman, B. J., & Baumeister, R. F. (2002). Does self-love or self-hate lead to violence? *Journal of Research in Personality, 36*, 543–545.

Bushman, B. J., Bonacci, A. M., van Dijk, M., & Baumeister, R. F. (2003). Narcissism, sexual refusal, and aggression: Testing a narcissistic reactance model of sexual coercion. *Journal of Personality and Social Psychology, 84*, 1027–1040.

Buss, D. M., & Chiodo, L. M. (1991). Narcissistic acts in everyday life. *Journal of Personality, 59*, 179–215.

Buss, D. M., & Shackelford, T. K. (1997). Susceptibility to infidelity in the first year of marriage. *Journal of Research in Personality, 31*, 193–221.

Campbell, W. K. (1999). Narcissism and romantic attraction. *Journal of Personality and Social Psychology, 77*, 1254–1270.

Campbell, W. K. (2001). Is narcissism really so bad? *Psychological Inquiry, 12*, 214–216.

Campbell, W. K., & Baumeister, R. F. (in press). Narcissistic personality disorder. In J. E. Fisher & W. O'Donohue (Eds.), *Practitioners' guide to evidence-based psychotherapy*. New York: Kluwer Academic/Plenum Press.

Campbell, W. K., Bonacci, A. M., Shelton, J., Exline, J. J., & Bushman, B. J. (2004). Psychological entitlement: Interpersonal consequences and validation of a new self-report measure. *Journal of Personality Assessment, 83*, 29–45.

Campbell, W. K., Bush, C. P., Brunell, A. B., & Shelton, J. (2005). Understanding the social costs of narcissism: The case of the tragedy of the commons. *Personality and Social Psychology Bulletin, 31*, 1358–1368.

Campbell, W. K., Finkel, E. J., Kumashiro, M., & Rusbult, C. E. (2004). *The metamor-*

phosis of Narcissus: Narcissism and commitment in marriage. Unpublished manuscript, University of Georgia, Department of Psychology.

Campbell, W. K., & Foster, C. A. (2002). Narcissism and commitment in romantic relationships: An investment model analysis. *Personality and Social Psychology Bulletin, 28,* 484–495.

Campbell, W. K., Foster, C. A., & Finkel, E. J. (2002). Does self-love lead to love for others?: A story of narcissistic game playing. *Journal of Personality and Social Psychology, 83,* 340–354.

Campbell, W. K., Goodie, A. S., & Foster, J. D. (2004). Narcissism, overconfidence, and risk attitude. *Journal of Behavioral Decision Making, 17,* 297–311.

Campbell, W. K., Reeder, G. D., Sedikides, C., & Elliot, A. J. (2000). Narcissism and comparative self-enhancement strategies. *Journal of Research in Personality, 34,* 329–347.

Campbell, W. K., Rudich, E., & Sedikides, C. (2002). Narcissism, self-esteem, and the positivity of self-views: Two portraits of self-love. *Personality and Social Psychology Bulletin, 28,* 358–368.

Carlson, K. S. (2002). *Dismissing attachment and narcissism: Examining two constructs in terms of personality similarities and differences over a 20-year period.* Unpublished doctoral dissertation: University of California at Santa Cruz.

Carroll, L. (1987). A study of narcissism, affiliation, intimacy, and power motives among students in business administration. *Psychological Reports, 61,* 355–358.

Cialdini, R. B., Borden, R. J., Thorne, A., Walker, M. R., Freeman, S., & Sloan, L. R. (1976). Basking in reflected glory: Three (football) field studies. *Journal of Personality and Social Psychology, 34,* 366–375.

Clark, R. D., & Hatfield, E. (1989). Gender differences in receptivity to sexual offers. *Journal of Psychology and Human Sexuality, 2,* 39–55.

Digman, J. M. (1997). Higher-order factors of the Big Five. *Journal of Personality and Social Psychology, 73,* 1246–1256.

Drigotas, S. M., Rusbult, C. E., Wieselquist, J., & Whitton, S. W. (1999). Close partner as sculptor of the ideal self: Behavioral affirmation and the Michelangelo phenomenon. *Journal of Personality and Social Psychology, 77,* 293–323.

Ellis, H. (1898). Auto-erotism: A psychological study. *Alienist and Neurologist, 19,* 260–299.

Emmons, R. A. (1984). Factor analysis and construct validity of the Narcissistic Personality Inventory. *Journal of Personality Assessment, 48,* 291–300.

Emmons, R. A. (1987). Narcissism: Theory and measurement. *Journal of Personality and Social Psychology, 52,* 11–17.

Emmons, R. A. (1991). Relationship between narcissism and sensation seeking. *Journal of Social Behavior and Personality, 6,* 943–954.

Farwell, L., & Wohlwend-Lloyd, R. (1998). Narcissistic processes: Optimistic expectations, favorable self-evaluations, and self-enhancing attributions. *Journal of Personality, 66,* 65–83.

Foster, J. D., Campbell, W. K., & Twenge, J. M. (2003). Individual differences in narcissism: Inflated self-views across the lifespan and around the world. *Journal of Research in Personality, 37,* 469–486.

Foster, J. D., Shrira, I., & Campbell, W. K. (2003, June). *The trajectory of relationships involving narcissists and non-narcissists.* Poster presented at the annual meeting of the American Psychological Society, Atlanta, GA.

Foster, J. D., Shrira, I., & Campbell, W. K. (2004, February). *Exploring relationships that result when a partner is attracted away from a previous partner.* Poster presented at the annual meeting of the Society for Personality and Social Psychology, Austin, TX.

Foster, J. D., Shrira, I., & Campbell, W. K. (in press). Narcissism and sociosexuality: The triumph of ego over intimacy. *Journal of Social and Personal Relationships.*

Freud, S. (1957). On narcissism: An introduction. In J. Strachey (Ed. & Trans.), *The standard edition of the complete psychological works of Sigmund Freud* (Vol. 14, pp. 67–104). London: Hogarth Press. (Original work published 1914)

Freud, S. (1950). Libidinal types. In J. Strachey (Ed. & Trans.), *The standard edition of the complete psychological works of Sigmund Freud* (Vol. 21, pp. 217–220). London: Hogarth Press. (Original work published 1931)

Gabriel, M. T., Critelli, J. W., & Ee, J. S. (1994). Narcissistic illusions in self-evaluations of intelligence and attractiveness. *Journal of Personality, 62,* 143–155.

Gosling, S. D., John, O. P., Craik, K. H., & Robins, R. W. (1998). Do people know how they behave?: Self-reported act frequencies compared with on-line codings by observers. *Journal of Personality and Social Psychology, 74,* 1337–1349.

Gramzow, R., & Tangney, J. P. (1992). Proness to shame and the narcissistic personality. *Personality and Social Psychology Bulletin, 18,* 369–376.

Greenberg, J. R., & Mitchell, S. A. (1983). *Object relations in psychoanalytic theory.* Cambridge, MA: Harvard University Press.

Hendrick, C., & Hendrick, S. S. (1986). A theory and method of love. *Journal of Personality and Social Psychology, 50,* 392–402.

Hogan, R. (1983). A socioanalytic theory of personality. In M. M. Page (Ed.), *Nebraska Symposium on Motivation, 1982* (pp. 55–89). Lincoln: University of Nebraska Press.

Hogan, R., & Hogan, J. (2002). Assessing leadership: A view from the dark side. *International Journal of Selection and Assessment, 9,* 40–51.

Horney, K. (1937). *The neurotic personality of our time.* New York: Norton.

Horton, R. S., Bleau, G., & Drwecki, B. (in press). Parenting Narcissus: Does parenting contribute to the development of narcissism? *Journal of Personality.*

Le, T. (in press). Cultural syndromes and love styles. *Journal of Social and Personal Relationships.*

John, O. P., & Robins, R. W. (1994). Accuracy and bias in self-perception: Individual differences in self-enhancement and the role of narcissism. *Journal of Personality and Social Psychology, 66,* 206–219.

Kelsey, R. M., Ornduff, S. R., McCann, C. M., & Reiff, S. (2001). Psychophysiological characteristics of narcissism during active and passive coping. *Psychophysiology, 38,* 292–303.

Kernberg, O. (1974). Barriers to falling and remaining in love. *Journal of the American Psychoanalytic Association, 22,* 486–511.

Kernberg, O. (1975). *Borderline conditions and pathological narcissism.* New York: Jason Aronson.

Kohut, H. (1977). *The restoration of the self*. New York: International Universities Press.

Krueger, R. F., Moffitt, T. E., Caspi, A., Bleske, A. L., & Silva, P. A. (1998). Assortative mating for antisocial behavior: Developmental and methodological implications. *Behavior Genetics, 28*, 173–186.

Leary, T. (1957). *Interpersonal diagnosis of personality*. New York: Ronald Press.

McCullough, M. E., Emmons, R. A., Kilpatrick, S. D., & Mooney, C. N. (2003). Narcissists as "victims": The role of narcissism in the perception of transgressions. *Personality and Social Psychology Bulletin, 29*, 885–893.

Miller, R. S. (1997). Inattentive and contented: Relationship commitment and attention to alternatives. *Journal of Personality and Social Psychology, 73*, 758–766.

Morf, C. C., & Rhodewalt, F. (2001). Unraveling the paradoxes of narcissism: A dynamic self-regulatory processing model. *Psychological Inquiry, 12*, 177–196.

Murray, H. A. (1938). *Explorations in personality: A clinical and experimental study of fifty men of college age*. New York: Oxford University Press.

Murray, S. L., Holmes, J. G., & Griffin, D. W. (1996). The benefit of positive illusions: Idealization and the construction of satisfaction in close relationships. *Journal of Personality and Social Psychology, 70*, 79–98.

Murray, S. L., Holmes, J. G., Griffin, D. W., Bellavia, G., & Rose, P. (2001). The mismeasure of love: How self-doubt contaminates relationship beliefs. *Personality and Social Psychology Bulletin, 27*, 423–436.

Neumann, E., & Bierhoff, H. W. (2004). Narzissmus im Zusammenhang mit Bindung und Liebesstilen [Egotism versus love in romantic relationships: Narcissism related to attachment and love styles]. *Zeitschrift für Sozialpsychologie, 35*, 33–44.

Oltmanns, T. F., Friedman, J. N., Fiedler, E. R., & Turkheimer, E. (2004). Perceptions of people with personality disorders based on thin slices of behavior. *Journal of Research in Personality, 38*, 216–229.

Paulhus, D. L. (1998). Interpersonal and intrapsychic adaptiveness of trait self-enhancement: A mixed blessing? *Journal of Personality and Social Psychology, 74*, 1197–1208.

Paulhus, D. L. (2001). Normal narcissism: Two minimalist views. *Psychological Inquiry, 12*, 228–230.

Paulhus, D. L., & John, O. P. (1998). Egoistic and moralistic biases in self-perception: The interplay of self-deceptive styles with basic traits and motives. *Journal of Personality, 66*, 1025–1060.

Paulhus, D. L., & Williams, K. M. (2002). The dark triad: Narcissism, Machiavellianism, and psychopathy. *Journal of Research in Personality, 36*, 556–563.

Penney, L. M., & Spector, P. E. (2002). Narcissism and counterproductive work behavior: Do bigger egos mean bigger problems? International *Journal of Selection and Assessment, 10*, 126–134.

Raskin, R. N., & Hall, C. S. (1979). A narcissistic personality inventory. *Psychological Reports, 45*, 590.

Raskin, R. N., & Novacek, J. (1989). An MMPI description of the narcissistic personality. *Journal of Personality Assessment, 53*, 66–80.

Raskin, R. N., & Novacek, J. (1991). Narcissism and the use of fantasy. *Journal of Clinical Psychology, 47*, 490–499.

Raskin, R. N., Novacek, J., & Hogan, R. (1991). Narcissistic self-esteem management. *Journal of Personality and Social Psychology, 60,* 911–918.

Raskin, R. N., & Shaw, R. (1988). Narcissism and the use of personal pronouns. *Journal of Personality, 56,* 393–404.

Raskin, R. N., & Terry, H. (1988). A principle components analysis of the Narcissistic Personality Inventory and further evidence of its construct validity. *Journal of Personality and Social Psychology, 54,* 890–902.

Reich, W. (1949). *Character analysis* (3rd ed.). New York: Farrar, Straus, & Giroux.

Reis, H. T., & Shaver, P. (1988). Intimacy as an interpersonal process. In S. W. Duck (Ed.), *Handbook of personal relationships* (pp. 367–389). New York: Wiley.

Rhodewalt, F., & Eddings, S. K. (2002). Narcissus reflects: Memory distortion in response to ego relevant feedback in high and low narcissistic men. *Journal of Research in Personality, 36,* 97–116.

Rhodewalt, F., & Morf, C. C. (1995). Self and interpersonal correlates of the Narcissistic Personality Inventory. *Journal of Research in Personality, 29,* 1–23.

Robins, R. W., & Beer, J. S. (2001). Positive illusions about the self: Short-term benefits and long-term costs. *Journal of Personality and Social Psychology, 80,* 340–352.

Rose, P., & Campbell, W. K. (2004). Greatness feels good: A telic model of narcissism and subjective well-being. In S. P. Shohov (Ed.), *Advances in Psychology Research* (pp. 103–123). Hauppauge, NY: Nova.

Rusbult, C. E. (1980). Commitment and satisfaction in romantic associations: A test of the investment model. *Journal of Experimental Social Psychology, 16,* 172–186.

Rusbult, C. E. (1983). A longitudinal test of the investment model: The development (and deterioration) of satisfaction and commitment in heterosexual involvements. *Journal of Personality and Social Psychology, 45,* 101–117.

Schmitt, D. P., & Buss, D. M. (2001). Human mate poaching: Tactics and temptations for infiltrating existing mateships. *Journal of Personality and Social Psychology, 80,* 894–917.

Sedikides, C., Campbell, W. K., Reeder, G. D., & Elliot, A. J. (1998). The self-serving bias in relational context. *Journal of Personality and Social Psychology, 74,* 378–386.

Sedikides, C., Campbell, W. K., Reeder, G., Elliot, A. J., & Gregg, A. P. (2002). Do other persons bring out the worst in narcissists?: The "others exist for me" illusion. In Y. Kashima, M. Foddy, & M. Platow (Eds.), *Self and identity: Personal, social, and symbolic* (pp. 103–123). Mahwah, NJ: Erlbaum.

Sedikides, C., Oliver, M. B., & Campbell, W. K. (1994). Perceived benefits and costs of romantic relationships for women and men: Implications for exchange theory. *Personal Relationships, 1,* 5–21.

Stucke, T. S. (2003). Who's to blame?: Narcissism and self-serving attributions following feedback. *European Journal of Personality, 17,* 465–478.

Sullivan, H. S. (1953). *The interpersonal theory of psychiatry.* New York: Norton.

Tesser, A. (1988). Toward a self-evaluation maintenance model of social behavior. In L. Berkowitz (Ed.), *Advances in experimental social psychology* (Vol. 21, pp. 181–227). New York: Academic Press.

Thibaut, J. W., & Kelley, H. H. (1959). *The social psychology of groups.* New York: Wiley.

Tracy, J. L., & Robins, R. W. (2004). Putting the self into self-conscious emotions: A theoretical model. *Psychological Inquiry, 15*, 103–125.

Tschanz, B. T., Morf, C.C., & Turner, C. W. (1998). Gender differences in the structure of narcissism: A multi-sample analysis of the Narcissistic Personality Inventory. *Sex Roles, 38*, 863–870.

Twenge, J., & Campbell, W. K. (2003). "Isn't it fun to get the respect that we're going to deserve?": Narcissism, social rejection, and aggression. *Personality and Social Psychology Bulletin, 29*, 261–272.

Vangelisti, A., Knapp, M. L., & Daly, J. A. (1990). Conversational narcissism. *Communication Monographs, 57*, 251–274.

Vohs, K. D., & Campbell, W. K. (2004). *Narcissism and materialism*. Unpublished data, University of British Columbia, Department of Marketing.

Wallace, H. M., & Baumeister, R. F. (2002). The performance of narcissists rises and falls with perceived opportunity for glory. *Journal of Personality and Social Psychology, 82*, 819–834.

Waller, W. (1938). *The family: A dynamic interpretation*. New York: Dryden Press.

Watson, P. J., Grisham, S. O., Trotter, M. V., & Biderman, M. D. (1984). Narcissism and empathy: Validity evidence for the Narcissistic Personality Inventory. *Journal of Personality Assessment, 45*, 159–162.

Wiggins, J. S. (1991). Agency and communion as conceptual coordinates for the understanding and measurement of interpersonal behavior. In W. M. Grove & D. Ciccetti (Eds.), *Thinking clearly about psychology: Vol. 2. Personality and psychopathology* (pp. 89–113). Minneapolis: University of Minnesota Press.

Contingencies of Self-Worth and Self-Validation Goals

Implications for Close Relationships

LORA E. PARK

JENNIFER CROCKER

KATHLEEN D. VOHS

Of all the needs that humans possess, one of the most fundamental is the need for relatedness: the need to have close, mutually caring, and supportive relationships with others (see Baumeister & Leary, 1995, for a review; see also Blackhart, Baumeister, & Twenge, Chapter 12, this volume; Deci & Ryan, 2000). Close relationships serve as a safe haven, thereby alleviating distress and providing comfort and support in times of need (Bowlby, 1969; Collins & Feeney, 2000; see also Feeney, Chapter 7, this volume). Close relationships also serve as a secure base from which people can confidently explore their environment and develop autonomous, integrated personalities (Green & Campbell, 2000). Although relationships are meant to provide a sense of safety and security, certain intrapersonal processes may interfere with people's ability to form and maintain such relationships. In this chapter, we propose that people's *contingencies of self-worth*, or bases of self-esteem, and *self-validation goals*, the desire to prove that one possesses qualities on which self-esteem is based, may ultimately hinder people from sustaining quality relationships with others.

People differ in the domains on which they base their self-worth; some derive self-worth from being virtuous, having God's love, or experiencing support from their family, whereas others may base their self-worth on excelling academically, outdoing others in competition, obtaining others' approval, or being physically attractive (Crocker, Luhtanen, Cooper, & Bouvrette, 2003). Contingencies of self-worth (CSWs; Crocker & Wolfe, 2001), in turn, may influence feelings of closeness and security in relationships, and distinguish between those who are satisfied versus relatively dissatisfied in their relationships.

One mechanism by which people's CSWs may affect relationship outcomes is through the kinds of goals people adopt in their relationships. Specifically, people adopt *self-validation goals* to prove, demonstrate, and confirm that they possess certain qualities in domains on which their self-worth is staked (Crocker & Park, 2004). For example, a person who bases his self-esteem on gaining others' approval may adopt the goal of proving that he is likeable. Although pursuing self-validation goals is highly motivating, the motivation to prove qualities about the self may ultimately undermine close relationships because the focus is on the self, not on the relationship. Indeed, much of the existing literature on the effects of intrapersonal processes on interpersonal outcomes can be integrated in the larger framework of CSWs and self-validation goals. Consistent with the literature, certain individuals may be more vulnerable to experiencing negative relationship outcomes than others. Specifically, people who are highly rejection-sensitive, possess insecure attachment styles, have high, fragile self-esteem, or low self-esteem are likely to pursue self-validation goals in such a way that others are driven away, thereby hindering them from building close relationships with others.

We begin this chapter with a discussion of how childhood experiences and sociocultural factors shape people's CSWs and self-validation goals. We then examine how contingencies and self-validation goals create problems in interpersonal relationships for people with high rejection sensitivity, insecure attachment styles, high, fragile self-esteem, and low self-esteem. Finally, we propose directions for future research regarding the role of CSWs and self-validation goals in relationship outcomes and conclude with a discussion of alternatives to the pursuit of self-esteem. In short, our goal is to outline the ways in which CSWs have a direct effect on the quality of interpersonal relationships and then describe how relationships have a reciprocal influence on CSWs and self-validation goals.

ORIGINS OF CONTINGENCIES OF SELF-WORTH AND SELF-VALIDATION GOALS

In childhood, people experience events, such as being abandoned, rejected, or criticized, that threaten their sense of safety and security. In response, children draw conclusions about how others will respond to them (e.g., they won't be there for me, they will reject me, they will humiliate me), and what they must be or do to avoid these negative responses in the future. These conclusions take the form of specific beliefs, or CSWs, regarding what one must be or do to be a person of worth. Consequently, people are motivated to prove to themselves and to others that they have worth and value (i.e., that they satisfy their contingencies). These self-validation goals involve proving or demonstrating that one possesses certain qualities in domains of contingency. The pursuit of self-validation goals, in turn, regulates anxiety and ensures that fears (e.g., of criticism, of rejection) are kept at bay (see Crocker & Park, 2004). In sum, although CSWs and self-validation goals vary as a function of life experiences, the underlying motivation is to regulate anxiety, feel secure in relationships, and achieve the emotional high that accompanies success in domains of contingency.

Specific events in childhood are likely to overgeneralize to other settings in adulthood. For example, a child who felt abandoned may anticipate or perceive potential abandonment in future interpersonal situations, such as in the context of romantic relationships. Because people are anxious that the distressing event (e.g., abandonment) could occur again, they become vigilant for this possibility and readily interpret ambiguous events in ways that reinforce their expectations. To protect themselves from potential danger, people react in various ways, ranging from withdrawing and distancing themselves from others, to seeking excessive reassurance, to criticizing others. Although these reactions temporarily relieve anxiety, the anxiety and subsequent vigilance are likely to return. Reactions to potential threats become stronger as people increase their efforts to prevent the event from occurring again. Ultimately, this maladaptive interpersonal cycle is likely to disconnect people from others and undermine their sense of interpersonal safety and security.

Social Interactions

Interactions with peers, family members, teachers, and others may shape people's CSWs. In one study, 130 college students were asked to retrospectively report on their childhood experiences of peer acceptance versus peer rejection when they succeeded or failed in domains of contingency (Park, Montgomery, & Crocker, 2005). Specifically, participants were asked to think back to when they were a child and report how often they felt their peers acted positively versus negatively toward them when they succeeded versus failed in the domains of academics, physical appearance, and virtue.

Results showed that the more participants reported having been teased, rejected, or looked down upon by their peers when they performed poorly at school, the more likely they were to base their current self-esteem on academic competence and to possess academic self-validation goals. Importantly, the effects of negative perceived peer reactions on current academic CSW and self-validation goals were mediated by participants' anxiety in childhood about being smart when they were with their peers. A similar mediation process was found with the virtue CSW. Participants who reported negative peer reactions for not acting virtuously were more likely to base their current self-esteem on virtue. Furthermore, this relationship was significantly mediated by participants' anxiety in childhood about being virtuous when they were with their peers. Finally, for the appearance CSW, *positive* peer reactions to being attractive in childhood predicted basing one's current self-esteem on appearance and having the goal of validating one's attractiveness. These effects, however, were not mediated by anxiety in childhood about being attractive to one's peers.

Taken together, these findings suggest that positive versus negative peer interactions in childhood influence people's current CSWs and self-validation goals. Importantly, childhood anxiety about being X (e.g., competent, virtuous) mediated the relationship between negative peer reactions and CSWs. Finally, people do not simply base their self-esteem in domains that they are good at; for example, basing self-worth on academic competence was not significantly related to domain-specific self-esteem in the academic domain ($r = -.08$) (Park et al., 2005). Instead, people base their self-esteem in domains that are associated with anxiety. Anxiety about being smart or virtuous with one's peers may reflect underlying anxiety about being accepted versus rejected and feeling safe and secure in one's relationships.

Cultural Influences

In addition to being shaped by social influences and interactions, CSWs may also develop in response to prevailing cultural norms and values. For example, according to self-objectification theory, women in North American culture come to adopt an observer's perspective on their bodies as a result of living in a culture that objectifies women (Fredrickson & Roberts, 1997). Having an externalized perspective, in turn, may lead women to base their self-worth on domains that depend on others' feedback and validation, such as others' approval and physical attractiveness. Indeed, Crocker and colleagues (2003) found that college women tended to base their self-esteem more on others' approval and their appearance than did men. Moreover, for young women, being highly aware of one's body as an object was related to basing self-worth more on interpersonally contingent domains, such as others' approval and physical appearance, and less on domains such as God's love or virtue (Crocker, Stein, & Luhtanen, 2004). In sum, the objectification of women may lead them to be contingent on sources of self-worth that depend on others' reactions and feedback, such as being physically attractive or likeable.

Cultural values of independence and interdependence may also play a role in the development of specific CSWs. In individualistic cultures, such as the United States, the self is defined by independence, distinctiveness from others, and personal freedom (Markus & Kitayama, 1991). In contrast, in interdependent cultures, such as Japan, the self is defined by one's relationships, group memberships, and connections with others (Heine, Lehman, Markus, & Kitayama, 1999; Markus & Kitayama, 1991). In Japan, maintaining a sense of belongingness and harmonious relations is of paramount importance. Japanese people possess a strong external frame of reference; they view themselves through the eyes of others and strive to maintain "face" and avoid shame. Because of their heightened sensitivity to external cues of approval and disapproval, people in interdependent cultures may possess CSWs that are contingent on others' reactions, such as others' approval, being a good friend, or being a loyal group member. Indeed, research has shown that the Japanese are highly attuned to others' opinions and expectations (Kuwayama, 1992) and are guided less by internal attitudes or desires and more by social cues, such as social roles and norms (Markus & Kitayama, 1991). People in individualistic cultures may also have CSWs related to relational concerns, but because of cultural values stressing independence may derive their sense of self-worth more from being independent and unique.

When self-esteem is contingent on a domain, people typically adopt self-validation goals to prove their worth in those domains. For example, basing self-esteem on academic performance is strongly correlated with the goal of validating one's intelligence through schoolwork (Crocker, 2003), basing self-esteem on others' approval is strongly correlated with the goal of validating one's likeability, and basing self-esteem on physical appearance is strongly correlated with the goal of validating one's attractiveness (Park & Crocker, 2004a). Thus we assume that most people, most of the time, pursue self-validation goals in domains of contingency, with implications for interpersonal relationships.

CONTINGENCIES, SELF-VALIDATION GOALS, AND RELATIONSHIP OUTCOMES

CSWs and self-validation goals are likely to guide interpersonal behavior. In domains of contingent self-worth, people may have the goal of proving something about themselves, which they may do at the expense of others' needs or well-being. That is, when people are highly focused on proving their worth in domains of contingency, they are likely to become preoccupied with themselves, hindering them from forging close connections with others.

Several programs of research provide suggestive evidence for the role of CSWs and self-validation goals in dysfunctional relationship cycles. In the next section, we discuss personality traits that convey interpersonal insecurities in terms of their underlying CSWs.

Rejection Sensitivity

Rejection sensitivity refers to a cognitive-affective processing system in which people anxiously expect and readily perceive rejection from others (Downey & Feldman, 1996). Early experiences of conditional love by parents, emotional neglect, harsh disciplining, and exposure to family violence are associated with anxious expectations of rejection (Downey & Feldman, 1996; Downey, Khouri, & Feldman, 1997). In order to prevent rejection, high rejection-sensitive people are hypervigilant for signs of being abandoned; they anxiously expect, readily perceive, and overreact to signs of rejection (Downey & Feldman, 1996). Indeed, given their highly interpersonal focus, high rejection-sensitive people are likely to base their self-esteem on domains that are interpersonally based, such as physical attractiveness, and be sensitive to rejection based on their appearance (Park, 2005).

For high rejection-sensitive people, having interpersonal CSWs may serve a self-regulatory function; for example, basing self-esteem on being attractive or likeable may be a means to prevent rejection and maintain close relationships. Having interpersonal CSWs may then lead high rejection-sensitive people to be "on guard" in their relationships, seeking to prove that they are attractive and likeable, and not unattractive or unlikable, to prevent rejection. Along these lines, Downey and colleagues have proposed that rejection sensitivity operates as a defensive motivational system (Downey, Mugious, Ayduk, London, & Shoda, 2004). Situations where high rejection-sensitive people expect rejection (e.g., conflict) activate this system, leading them to vigilantly monitor signs of interpersonal negativity and rejection. To avoid rejection, high rejection-sensitive people overaccommodate, ingratiate, and self-silence in order to be liked and to maintain important relationships (Purdie & Downey, 2000).

The kinds of behaviors that high rejection-sensitive people engage in to prevent rejection may differ depending on their CSWs. For example, someone who is highly rejection-sensitive and bases her self-esteem on physical appearance may engage in excessive dieting or exercising in order to appear more attractive to her partner and avoid rejection. Indeed, research has shown that basing self-esteem on one's appearance predicts symptoms of disordered eating, especially among women (Egnatios, Park, & Crocker, 2004; Sanchez & Crocker, 2005) and being rejection-sensitive based on appearance also uniquely predicts eating disorder symptoms (Park, 2005). Thus knowing high rejection-sensitive people's CSWs may help predict the specific kinds of behaviors they might engage in to prevent rejection in their close relationships.

In sum, high rejection-sensitive people may invest a great deal of time and energy into satisfying their CSWs in order to maintain their relationships. Although heightened efforts to fulfill CSWs may temporarily assuage anxieties about rejection, this may eventually give way to overreactions of hostility, depression, and other negative mental health outcomes when rejection has occurred. Ultimately, anxiety and vigilance about rejection are likely to return, and efforts to validate self-worth and prevent future rejection are likely to escalate. Thus, when people are caught in the cycle of validating self-worth in contingent domains, they may end up creating the opposite of what they want, which is to feel secure in their relationships.

Insecure Attachment Style

Through interactions with attachment figures, children come to develop mental models of the self, beliefs about their lovability and worthiness of care and attention, and mental models of others, beliefs about how emotionally available and responsive others will be toward their needs (Bartholomew & Horowitz, 1991; Bowlby, 1969; Collins, 1996). We propose that people's attachment styles, stemming from childhood and continuing into adulthood, affect the types of CSWs and self-validation goals they pursue, with implications for interpersonal relationships.

Preoccupied Attachment Style

People with a preoccupied/anxious attachment style are highly dependent on others and seek excessive closeness with others, but simultaneously worry that their partners will not want to be as close to them as they would like (Collins & Read, 1990; Simpson, Rholes, & Nelligan, 1992). People with a preoccupied attachment style are likely to have had caregivers who conveyed messages of conditional acceptance and rejection, leading them to internalize a negative view of the self and a positive view of others (Bartholomew & Horowitz, 1991; Levy, Blatt, & Shaver, 1998). Preoccupied people's deepseated doubts about their lovability and worth lead them to look to others for validation (Bartholomew, 1990). Indeed, research has shown that preoccupied people possess self-esteem that fluctuates dramatically in response to perceived approval or rejection by others (Collins & Read, 1990). In a study of over 700 college students, Park and colleagues (2004) found that basing self-esteem on physical attractiveness was related to having a preoccupied attachment style. Because physical attractiveness plays an important role in interpersonal attraction and relationships, preoccupied people are likely to invest their self-worth in this domain to gain others' approval and adopt self-validation goals aimed at proving their attractiveness to others (Park, 2005).

When preoccupied people experience anxiety, they react in ways that temporarily relieve anxiety but ultimately strain their close relationships. Indeed, research has shown that preoccupied people tend to be clingy, dependent, emotionally unstable, and jealous in their romantic relationships, which is likely to drive partners away (Bartholomew & Horowitz, 1991; Griffin & Bartholomew, 1994). Preoccupied people also react to anxiety by caring for their partners in a compulsive, inconsistent, controlling manner, overwhelming their partners with care and support even when it is unwanted in order to keep their partners close and committed to the relationship (Feeney & Collins, 2001). Not surprisingly, people with a preoccupied/anxious attachment style report experiencing more negative emotions in their relationships and less relationship closeness, satisfaction, or commitment than securely attached people (Simpson, 1990). These and other negative relationship outcomes may be due, in part, to preoccupied people's desire to validate their worth in interpersonal domains—to prove that they are likeable, attractive relationship partners. Although attempts to prove one's worth to others may temporarily relieve anxiety, this may ultimately hinder feelings of safety and security because the focus is on validating the self rather than on strengthening connections with others. Future research is needed to test this possibility.

Fearful Attachment Style

People with a fearful attachment style are likely to have had caregivers who were rejecting, malevolent, and punitive (Levy et al., 1998). These experiences lead fearfully attached people to conclude that they are unlovable and that others are uncaring and unavailable to meet their needs (Bartholomew & Horowitz, 1991). To prevent negative responses from others, fearfully attached people are likely to base their self-worth on interpersonal domains, such as physical attractiveness, that enable them to indirectly gain acceptance from others without risking overt rejection (Park et al., 2004). Given that people like others who are attractive, fearfully attached people, who desire acceptance yet fear rejection, may adopt self-validation goals aimed at validating their attractiveness. Future research is needed to examine the potential mediating role of CSWs and self-validation goals in producing maladaptive relationship outcomes associated with fearful attachment, such as jealousy, "intimacy anger," and verbal/physical abuse toward partners (Dutton, Saunders, Starzomswki, & Bartholomew, 1994).

Dismissive Attachment Style

Based on their early attachment experiences with unreliable, unresponsive, neglectful caregivers (Levy et al., 1998), people with a dismissive/avoidant attachment style conclude that others are not available to meet their needs, so they must rely on themselves. Dismissive individuals possess a positive mental model of the self and a negative mental model of others (Bartholomew, 1990; Levy et al., 1998), preferring to be self-sufficient and independent rather than rely on others' feedback or support (Brennan & Bosson, 1998; Brennan & Morris, 1998).

People with a dismissive attachment style maintain emotional distance from others; they show little interest in forming close relationships, fall in love less often (Feeney & Noller, 1990), avoid others' support (Collins & Feeney, 2000), and self-disclose less than people with a secure attachment style (Mikulincer & Nachshon, 1991). These interpersonal responses may reflect an underlying desire to regulate anxiety and needs for safety and security. Indeed, Park and colleagues (2004) found that people with a dismissive attachment style were *less* likely to base their self-esteem on domains that depended on others, such as others' approval, family support, and God's love. Dismissive people may instead derive their self-worth from being independent and self-reliant and adopt self-validation goals in these domains. Consequently, negative relationship outcomes for dismissive people may result from their CSWs and self-validation goals aimed at demonstrating their independence and self-reliance rather than strengthening relationships.

Indeed, research has shown that the dismissive/avoidant attachment style is associated with low interdependence, trust, commitment, and satisfaction in relationships (Simpson, 1990). Furthermore, people with this attachment style feel uncomfortable in caregiving and support-seeking roles: avoidant men tend to be unresponsive to their partners' needs, especially when their partners express a need for support; avoidant women seek less support from partners the more anxious they feel (Feeney & Collins, 2001; Simpson et al., 1992). In both of these cases, the link between avoidant attachment and ineffective caregiving and support seeking may be mediated, in part, by dismissive/avoidant people's CSWs and self-validation goals (e.g., independence from others, self-reliance). Although validating these qualities may help alleviate dismissive people's anxiety under threatening conditions, this may ultimately drive others away, hindering the development of close, mutually caring relationships.

In sum, we propose that negative relationship outcomes resulting from insecure attachment styles may be due, in part, to people's CSWs and self-validation goals aimed at proving qualities in contingent domains. Although the specific content of CSWs and self-validation goals may differ from person to person, we think that the underlying goal—to manage anxiety and protect the self from dangers experienced in childhood—is the same. Moreover, people's attempts to manage anxiety, via CSWs and self-validation goals, may ultimately create and perpetuate a dysfunctional cycle of relationship functioning.

High, Fragile Self-Esteem

Although high self-esteem (HSE) signals positive self-evaluations (Baumeister, 1998; Baumeister, Tice, & Hutton, 1989), self-concept clarity (Campbell, 1990), and feeling socially accepted by others (Leary & Baumeister, 2000), researchers have distinguished between different types of HSE that are likely to affect relationship outcomes. In particular, researchers have distinguished between HSE that is stable, secure, and "true," versus HSE that is unstable, fragile, defensive, or contingent (e.g., Deci & Ryan, 2000; Kernis & Waschull, 1995). Compared with people who have stable HSE, those with fragile HSE tend to experience greater fluctuations in self-feelings in response to daily events (Kernis & Waschull, 1995) and are highly ego involved in everyday activities, chronically perceiving that their self-worth is "on the line" (Kernis, Cornell, Sun, Berry, & Harlow, 1993).

Although it is unclear where fragile HSE comes from, one possibility is that early attachment experiences in which caregivers were inconsistent or unreliable may lead people to conclude that others cannot be trusted, and therefore, they must be self-reliant. In attachment terms, this translates into having a positive mental model of the self and a negative mental model of others, which characterizes the dismissive attachment style (Bartholomew, 1990). Although dismissive people typically report having HSE, their self-esteem is likely to be defensive and fragile; dismissive people refuse to acknowledge personal weaknesses that might expose their flaws to others and make them vulnerable to rejection (Mikulincer, 1995). Furthermore, they frequently engage in defensive projection by suppressing their flaws and projecting them onto others, and maintain interpersonal distance by being averse to others' feedback or support (Mikulincer & Horesh, 1999; Brennan & Bosson, 1998; Brennan & Morris, 1998). Accordingly, people with fragile HSE (e.g., a dismissive attachment style) may base their self-worth on domains that emphasize competence and self-reliance. Along these lines, research has shown that after ego threat, HSE people become more independent in their self-construal, focusing on their competencies and unique traits (Vohs & Heatherton, 2001).

Previous research by Heatherton and Vohs (2000) found that after an ego threat (e.g., negative feedback on the Remote Associates Test) HSE people were rated as more antagonistic and unlikable by others in the context of a structured dyadic interaction. A series of follow-up studies by Vohs and Heatherton (2001) showed that differences in likability following threat were due to HSE people's increased focus on personal versus interpersonal aspects of the self. HSE people who received an ego threat sought competency feedback (e.g., "What areas of intellectual performance do I excel in?") over interpersonal feedback (e.g., "How do others really see me?"), and adopted an independent self-construal, which statistically accounted for HSE people's decreased likeability following threat.

Although these effects occurred broadly in the group of HSE people (i.e., stability of self-esteem was not measured in these studies), administering an ego threat among people with fragile HSE is likely to result in even stronger effects (Kernis et al., 1993). Indeed, studies have shown that people with fragile HSE react to ego threat with defensiveness, anger, and hostility toward others (Kernis et al., 1993; Kernis, Grannemann, & Barclay, 1989).

Along these lines, Park and Crocker (2005d) showed that it is not just level of self-esteem that matters, but CSWs *interacting* with self-esteem level and ego threat that influences likeability and interpersonal perceptions. Specifically, Park and Crocker examined the effects of receiving a threat to a contingent domain (i.e., academics) on people's ability to attend to the needs and feelings of others. In their study, two unacquainted, same-sex students participated in each experimental session. One of the participants (partner) wrote an essay about a personal problem while the other participant (target) completed either a Graduate Record Exam (GRE) test and received failure feedback or completed a non-GRE word associations task and received no feedback. In the second half of the experiment, the essay partner discussed his or her personal problem with the target. Afterwards, partners rated targets on various interpersonal qualities, including how supportive, compassionate, understanding, preoccupied, and bored. the target seemed, and indicated how much they liked the target, wanted to interact with him or her again, and disclose a personal problem to him or her in the future.

Results showed that for targets in the failure feedback condition, the combination of having HSE and highly contingent on academic competence was related to being perceived by their partners as being less supportive, caring, and concerned, and more preoccupied, interrupting, and bored with the partner's personal problem. In addition, HSE, highly contingent targets who failed were rated as less likable and less desirable for future interactions or to discuss one's problems with in the future. Under no threat, HSE, highly contingent targets were not rated negatively or disliked by their partners. These findings suggest that HSE people, but only those whose self-worth is at stake, may have difficulty disengaging from the pursuit of self-esteem following threat, hindering them from providing support to others. Over time, these self-focused reactions to ego threat could interfere with people's ability to form and maintain close, mutually supportive relationships with others.

Low Self-Esteem

Low self-esteem (LSE) people possess relatively unfavorable self-evaluations relative to HSE people (Campbell, 1990). As a result of early experiences characterized by failures and low feelings of self-efficacy, LSE people conclude that they are unlikely to meet others' standards for acceptance. According to sociometer theory (Leary et al., 1995; see also Leary, Chapter 12, this volume), LSE people operate at an "inclusion deficit." Because they do not feel included by others, they are highly attuned to signs of potential acceptance and rejection by others, even if the "other" is a stranger (Nezlek, Kowalski, Leary, Blevins, & Holgate, 1997), and prefer to interact with someone who wants to form a relationship, regardless of how positively they are evaluated by them (Rudich & Vallacher, 1999).

In order to compensate for their perceived deficiencies, LSE people look to others to validate their impoverished self. Along these lines, research has shown that LSE people tend to base their self-worth on interpersonally contingent domains that depend on others' reactions and feedback, such as others' approval and physical appearance (Crocker et al., 2003). Accordingly, we would expect LSE people to have self-validation goals aimed at proving their likeability, attractiveness, and other interpersonal qualities. Indeed, Park and Crocker (2005c) found that LSE people were likely to have self-validation goals in the domains of others' approval and appearance. Further evidence for this hypothesis comes from research showing that after ego threat, LSE people are more likeable (Heatherton & Vohs, 2000). In fact, Vohs and Heatherton (2001) found that LSE people's tendency to construe the self as interdependent following threat led them to be more likeable. Similarly, Park and Crocker (2005d) found a trend for LSE people who were highly contingent on academics to become more supportive toward another's personal problem and more likeable following threat.

Because LSE people have less positive self-views and are less certain of their competencies than are HSE people, they are less effective at refuting threats directly when they occur. Instead, they react with indirect strategies by withdrawing from the situation, becoming risk-averse, self-protective, and more interpersonally focused in order to repair self-esteem (Blaine & Crocker, 1993; Vohs & Heatherton, 2001). At first glance, becoming more relational and likeable after threat may appear to be an effective strategy for fulfilling one's need for relatedness. However, studies of ongoing, close relationships reveal that LSE people often react in ways that undermine their relationships with others. After ego threat, LSE people distrust their partners' expressions of love and support, perceive fewer positive qualities in their partners, and report less satisfaction or optimism about the future than their partner's feelings of love and commitment warrant (Murray, Griffin, Rose, Bellavia, & Holmes, 2001; Murray, Rose, Bellavia, Holmes, & Kusche, 2002). Indeed, Murray and colleagues propose that LSE people possess relational contingencies of self-esteem, or self-esteem that is contingent on gaining acceptance/ avoiding rejection (Murray, Griffin, Rose, & Bellavia, 2003).

Baldwin and colleagues have also posited that LSE people possess relational schemas of "If . . . then" contingencies of interpersonal acceptance, such as "If I fail, then I will be rejected" (Baldwin, 1992, 1997; Baldwin & Sinclair, 1996). Indeed, when LSE people experience a threat, or even when simply primed with failure-related words ("lose," "incompetent"), this is likely to automatically activate thoughts of rejection (disliked, ridiculed). Along these lines, we propose that LSE people's negative relationship outcomes may be mediated by the extent to which they base their self-worth on interpersonally contingent sources (others' approval, appearance) and their desire to self-validate in these domains following threat. In a one-time interaction with strangers, LSE people may be able to satisfy their CSWs and self-validation goals, as reflected by their increased likeability following threat. However, in an ongoing relationship, their self-validation goals may interfere with LSE people's ability to maintain mutually caring, supportive relationships.

In sum, early experiences characterized by feelings of low self-regard and low self-efficacy lead LSE people to conclude that they must be likeable to be accepted by others. Consequently, LSE people base their self-worth on and pursue self-validation goals in interpersonal domains (Crocker et al., 2003; Park & Crocker, 2005c). When LSE people encounter threats, they react in self-protective ways, such as withdrawing and distancing themselves, that temporary relieve anxiety in the short term, but may undermine their close relationships with others in the long term. Future research is needed to investigate the mediating effects of interpersonal CSWs and self-validation goals on relationship outcomes among LSE people.

FUTURE DIRECTIONS

In this chapter, we proposed a theoretical model to explain why some people frequently experience negative outcomes in their relationships. We suggested that significant childhood experiences lead people to draw conclusions about the social world. In response, people adopt specific CSWs about what they must be or do to be a person of worth and adopt self-validation goals to prove their worth in domains of contingency, thereby protecting themselves from rejection, abandonment, criticism, and so on. The manner in which people regulate their anxiety and needs for safety and security may vary as a function of rejection sensitivity, attachment style, self-esteem level, and self-esteem stability. Although research has established associations between CSWs and attachment styles (Park et al., 2004), CSWs and self-esteem level (Crocker et al., 2003), and CSWs and self-validation goals (Park & Crocker, 2005c), further research is needed to examine the associations between CSWs and self-validation goals with rejection sensitivity and stability of self-esteem. Furthermore, in order to test the mediating role of CSWs and self-validation goals in producing relationship outcomes as a function of individual differences, researchers must first examine the associations among CSWs and self-validation goals with specific relationship outcomes, such as caregiving and support seeking, interpersonal conflict, relationship closeness, satisfaction, and other outcomes of interest.

Preliminary evidence suggests that specific contingencies are associated with specific relationship outcomes. For example, a study of over 400 college students showed that the more students based their self-esteem on physical appearance, the more romantic breakups they reported experiencing, whereas basing self-worth on family love and support predicted fewer romantic breakups (Park & Crocker, 2004). These effects were found even after controlling for number of romantic relationships, self-esteem level, and attachment styles. These data suggest that people's bases of self-esteem predict important relationship outcomes; future research is needed to determine *why* basing self-worth on certain domains leads to certain relationship outcomes and not others.

Reactions to threat may assuage anxiety temporarily, but produce long-term costs to the self and to others (Crocker, Lee, & Park, 2004; Crocker & Park, 2003, 2004a). Anxiety and vigilance about the potential danger is likely to return, and reactions to the threat may be exacerbated as people increase their efforts to validate the self and manage their anxiety. Ultimately, this pattern may result in a dysfunctional cycle in which people feel increasingly disconnected from others, undermining their ability to form and sustain close, caring relationships with others. Although several programs of research have shown that people respond to threats in ways that undermine their interpersonal functioning (Downey & Feldman, 1996; Murray et al., 2001, 2002, 2003; Vohs & Heatherton, 2001), studies have yet to examine whether people's CSWs and self-validation goals, especially in interpersonally contingent domains, lead to negative relationship outcomes as we have hypothesized.

Future research is also needed to investigate chronic versus state-specific aspects of CSWs and self-validation goals. Contingencies have been shown to be relatively stable over time (Crocker et al., 2003), and the pursuit of self-validation goals in domains of contingency are thought to be the default goal pursuit for most people most of the time (Crocker & Park, 2004a, 2004b). However, recent research has shown that after a threat in a contingent domain, HSE, highly contingent people continue to have the goal to self-validate, whereas LSE, highly contingent people tend to disengage their contingency from their self-validation goals, saying it is less important for them to be likeable after an academic ego threat (Park & Crocker, 2005a), but say it is more important to be perceived as attractive (and less important to be viewed as warm/caring/kind) following interpersonal rejection (Park & Crocker, 2005d).

Experiences in close relationships may also affect the pursuit of self-validation goals. For example, although attachment styles are present at the chronic trait level, they are also present at the state level, varying across relationships and as a function of availability and accessibility of relationships (Baldwin, Keelan, Fehr, Enns, & Rangarajoo, 1996). Similarly, in the context of secure, unconditionally accepting relationships, people may be less contingent on domains that depend on others' reactions and less intent on proving their worth in these domains. In other words, being in a close, mutually caring relationship may lower anxiety and thereby reduce people's need to validate themselves in domains of contingency. In contrast, in insecure, conditionally accepting relationships, people may become more contingent on interpersonal domains and strive to validate their worth in those domains to manage their anxiety and feel secure. Thus future research could examine how people's CSWs and self-validation goals change in response to being in unconditional versus conditionally accepting relationships.

Finally, research is needed to disentangle the effects of CSWs from the effects of other personality variables on relationship outcomes. We propose that the CSWs and self-validation goals framework can provide an integrative framework that emphasizes the common core of diverse personality traits. In particular, CSWs and self-validation goals may mediate the relationships between specific personality variables and relationship outcomes. For example, people with a dismissive attachment style may experience less relationship closeness and commitment because they base self-worth on being independent and self-reliant and have the goal of validating these qualities. High rejection-sensitive people may experience more interpersonal conflicts and less relationship satisfaction the more contingent they are on domains that require validation and reassurance from others, such as being attractive or likeable. In sum, when people's self-esteem is invested in a domain and they have the goal of validating the self in that domain, other goals, such as strengthening connections with others, may be sacrificed.

ALTERNATIVES TO THE PURSUIT OF SELF-ESTEEM

Given the potentially negative effects of CSWs and self-validation goals on relationship outcomes, what, if anything, can be done to attenuate these effects? Although CSWs and self-validation goals are highly correlated (Park & Crocker, 2004c), we do not think that having CSWs necessitates that people pursue self-validation goals. This point reflects our earlier discussion of the distinction between trait and state-specific CSWs and self-validation goals. Whereas CSWs are relatively stable, we think that self-validation goals are more malleable; at any given moment, people can have the goal of validating their self-worth, or they can adopt a different goal (Crocker & Park, 2004a, 2004b). Thus, whereas CSWs are relatively stable and difficult to change, self-validation goals are more situation-specific and can be consciously chosen by the individual. For example, someone who bases his or her self-esteem on academic competence can be focused on proving that he or she is smart, or he or she can adopt an alternative goal, such as being open to feedback and learning from mistakes.

Along these lines, we argue that people who are highly contingent can consciously decide to adopt a goal that is larger than themselves and includes others, such as wanting to create a mutually caring and supportive relationship, rather than validating their likeability or attractiveness. By adopting goals that are beneficial to both the self and to others, people can learn to act autonomously instead of being controlled by external feedback. Over time, choosing goals that include the self with others may reduce people's automatic associations between threat and rejection, thereby minimizing the impact of external feedback on self-worth and enabling people to create close, mutually caring relationships with others.

ACKNOWLEDGMENTS

The research reported in this chapter was supported by a National Science Foundation Graduate Research Fellowship awarded to Lora Park while at the University of Michigan and by National Institute of Mental Health Grant Nos. R01 MH58869 and K02 MH01747 awarded to Jennifer Crocker.

REFERENCES

Baldwin, M. W. (1992). Relational schemas and the processing of social information. *Psychological Bulletin, 112*, 461–484.

Baldwin, M. W. (1997). Relational schemas as a source of if-then self-inference procedures. *Review of General Psychology, 1*, 326–335.

Baldwin, M. W., Keelan, J. P. R., Fehr, B., Enns, V., & Koh-Rangarajoo, E. (1996). Social-cognitive conceptualization of attachment working models: Availability and accessibility effects. *Journal of Personality and Social Psychology, 71*, 94–109.

Baldwin, M. W., & Sinclair, L. (1996). Self-esteem and "If . . . then" contingencies of interpersonal acceptance. *Journal of Personality and Social Psychology, 71*, 1130–1141.

Bartholomew, K. (1990). Avoidance of intimacy: An attachment perspective. *Journal of Social and Personal Relationships, 7*, 147–178.

Bartholomew, K., & Horowitz, L. M. (1991). Attachment styles among young adults: A test of a four-category model. *Journal of Personality and Social Psychology, 61*, 226–244.

Baumeister, R. F. (1998). The self. In D. T. Gilbert, S. T. Fiske, & G. Lindzey (Eds.), *Handbook of social psychology* (4th ed., Vol. 2, pp. 680–740). New York: McGraw-Hill.

Baumeister, R. F., & Leary, M. R. (1995). The need to belong: Desire for interpersonal attachments as a fundamental human motivation. *Psychological Bulletin, 111*, 497–529.

Baumeister, R. F., Tice, D. M., & Hutton, D. G. (1989). Self-presentational motivations and personality differences in self-esteem. *Journal of Personality, 57*, 547–579.

Blaine, B., & Crocker, J. (1993). Self-esteem and self-serving biases in reactions to positive and negative events: An integrative review. In R. F. Baumeister (Ed.), *Self-esteem: The puzzle of low self-regard* (pp. 55–85). Hillsdale, NJ: Erlbaum.

Bowlby, J. (1969). *Attachment and loss: Vol. 1. Attachment* (2nd ed.) New York: Basic Books.

Brennan, K. A., & Bosson, J. K. (1998). Attachment-style differences in attitudes toward and reactions to feedback from romantic partners: An exploration of the relational bases of self-esteem. *Personality and Social Psychology Bulletin, 24,* 699–714.

Brennan, K. A., & Morris, K. A. (1998). Attachment styles, self-esteem, and patterns of seeking feedback from romantic partners. *Personality and Social Psychology Bulletin, 23,* 23–31.

Campbell, J. D. (1990). Self-esteem and clarity of the self-concept. *Journal of Personality and Social Psychology, 59,* 538–549.

Collins, N. L. (1996). Working models of attachment: Implications for explanation, emotion, and behavior. *Journal of Personality and Social Psychology, 571,* 810–832.

Collins, N. L., & Feeney, B. (2000). A safe haven: An attachment theory perspective on support seeking and care giving in close relationships. *Journal of Personality and Social Psychology, 78,* 1053–1073.

Collins, N. L., & Read, S. J. (1990). Adult attachment, working models, and relationship quality in dating couples. *Journal of Personality and Social Psychology, 58,* 644–663.

Crocker, J. (2003). *Academic contingency of self-worth and self-validation goals.* Unpublished data, Department of Psychology, University of Michigan, Ann Arbor.

Crocker, J., Lee, S. J., & Park, L. E. (2004). The pursuit of self-esteem: Implications for good and evil. In A. G. Miller (Ed.), *The social psychology of good and evil* (pp. 271–302). New York: Guilford Press.

Crocker, J., Luhtanen, R., Cooper, M. L., & Bouvrette, S. A. (2003). Contingencies of self-worth in college students: Measurement and theory. *Journal of Personality and Social Psychology, 85,* 894–908.

Crocker, J., & Park, L. E. (2003). Seeking self-esteem: Construction, maintenance, and protection of self-worth. In M. R. Leary & J. P. Tangney (Eds.), *Handbook of self and identity* (pp. 291–313). New York: Guilford Press.

Crocker, J., & Park, L. E. (2004a). The costly pursuit of self-esteem. *Psychological Bulletin, 130,* 392–414.

Crocker, J., & Park, L. E. (2004b). Reaping the benefits of self-esteem without the costs? Response to comments on Crocker & Park (2004a). *Psychological Bulletin, 30,* 430–434.

Crocker, J., Stein, K. F., & Luhtanen, R. K. (2004). *Objectified body consciousness and contingent self-worth.* Unpublished data, Department of Psychology, University of Michigan, Ann Arbor.

Crocker, J., & Wolfe, C. T. (2001). *Contingencies of self-worth. Psychological Review, 108,* 593–623.

Deci, E. L., & Ryan, R. M. (2000). The "what" and "why" of goal pursuits: Human needs and the self-determination of behavior. *Psychological Inquiry, 11,* 227–268.

Downey, G., & Feldman, S. (1996). Implications of rejection sensitivity for intimate relationships. *Journal of Personality and Social Psychology, 70,* 1327–1343.

Downey, G., Khouri, H., & Feldman, S. (1997). Early interpersonal trauma and adult

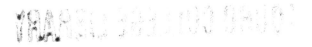

adjustment: The mediational role of rejection sensitivity. In D. Cicchetti & S. Toth (Eds.), *Rochester Symposium on Developmental Psychopathology: Vol. VIII. The effects of trauma on the developmental process* (pp. 85–114). Rochester, NY: University of Rochester Press.

Downey, G., Mugious, V., Ayduk, O., London, B., & Shoda, Y. (2004). Rejection sensitivity and the startle response to rejection cues: A defense motivational system. *Psychological Science, 15,* 668–673.

Dutton, D. G., Saunders, K., Starzomswki, A., & Bartholomew, K. (1994). Intimacy–anger and insecure attachment as precursors of abuse in intimate relationships. *Journal of Applied Social Psychology, 24,* 1367–1386.

Egnatios, N., Park, L. E., & Crocker, J. (2004). *Differences among sisters: Reasons for joining the Greek system, contingencies of self-worth, and risk behaviors among sorority members.* Unpublished manuscript, Department of Psychology, University of Michigan, Ann Arbor.

Feeney, B. C., & Collins, N. L. (2001). Predictors of caregiving in adult intimate relationships: An attachment theoretical perspective. *Journal of Personality and Social Psychology, 80,* 972–994.

Feeney, J. A., & Noller, P. (1990). Attachment style as a predictor of adult romantic relationships. *Journal of Personality and Social Psychology, 58,* 281–291.

Fredrickson, B. L., & Roberts, T. A. (1997). Objectification theory: Toward understanding women's lived experiences and mental health risks. *Psychology of Women Quarterly, 21,* 173–206.

Green, J. D., & Campbell, W. K. (2000). Attachment and exploration in adults: Chronic and contextual accessibility. *Personality and Social Psychology Bulletin, 26,* 452–461.

Griffin, D. W., & Bartholomew, K. (1994). The metaphysics of measurement: The case of adult attachment. In K. Bartholomew & D. Perlman (Eds.), *Advances in personal relationships: Vol. 5. Attachment processes in adulthood* (pp. 17–52). London: Kingsley.

Heatherton, T. F., & Vohs, K. D. (2000). Interpersonal evaluations following threat to self. *Journal of Personality and Social Psychology, 78,* 725–736.

Heine, S. J., Lehman, D. R., Markus, H. R., & Kitayama, S. (1999). Is there a universal need for positive self-regard? *Psychological Review, 106,* 766–795.

Kernis, M. H., Cornell, D. P., Sun, C., Berry, A., & Harlow, T. (1993). There's more to self-esteem than whether it is high or low: The importance of stability of self-esteem. *Journal of Personality and Social Psychology, 65,* 1190–1204.

Kernis, M. H., Grannemann, B. D., & Barclay, L. C. (1989). Stability and level of self-esteem as predictors of anger arousal and hostility. *Journal of Personality and Social Psychology, 56,* 1013–1022.

Kernis, M. H., & Waschull, S. B. (1995). The interactive roles of stability and level of self-esteem: Research and theory. In M. P. Zanna (Ed.), *Advances in experimental social psychology* (Vol. 27, pp. 93–141). San Diego, CA: Academic Press.

Kuwayama, T. (1992). The reference other orientation. In N. R. Rosenberger (Ed.), *Japanese sense of self* (pp. 121–149). Cambridge, UK: Cambridge University Press.

Leary, M. R., & Baumeister, R. F. (2000). The nature and function of self-esteem: Sociometer theory. *Advances in Experimental Social Psychology, 32,* 25–51.

Levy, K. N., Blatt, S. J., & Shaver, P. R. (1998). Attachment styles and parental representations. *Journal of Personality and Social Psychology, 74,* 407–419.

Markus, H. R., & Kitayama, S. (1991). Culture and the self: Implications for cognition,
emotion, and motivation. *Psychological Review, 98,* 224–253.

Mikulincer, M. (1995). Attachment style and the mental representation of the self.
Journal of Personality and Social Psychology, 69, 1203–1215.

Mikulincer, M., & Horesh, N. (1999). Adult attachment style and the perception of
others: The role of projective mechanisms. *Journal of Personality and Social Psychology, 76,* 1022–1034.

Mikulincer, M., & Nachshon, O. (1991). Attachment style and patterns of self-
disclosure. *Journal of Personality and Social Psychology, 61,* 321–331.

Murray, S. L., Griffin, D. W., Rose, P., & Bellavia, G. (2003). Calibrating the
sociometer: The relational contingencies of self-esteem. *Journal of Personality
and Social Psychology, 85,* 61–84.

Murray, S. L., Griffin, D. W., Rose, P., Bellavia, G., & Holmes, J. G., (2001). The
mismeasure of love: How self-doubt contaminates relationship beliefs. *Personality and Social Psychology Bulletin, 27,* 423–436

Murray, S. L., Rose, P., Bellavia, G., Holmes, J., & Kusche, A. (2002). When rejection
stings: How self-esteem constrains relationship-enhancement processes. *Journal
of Personality and Social Psychology, 83,* 556–573.

Nezlek, J. B., Kowalski, R. M., Leary, M. R., Blevins, T., & Holgate, S. (1997). Personality moderators of reactions to interpersonal rejection: Depression and trait self-
esteem. *Personality and Social Psychology Bulletin, 23,* 1235–1244.

Park, L. E. (2005). *Appearance-based rejection sensitivity: Implications for mental and
physical health, affect, and motivation.* Manuscript in preparation, Department of
Psychology, University at Buffalo, The State University of New York.

Park, L. E., & Crocker, J. (2004, January). *Friends, lovers, and breakups: The effects of
contingencies of self-worth and attachment styles on relationship outcomes.* Poster
presented at the annual meeting of the Society for Personality and Social Psychology, Austin, TX.

Park, L. E., & Crocker, J. (2005a). *Contingencies of self-worth, academic failure, and
self-validation goals.* Manuscript submitted for publication.

Park, L. E., & Crocker, J. (2005b). *Contingencies of self-worth and rejection: Implications for self-esteem, affect, and goal pursuit.* Manuscript submitted for publication.

Park, L. E., & Crocker, J. (2005c). *Contingencies of self-worth and self-validation goals.*
Unpublished manuscript, Department of Psychology, University of Michigan.

Park, L. E., & Crocker, J. (2005d). Interpersonal consequences of seeking self-esteem.
Personality and Social Psychology Bulletin, 11, 1587–1598.

Park, L. E., Crocker, J., & Mickelson, K. D. (2004). Attachment styles and contingencies of self-worth. *Personality and Social Psychology Bulletin, 30,* 1243–1254.

Park, L. E., Montgomery, B., & Crocker, J. (2005). *Effects of peer influence on contingencies of self-worth and self-validation goals.* Unpublished manuscript. Department of Psychology, University of Michigan.

Purdie, V., & Downey, G. (2000). Rejection sensitivity and adolescent girls' vulnerability to relationship-centered difficulties. *Child Maltreatment, 5,* 338–350.

Rudich, E. A., & Vallacher, R. R. (1999). To belong or to self-enhance?: Motivational bases for choosing interaction partners. *Personality and Social Psychology Bulletin, 25,* 1387–1405.

Sanchez, D. T., & Crocker, J. (2005). How investment in gender ideals affects well-being: The role of external contingencies of self-worth. *Psychology of Women Quarterly, 29,* 63–77.

Simpson, J. A. (1990). Influence of attachment styles on romantic relationships. *Journal of Personality and Social Psychology, 59,* 971–980.

Simpson, J. A., Rholes, W. S., & Nelligan, J. S. (1992). Support-seeking and support-giving within couple members in an anxiety-provoking situation: The role of attachment styles. *Journal of Personality and Social Psychology, 62,* 434–446.

Vohs, K. D., & Heatherton, T. F. (2001). Self-esteem and threats to self: Implications for self-construals and interpersonal perceptions. *Journal of Personality and Social Psychology, 81,* 1103–1118.

The Inner and Outer Turmoil of Excessive Reassurance Seeking

From Self-Doubts to Social Rejection

KIMBERLY A. VAN ORDEN
THOMAS E. JOINER, JR.

> Reassurance is the safest, least expensive Band-Aid for worry that we have, but it is only a Band-Aid and does not solve any underlying problems.
> —HOLLOWELL (1997, p. 267)

One of the most basic, yet arguably fundamental, formulations of human motivation was set forth by Freud (1920/1950). His "pleasure principle" states that human beings are motivated to attain pleasure and avoid pain. Extending this idea to the emotional domain, we have the following corollary: human beings want to feel good (so we strive to attain pleasure), and do not want to feel bad (so we strive to avoid pain). However, this formulation of motivation in no way suggests that all of our strategies will be effective or useful for us. Sometimes we may want to feel better quickly and easily and may resort to a "Band-Aid method" of emotion regulation (i.e., a quick-fix emotional solution that will only work temporarily). Sometimes Band-Aids can even make the problem worse: consider a situation in which a nasty cut is quickly covered by a Band-Aid and forgotten about until it gets infected. Our "solutions" can sometimes create even bigger problems. In this chapter we discuss the intrapersonal antecedents and interpersonal consequences of one type of "Band-Aid emotion regulation," excessive reassurance seeking. Excessive reassurance seeking involves persistently asking others for reassurance of worth, regardless of whether that feedback has already been provided (Joiner & Metalsky, 2001; Joiner, Metalsky, Katz, & Beach, 1999).

Research on excessive reassurance seeking developed out of Coyne's (1976) interpersonal characterization of depression. Coyne painted a picture of an individual with two intrapersonal vulnerabilities, mild dysphoria and self-doubts, who experiences a stressful life event. The individual then seeks to assuage the bad feelings and quell the self-doubt by asking others for reassurance of his or her worth. But this individual has merely put a Band-Aid on the bad feelings and soon the Band-Aid falls off: the individual's self-doubts that activated the need for reassurance lead the person to doubt the sincerity of the provided reassurance. So the individual tries again and seeks more reassurance, but no amount of reassurance will be enough. Joiner, Alfano, and Metalsky (1993) suggests why the provided reassurance will never be enough by integrating Coyne's model with self-verification theory (e.g., Swann, 1990). The self-verification framework posits that individuals seek both self-enhancing and self-confirming feedback (this theory is discussed in more depth later in the chapter). For individuals with self-doubts, this means both positive feedback about the self that disconfirms self-doubts and negative feedback about the self that confirms self-doubts. Seeking reassurance may function to disconfirm self-doubts temporarily, but doing so will likely activate needs for self-confirmation and thus the reassurance from others may be discounted. As a consequence of these competing motives, any reassurance given will never be enough and the individual, as well as the people in his or her life, becomes trapped in a vicious downward cycle that culminates in interpersonal disruptions (especially rejection) and more bad feelings all around.

A large literature exists that documents a relationship between depression and interpersonal problems (for a review, see Segrin & Dillard, 1992). Joiner, Metalsky, and colleagues (1999) posit that excessive reassurance seeking is the key construct in Coyne's interpersonal formulation of depression and functions as the "interpersonal vehicle" that transports the bad feelings inside a depressed person to the interpersonal context—with the end result being interpersonal problems. Excessive reassurance seeking cannot be understood outside of its interpersonal context: the reactions of the "other person" in the social exchange must be taken into account. The Reassurance-Seeking subscale of the Depressive Interpersonal Relationships Inventory (DIRI-RS; Joiner & Metalsky, 2001) is a commonly used assessment tool for measuring excessive reassurance seeking. The four items on the DIRI help to elucidate the interactional nature of the construct:

Do you find yourself often asking the people you feel close to how they *truly* feel about you?

Do you frequently seek reassurance from the people you feel close to as to whether they *really* care about you?

Do the people you feel close to sometimes become irritated with you for seeking reassurance from them about whether they *really* care about you?

Do the people you feel close to sometimes get "fed up" with you for seeking reassurance from them about whether they *really* care about you?

The first two items tap the persistence with which an individual seeks reassurance from others, while the latter two items tap the negative emotional reactions of the interaction partner(s). Despite the slightly different emphasis on persistence versus negative reactions, the four items are clearly unitary and cohesive.

Joiner and Metalsky (2001) report that scores on the DIRI-RS correlate with actual reassurance-seeking behaviors in the laboratory. Undergraduate students and their same-sex roommates were brought into the lab and told that they would participate in a project to help clinical psychology students improve their test interpretation skills. Both partners completed brief questionnaires they believed would be interpreted by a clinical psychology student. The experimenter gave both roommates bogus feedback on the questionnaire in the form of personality descriptors, such as "active" and "edgy." The roommates were then told to get detailed information from each other on one another's opinions of the ratings. Participants were videotaped as they discussed the feedback and judges later rated the target participants' questions to determine if they met criteria for reassurance seeking. The judges' ratings of participants' reassurance-seeking behaviors in the lab and participants scores on the DIRI-RS were positively correlated, supporting the construct validity of the DIRI-RS, as well as suggesting a domain in which individuals may tend to seek reassurance: when faced with ambiguous and potentially negative self-relevant feedback.

An individual engaging in excessive reassurance seeking does so frequently and persistently to the point that the people in his or her life become irritated and frustrated. The DIRI-RS measures individuals' perceptions of the presence of these qualities in their interpersonal worlds; it does *not* measure the full continuum of reassurance-seeking behaviors (i.e., from the healthy end of seeking of social support to the maladaptive end of excessive reassurance seeking) and thus does not use cutoff scores to define "excessive." Excessive reassurance seeking is conceptualized as a stable tendency to seek reassurance from others of one's worth even if that reassurance has already been provided, but it is not hypothesized to be a stable trait that will exert influence on behavior in all situations. Rather, excessive reassurance seeking is best conceptualized within a social-cognitive model of personality (e.g., Mischel & Shoda, 1995): individuals who tend to excessively seek reassurance will do so in particular situations (i.e., when doubts about the self are activated). These situations will differ from person to person, but are likely to include situations involving competence (e.g., failing an exam) or social acceptance (e.g., fight with a significant other). Importantly, excessive reassurance seeking is also conceptualized as a behavior through which impaired intrapersonal functioning (e.g., self-doubt and worry) affects *interpersonal* functioning.

Excessive reassurance seeking has been found to moderate the relationship between depression and social rejection such that depression results in social rejection most often when individuals engage in excessive reassurance seeking (Joiner, Alfano, & Metalsky, 1992; Joiner & Metalsky, 1995; Katz & Beach, 1997). This relationship has received support in samples of both adults and children (Joiner, 1999). We suggest that, in addition to depression, the intrapersonal components that likely give rise to reassurance-seeking behaviors are increased anxiety and lowered self-esteem following a negative life event. Joiner, Katz, and Lew (1999) found that increased anxiety and lowered self-esteem mediated the relationship between negative life events and increases in reassurance seeking. In this chapter, we focus on these three intrapersonal components (i.e., depression, lowered self-esteem, and increased anxiety) as precursors of excessive reassurance seeking, a behavior that in turn elicits negative interpersonal interactions (e.g., frustration and feeling misunderstood) from others and ends finally with social rejection. The negative feelings resulting from rejection then set the system in motion again (i.e., heightened doubts about the self) and a vicious cycle begins. Following a discussion of both the intrapersonal and interpersonal processes involved, we then elaborate our description of the process of excessive reassurance seeking and suggest possible mechanisms for the relation between the intrapersonal vulnerabilities and the interpersonal outcome of rejection. We then discuss how an understanding of this bidirectional interpersonal cycle can inform research on both the self and interpersonal processes, as well as research at the intersection of the two.

INTRAPERSONAL PROCESSES: WORRIES ABOUT THE SELF AND THE FUTURE

Excessive reassurance seeking is an interpersonal strategy used to cope with doubts and worries resulting from stressful life events (see, e.g., Joiner, Katz, & Lew, 1999). Unfortunately, it is a maladaptive strategy, with negative interpersonal consequences (e.g., social rejection). Why might someone persistently ask others if they truly care? Joiner, Katz, and Lew (1999) posited that negative life events bring up doubts about the worthiness of the self (e.g., "Am I worthy of others' love?") as well as worries about safety and about what the future holds (e.g., "Will others be there to support me?"). They further predicted that increases in doubts about the self (i.e., lowered self-esteem) and increases in worries about the future (i.e., increases in anxiety) would mediate the relationship between the occurrence of negative life events and changes in reassurance-seeking behaviors such that individuals engage in reassurance seeking to assuage self-doubts and quell worries about the future. Doubts about the self were measured with the Rosenberg Self-Esteem Scale (Rosenberg, 1965). This measure of self-esteem could perhaps be more aptly described as a measure of self-worth due to the content of its items, including "I feel that I'm a person of worth, at least on an equal plane with others" and "On the whole, I am satisfied with myself." Worries about the future were tapped by participants' endorsement of anxious symptoms on the Beck Anxiety Inventory (Beck, Epstein, Brown, & Steer, 1988). Participants completed the measures of self-esteem and anxiety, as well as self-report measures of reassurance seeking (Depressive Interpersonal Relationships Inventory; Joiner & Metalsky, 2001), depressive symptomatology (Beck Depression Inventory [BDI]; Beck, Rush, Shaw, & Emery, 1979; Beck & Steer, 1987), and negative life events (Negative Life Events Questionnaire; Metalsky & Joiner, 1992) at time 1 and again at time 2, 3 weeks later. Results supported the mediational hypothesis that stressful negative life events lead to decreases in self-esteem and increases in anxiety, which in turn lead to increases in reassurance seeking. Negative life events at time 2 predicted changes in self-esteem and changes in anxiety beyond effects attributable to depression. Furthermore, negative life events at time 2 predicted changes in reassurance seeking. Finally, negative life events no longer predicted changes in reassurance seeking when anxiety and self-esteem were accounted for. These results are consistent with the hypothesis that changes in reassurance seeking following stressful negative life events are motivated by drops in self-esteem (i.e., doubts about self-worth) and increases in anxiety (i.e., worries about the future). Thus individuals who engage in the interpersonal behavior of reassurance seeking are likely doing so due to intrapersonal turmoil, doubts about the self's worth and security.

It should be noted that although depression is a key intrapersonal construct in the relation between reassurance seeking and social rejection, it was not predicted to be (nor was it found to be) a mediator between the occurrence of negative life events and changes in reassurance seeking. Joiner, Katz, and Lew (1999) posited that individuals seek reassurance in response to doubts about self-worth and self-security, not in response to the experience of becoming depressed. Depression would only be involved in predicting reassurance seeking insofar as lowered self-esteem is a symptom of depression; thus level of depressive symptoms were controlled for when using self-esteem to predict reassurance seeking. Although depression is not a mediator of the stressful life event–reassurance-seeking link, depression does predict *when* reassurance seeking will relate to negative interpersonal outcomes (e.g., social rejection). In other words, depression has consistently been found to moderate the relationship between reassurance seeking and rejection in college roommates (Joiner et al., 1992; Joiner, Alfano, & Metalsky, 1993; Joiner & Metalsky, 1995, 2001), heterosexual dating pairs (Katz & Beach, 1997), childhood peer relationships (Joiner, 1999), and married couples (Benazon, 2000).

Why might the presence of depressive symptomatology play a role in the relationship between reassurance seeking and social rejection? Joiner and colleagues (1993) found that a three-way interaction of depressive symptomatology, negative feedback seeking (this construct and its relation to reassurance seeking is discussed below), and reassurance seeking predicted social rejection. However, the two-way interaction of negative feedback seeking and reassurance seeking did *not* predict rejection—the presence of depressive symptomatology was necessary to obtain the effect. The authors suggest that depression "toxifies information-seeking behaviors [i.e., reassurance-seeking] by adding a quality of distress which others find particularly aversive" (p. 128). The authors also suggest that reassurance seeking in nondepressed individuals may seem less desperate and thus be less aversive to interaction partners. However, an empirical investigation of differential interpersonal consequences of reassurance seeking in depressed versus nondepressed individuals awaits future research.

In line with Coyne's (1976) formulation of depression as inseparable from its interpersonal context, differences in the aversive quality of reassurance seeking between depressed and nondepressed individuals may be best understood by also focusing on processes within interaction partners of depressed individuals. Perhaps interaction partners of reassurance-seeking individuals make more stable, dispositional, and controllable attributions about reassurance-seeking behavior for depressed individuals than for nondepressed individuals, such that reassurance seeking is perceived as more aversive when done by depressed individuals (Sacco & Nicholson, 1999). In support of this explanation, Sacco and Dunn (1990) found that observers made more dispositional and controllable attributions about the cause of a problem that provoked help-seeking behaviors when the target was depressed than when then target was not depressed. These dispositional and controllable attributions mediated the extent of the observers' negative emotional reactions. Thus perhaps interaction partners of depressed individuals who excessively seek reassurance are perceived by their partners as people who will *always choose* to seek reassurance because they are "reassurance seekers." In contrast, the reassurance-seeking behaviors of a nondepressed individual might be attributed to the situation (e.g., "He [She] was having a particularly tough day") and will not be expected to recur.

It is also possible that interaction partners attribute different causes to the reassurance-seeking behaviors of depressed versus nondepressed individuals: perhaps reassurance seeking among depressed individuals is viewed as indicative of different underlying personality traits than those same behaviors among nondepressed individuals (Katz & Beach, 1997). Reassurance-seeking behaviors among depressed individuals may also suggest to interaction partners that, due to societal norms (i.e., we are expected to provide help to those in need), certain responses are appropriate or expected from them. Katz and Beach (1997) suggest that the interaction partners of nondepressed individuals may feel that their response to requests for reassurance will have less of an impact on the reassurance-seeking individual because "less is at stake" (p. 254). The toxicity of reassurance seeking done by depressed individuals may result from implications that the partner is somehow to blame for the emotional pain of the depressed individual (e.g., "You don't love me anymore, do you?") or is obligated to ameliorate the pain, such that the interaction partner feels overwhelmed (Joiner, Metalsky, et al., 1999). The relation of depression as an intrapersonal construct (insofar as it is experienced by targets and partners as a characteristic of an individual) to social rejection thus seems to depend on interpersonal factors, such as others' perceptions of an interpersonal behavior, like reassurance seeking.

Along with depression, self-esteem is another key intrapersonal player on the reassurance-seeking and social rejection stage. As described above, self-esteem helps explain why stressed individuals may seek reassurance. In addition, self-esteem (along with depression) helps predict *when* reassurance seeking will relate to negative interpersonal outcomes (e.g., social rejection). Negative feedback seeking is an example of an interpersonal behavior driven by an intrapersonal vulnerability: low self-esteem. Based in self-verification theory (e.g., Swann, 1990), negative feedback seeking involves the tendency for individuals with negative self-views (i.e., low self-esteem) to seek out negative feedback from others. Negative feedback can be elicited by selecting relational partners who will verify individuals' negative self-views (e.g., by providing criticism) or by interpreting evaluative information in a manner consistent with the self-concept (i.e., as negatively valenced).

Why would individuals seek out information that will make them feel badly about themselves? Research on self-verification theory (e.g., Swann, 1990) suggests that individuals are motivated to confirm self-perceptions, even if they are negative, because confirming feedback fosters a sense of prediction and control, whereas disconfirming feedback threatens individuals' most basic knowledge base: their own self-concepts. Disconfirming feedback about the self may leave individuals wondering, "If I don't know myself, what do I know?" Self-verification theory also posits that individuals are motivated to confirm self-perceptions out of pragmatic concerns: social interactions in which partners see themselves in the same manner as others see him or her are more likely to proceed smoothly. Self-verification theory also posits that individuals have needs for both positive self-feelings (enhancement needs) and consistent self-views (consistency needs; e.g., Swann, Wenzlaff, Krull, & Pelham, 1992). For individuals with low self-esteem, self-enhancement needs are in conflict with consistency needs such that these individuals need to feel good about themselves, yet they also need to garner feedback about their negative qualities to confirm their self-perceptions. Thus individuals with low self-esteem are stuck in the "cognitive-affective crossfire" (Swann, Griffin, Predmore, & Gaines, 1987).[1]

Joiner and colleagues (1992) found that mildly depressed male college students were rejected by their roommates when they excessively sought reassurance *and* had low self-esteem; however, the effect was not found for female participants. To understand this finding, the authors considered a construct related to low self-esteem, negative feedback seeking—an interpersonal behavior driven by an intrapersonal vulnerability (i.e., low self-esteem). They found that mildly depressed students (both men and women) were more likely to be rejected by their roommates when they excessively sought reassurance *and* engaged in negative feedback seeking (Joiner et al., 1993).

In a prospective test of the relation between rejection and the "cognitive-affective crossfire" in college roommates, Joiner and Metalsky (1995) measured reassurance-seeking and negative feedback-seeking tendencies, as well as the current extent of depressive symptomatology and rejection by participants' roommates at time 1, and then again at time 2, 3 weeks later. Thus, reassurance seeking, negative feedback seeking, and depressive symptoms were used to predict *increases* in rejection from time 1 to time 2. This methodology allows for stronger causal inferences than a cross-sectional design by providing support for the temporal antecedence criterion of a vulnerability factor (see Garber & Hollon, 1991, for a discussion of these criteria). In this case, reassurance seeking, negative feedback seeking, and depressive symptoms occurred *before* any increases in rejection, giving us some confidence in our hypothesized causal sequence and allowing us to infer that rejection cannot fully account for levels of reassurance seeking, negative feedback seeking, or depression. Joiner and Metalsky found that the combination of reassurance seeking, negative feedback seeking, depressive symptoms, and gender at time 1 significantly predicted increases in rejection (by the roommate) at time 2. An investigation of the form of this interaction revealed that no discernable pattern between the variables emerged for female participants. However, for male participants, increases in rejection from time 1 to time 2 did not occur regardless of the level of reassurance seeking or negative feedback seeking *if the target was not depressed*. In contrast, for male participants who were depressed, the combination of high reassurance seeking and high negative feedback seeking elicited increases in rejection by their roommates.[2] It is notable that the combination of high reassurance seeking, high negative feedback seeking and depression was required to elicit rejection.

For all of the intrapersonal vulnerabilities discussed thus far, depressive symptoms, anxiety, and self-esteem (tapped by both self-report questions and preferences for negative feedback), rejection was best predicted when an intrapersonal vulnerability was considered in combination with other intrapersonal vulnerabilities and maladaptive interpersonal behaviors.

INTERPERSONAL OUTCOMES: SOCIAL REJECTION

Thus far, evidence has been provided that depressed individuals with low self-esteem who also excessively seek reassurance from others tend to get rejected. In the following section we discuss the nature of the rejection and how it has been measured. Acceptance and rejection are often conceptualized (both in the psychological literature and colloquially) as a dichotomy such that one is either fully rejected or accepted (Leary, 2001; see also Leary, Chapter 11, this volume). For example, being dumped by a girlfriend or boyfriend would most likely be a salient example of rejection for many individuals. In this case the dividing line between rejection and acceptance is clear—or is it? Leary (2001) suggests that acceptance and rejection are often described as a dichotomy, but would be better described as a continuum, with varying degrees of acceptance and rejection. Leary's "Inclusionary-Status" continuum is based on the idea that individuals expend differing amounts of effort to include or exclude others and these differing amounts may represent degrees of acceptance and rejection. For example, it is very unlikely that dating partners experience relational bliss the day before one partner dumps the other. It is more likely that the breakup was preceded by increasing degrees of rejection, with corresponding declines in acceptance.

According to Leary, the most extreme form of exclusion involves physical efforts to reject, abandon, ostracize, or banish another person (e.g., dumping a boy-/girlfriend). A milder form involves efforts to avoid the individual (e.g., "I'm really busy this weekend"), while a still milder form involves efforts to ignore the individual (e.g., "Yes, sure, I was listening to you"). Leary (2001) further suggests that the psychological underpinning of these behaviors is "relational evaluation—the degree to which a person regards his or her relationship with another individual as valuable, important, or close" (p. 6). Thus *rejection* can be defined as instances of low relational evaluation in which one member of the relationship does not positively evaluate or significantly value the relationship (i.e., the relationship is not perceived as valuable, important, or close). Leary posits that only in extreme cases do individuals engage in behaviors such as exclusion or abandonment; a more common scenario involves individuals who value their relationships only slightly and thus invest little effort to improving or sustaining the relationship. In fact, one of the most painful forms of rejection may not involve extreme levels of exclusion, but rather a *relative decline* in relational evaluation: "Because the other person does not value the relationship as much as before, one experiences a deep feeling of rejection" (p. 7). Leary calls this painful form of rejection "relational devaluation."

Low relational evaluation is the manifestation of rejection measured in the studies on reassurance seeking discussed thus far. The instrument most commonly used is a modification of the Rosenberg Self-Esteem Scale (Rosenberg, 1965) developed by Swann and colleagues (1992) to assess a partner's evaluation of a target participant (hereafter referred to as the Rosenberg Partner Esteem Scale [RSE-P]). Partners answer the 10 questions on the RSE-P Scale, reworded to refer to the esteem in which the partner holds the target (e.g., "I feel that my roommate/girlfriend/boyfriend is a person of worth, at least on an equal plane with others"). The studies discussed thus far (Joiner et al., 1992, 1993; Joiner & Metalsky, 1995) utilized this measure, as did studies that are discussed below (Katz & Beach, 1997; Katz, Beach, & Joiner, 1998; Joiner & Metalsky, 2001, Study 5). Studies with prospective designs (e.g., Joiner & Metalsky, 1995) are able to address relational devaluation (as opposed to low levels of relational evaluation) because they measures changes in relational evaluation over time.

Some studies investigating the negative interpersonal outcomes of excessive reassurance seeking have used measures other than partner esteem (i.e., RSE-P) to tap points along the social rejection continuum. In an investigation of the "cognitive-affective crossfire" in heterosexual dating couples, Katz and Beach (1997) used reassurance seeking, negative feedback seeking, and depression to predict partner relationship satisfaction. They measured the women's interest in reassurance seeking and negative feedback as well as their depressive symptoms. They also measured the male partners' relationship satisfaction as the measure of social rejection. Men's relationship satisfaction was tapped by the Quality of Marriage Index (QMI; Norton, 1983), with the questions reworded to apply to dating (vs. spousal) relationships. Katz and Beach report that the QMI taps into the component of marital satisfaction that reflects partners' evaluation of their relationships. Thus this measure of social rejection maps cleanly onto Leary's (2001) concept of relational evaluation by measuring how much partners positively evaluate and value their relationships. Male partners reported the highest level of relationship dissatisfaction when their female partners reported higher depressive symptoms on the BDI in combination with higher levels of interest in both reassurance seeking and negative feedback seeking. The male partners' global evaluation of the women (as measured by the RSE-P) independently predicted male partner dating satisfaction and did not mediate the relationship between the three-way interaction (i.e., reassurance seeking, negative feedback seeking, and depression) and partner dissatisfaction. The authors suggest that these results point to type of relationship as a possible moderator of the link between depression and interpersonal problems (i.e., rejection). Thus, by integrating this study with those discussed previously, we can surmise that roommate and romantic relationships both seem to be adversely affected by the socially toxic intrapersonal combination of excessive reassurance seeking, negative feedback seeking, and depression, but the rejection that ensues may take different forms. For example, romantic partners may be more likely to negatively evaluate their relationships, whereas roommates may be more likely to negatively evaluate the worth of the other roommate.

In an investigation of the relationship between reassurance seeking, depression, and rejection with married couples, Benazon (2000) assessed spousal appraisal of depressed individuals and hypothesized that negative attitudes toward spouses of depressed individuals may be an appropriate indicator of interpersonal rejection in married couples. Spouse appraisal of the depressed individual was assessed with the Principal Index of Partner Appraisal (PPA; Pelham & Swann, 1989), a measure that asks one spouse to rate the other spouse in 10 dimensions the authors propose are key contributors to self-worth (e.g., intellectual capability, emotional stability). In that this measure and the RSE-P Scale both involve evaluations of the partner's global worth, we suggest that they are tapping similar points along the rejection–acceptance continuum. Target participants in the study were married individuals who were receiving treatment for major depressive disorder (MDD). What was found, consistent with past research, is that both reassurance seeking and depressed mood (measured by a depressive mood checklist) significantly predicted partner appraisal. When level of marital adjustment was controlled for, only reassurance seeking remained a significant predictor of partner appraisal. Thus the rejection experienced by depressed spouses cannot be attributed solely to partners' levels of marriage satisfaction— interpersonal variables, such as reassurance seeking, may also play an explanatory role.

The relationship between depression, reassurance seeking, and social rejection was also examined with children (Joiner, 1999) in a cross-sectional study of youth psychiatric inpatients. A new index of social rejection was devised for this sample. Five items related to rejection were compiled from the Children's Depression Inventory (CDI; Kovacs, 1992), including "I do not have any friends" and "Nobody really loves me." This measure of rejection is admittedly different from the others discussed thus far in that it focuses on the intrapersonal consequences of presumed interpersonal rejection and discord. This formulation of rejection was also found to be predicted by the interaction of depressive symptoms (as measured by a lack of positive affect) and reassurance seeking. The form of the interaction indicated that children with higher depression scores (i.e., low positive effect) but low reassurance-seeking scores did not report elevated social rejection scores. The combination of depression and reassurance seeking was again necessary to obtain the effect of elevated social rejection.

Thus the rejection experienced by depressed individuals who excessively seek reassurance (in combination with an intrapersonal vulnerability, such as low self-esteem or negative feedback seeking) has frequently been shown to take the form of lowered esteem in the eyes of their partners. Partner relationship satisfaction as well as the endorsement of items reflecting isolation and loneliness are also forms of rejection that have been found to be predicted by the depression and reassurance-seeking combination. It is a sad irony that the depressed, self-doubting individuals who ask for reassurance are the most likely to elicit the rejection they so desperately fear.

MECHANISMS FOR THE INTRAPERSONAL–INTERPERSONAL LINK

Individuals who feel insecure about themselves and worried about their future often seek reassurance. We have provided evidence that self-doubts and worries about the future predict changes in reassurance-seeking behavior and that excessive reassurance seeking can help explain *when* depressed individuals will experience rejection. Thus we have provided one example of how intrapersonal vulnerabilities lead to interpersonal turmoil. Thus far left unanswered is the question, Why is excessive reassurance seeking so interpersonally toxic as a self-soothing strategy? In short, using the Band-Aid metaphor, excessive reassurance seeking is interpersonally maladaptive because the Band-Aid continually falls off (and thus needs to be reapplied) and creates a kind of contagious interpersonal infection. In other words, we suggest that the reassurance is never enough, and, furthermore, it exacerbates bad feelings by sending aversive messages into the interpersonal sphere.

What are individuals doing to annoy their interaction partners when they engage in excessive reassurance seeking? Kowalski (2003) argues that interaction partners will perceive a behavior as obnoxious when it is performed repetitively and when it thwarts the partner's basic psychological needs—she posits that excessive reassurance seeking is one such annoying behavior.[3] In a description of what makes interacting with depressed individuals an aversive experience, Katz and Joiner (2001) argue that the interpersonal context of depression is only aversive when the intrapersonal distress of the depressed individual is clearly and persistently communicated to interaction partners. This is done in two ways: first, by overwhelming interaction partners with pleas for help to end personal distress, and second, by communicating to partners that the partners are part of the problem or that their relationship is no longer satisfying.

These two criteria for "aversiveness" help delineate how excessive reassurance seeking made Kowalski's list of annoying behaviors. First, excessive reassurance seeking is by definition excessive, and when placed in the context of Coyne's (1976) theory, performed repetitively, thus meeting Kowalski's (2003) criterion for repetitiveness. Excessive reassurance seeking is distinct from the benign and often necessary process of eliciting social support, which at times may take the form of reassurance seeking (Joiner, Metalsky, et al., 1999). However, for an individual engaging in *excessive* reassurance seeking, no matter how much reassurance has been provided, it will never be enough. The reassurance will be sought over and over again, with the same individuals, in the same situations. Elsewhere we have argued that individuals who engage in excessive reassurance seeking may enter interpersonal interactions with an interpersonal script containing the contingency, "When I feel bad, I ask others if I am okay" (Van Orden, Wingate, Gordon, & Joiner, 2005). A highly accessible interpersonal script of this sort could help account for the excessive and persistent nature of reassurance seeking in some individuals.

Admittedly, not all repetitive behaviors are annoying enough to eventuate in rejection. For example, an interaction partner may excessively and persistently tell the same bad joke over and over and over again. Perhaps we get tired of hearing the joke, but we may find the repetitive nature endearing at times. We suggest that a repetitive behavior must implicate the interaction partner in some way for its repetitiveness to be perceived as annoying or aversive. Katz and Joiner's (2001) first criterion for what makes interactions with depressed individuals aversive helps delineates how these interactions implicate the partners over and over again—namely, excessively asking for reassurance may overwhelm interaction partners with pleas for help. These pleas either explicitly or implicitly send the message, "I just wish someone could help me feel better" (Katz & Joiner, 2001, p. 118). Interaction partners may be overwhelmed by these pleas for help because they are so repetitive and nothing the interaction partner does is ever successful—no amount of reassurance will ever be enough.

These interaction partners get fed up, perhaps wondering, "Nothing I ever do helps, so why does he [she] keep asking?" Thus what might also be annoying due to the repetitiveness is that excessive reassurance seekers do not pick up on the frustration of their interaction partners. Hamilton and Deemer (1999) suggest that high levels of self-focus may play a role in the negative outcomes associated with excessive reassurance seeking. Thus individuals engaging in excessive reassurance seeking may be so focused on their own emotional pain that they do not pick up on the social cues indicating they should stop. If these individuals do not notice the frustration and helplessness of their interaction partners, their behaviors will most surely be guided by their own desires for reassurance that feel unsatisfied. Unfortunately, ignoring social cues is annoying and aversive for individuals on the receiving end.

Excessive reassurance seeking also meets Kowalski's (2003) second criterion for an annoying behavior—it thwarts partners' basic psychological needs—because of the aversive messages (posited by Katz & Joiner, 2001) that it sends to partners—namely, that the partners are part of the problem (e.g., "You don't care about me anymore, do you?") or that their relationship is no longer satisfying (e.g., "We aren't close anymore, are we?"). The latter message communicates a message of relational devaluation, as described by Leary (2001; see also Leary, Chapter 11, this volume). The perception of relational devaluation is painful, Leary (2001) posits, because human beings may have a "sociometer," which triggers negative affect when exclusion is detected—resulting in affiliative motives to increase inclusion in order to assuage the negative affect. Leary further argues that the sociometer may have evolutionary adaptive value (and thus individuals with the need to belong might have been more likely to survive and pass along their genes) because early human beings might have been better off when they lived in groups and worked together. Thus the sting of relational devaluation may result from the thwarting of a basic psychological need, described by Baumeister and Leary (1995) as the need to belong. Receiving a message (whether intended or not) from an interaction partner that your relationship is not as satisfying anymore may at least partially thwart the belongingness needs of the person on the receiving end of excessive reassurance seeking. After receiving this message over and over again, excessive reassurance-seeking efforts will likely be perceived as annoying, aversive, and hurtful.

In addition to an unmet need to belong, excessive reassurance-seeking behaviors may also thwart the self-consistency needs of the partner (Swann & Bosson, 1999). As described above, self-verification theory (e.g., Swann, 1990) posits that individuals are motivated to confirm their self-perceptions by seeking out self-consistent feedback. Doing so engenders a sense of prediction and control over one's life and fosters smooth social interactions because interaction partners are "on the same page." Thus far, self-consistency needs have been discussed in the context of individuals with low self-esteem who both desire to feel good (by receiving positive feedback to satisfy self-enhancement needs) and need to feel confirmed (by receiving negative feedback to satisfy self-consistency needs). For individuals with positive self-concepts, however, needs for enhancement and consistency are not in conflict. Thus negative feedback is neither enhancing nor confirming. Swann and Bosson (1999) suggest that clues to the aversive quality of excessive reassurance seeking must not focus solely on the person engaging in the behaviors; as an interpersonal process, the perspective and experiences of the interaction partners must be taken into account. This framework is reminiscent of Coyne's (1999) reflection on his (1976) interpersonal conceptualization of depression in which he argues that a key contribution of an interactional perspective on depression is that it prevents "the fundamental attributional error in depression theory and research" (p. 369). He posits that many conceptualizations of depression attribute causality for the symptoms of depression to "the person" rather than to "the situation," when, in fact, many processes in depression may be best understood as resulting from exchanges between a depressed person and his or her environment. Research on excessive reassurance seeking grew out of this interactional framework, and thus a full understanding of what makes excessive reassurance seeking annoying can only be achieved by examining the psychological experiences of both individuals in the interactions.

Swann and Bosson (1999) focus on the experience of the individual being bombarded with requests for reassurance to make a case for why excessive reassurance is annoying. They posit that self-verification theory can help make sense out of why individuals are upset by the fact that the distressed other is not reassured by them (as evidenced by repeated questioning despite having already provided reassurance). In short, when individuals keep asking for reassurance, they communicate to their partners that they are not convinced by his or her messages and that the sender of the messages is not a trustworthy or credible source of feedback. For nondepressed individuals with high self-esteem, this information will likely clash with self-beliefs and thus represent nonverifying feedback. Swann and Bosson assert that for the individuals on the receiving end of excessive reassurance seeking, "the unabated incredulity of depressed persons will represent a direct challenge to their beliefs about themselves" (p. 302). Left with inconsistent interpersonal feedback, these individuals may feel unsure about the veracity of their self-knowledge when engaging with the individual who excessively seeks reassurance. In this case, Swann and Bosson suggest that the relationship is no longer a source of self-verifying information and the partner may lose interest in remaining in the relationship. Although this hypothesis has not yet been tested (to our knowledge), it represents an intriguing avenue for future research that could further illuminate the mechanisms by which excessive reassurance seeking in depressed individuals often results in the unfortunate interpersonal outcome of social rejection.

A TRANSACTIONAL PROCESS: REASSURANCE SEEKING AS A VULNERABILITY FOR DEPRESSION

Our discussion of excessive reassurance seeking has thus far focused on intrapersonal vulnerabilities that may partially explain its occurrence, the common interpersonal outcome of engaging in the behavior (i.e., social rejection), as well as possible mechanisms for this negative outcome. However, this framework leaves much of the literature on excessive reassurance seeking untouched: a great deal of data suggests that in addition to serving as a *intrapersonal vulnerability* for the origination of reassurance-seeking behaviors, depression may also be an *intrapersonal consequence* of excessive reassurance seeking (e.g., Joiner & Metalsky, 2001). Excessive reassurance seeking is an interpersonal behavior embedded in a transactional process in which the antecedents and consequences mutually interact, such that at one point in the process what might be most aptly described as an antecedent factor may be most aptly described at a later point as a consequent factor. In this section, we briefly discuss the literature on excessive reassurance seeking as (1) a self-propagatory process that both maintains and exacerbates depression (e.g., Joiner, 2000), (2) a vulnerability factor for the development of depressive symptoms (e.g., Joiner & Metalsky, 2001), and (3) a vehicle for the transmission of depressive symptoms across the interpersonal sphere (e.g., Joiner, 1994).

We have described and elaborated the processes posited by Coyne's (1976) model, which lead a depressed individual down a path toward rejection. However, the model goes on to describe a later section of the path in which the rejection experienced by depressed individuals adds to their distress such that rejection may maintain or even exacerbate depressive symptoms (e.g., see Joiner, Metalsky, et al., 1999). Thus an interpersonal outcome of reassurance-seeking behaviors (i.e., rejection) may also function as a maintaining cause of depression—which was originally formulated as an intrapersonal vulnerability of reassurance seeking. Joiner (2000, 2002) posits that processes such as excessive reassurance seeking that both result from psychological pathology (e.g., depression) and fuel pathology, function as self-propagatory processes. These processes involve a set of intrapersonal vulnerabilities and interpersonal behaviors that "take on a life of their own" and consequently maintain or exacerbate current symptoms or rekindle past symptoms. Joiner (2000) explains that the label *self-propagatory* "is used in the sense that depression and its sequellae [i.e., rejection] induce one another and thus propagate themselves" (p. 205). The presence of interpersonal problems produced by the active behaviors involved in self-propagatory behaviors (i.e., reassurance seeking) can predict lengthened episodes of depression as well as future episodes (Joiner, 2000).

Before any claims could be made about excessive reassurance seeking as a vulnerability for the development of depressive symptoms, it was first shown that excessive reassurance seeking and depressive symptoms covary (e.g., see Joiner & Metalsky, 2001; Joiner, Metalsky, et al., 1999). This covariation of reassurance seeking (as measured by the DIRI) and depressive symptoms has been found in samples of college students (Davila, 2001; Joiner, 1994; Joiner et al., 1992, 1993; Joiner & Metalsky, 1995, 2001; Pothoff, Holahan, & Joiner, 1995), U.S. Air Force cadets (Joiner & Schmidt, 1998), clinically depressed undergraduates (Joiner & Metalsky, 2001), and women in heterosexual dating relationships (Katz & Beach, 1997; Katz et al., 1998).[4] The magnitude of the correlation between excessive reassurance seeking and depressive symptoms is relatively consistent given the diversity of the samples; the median correlation magnitude is approximately .36 (Katz & Joiner, 2001).

One way to demonstrate evidence for bidirectional causality among the variables in the reassurance-seeking process would be to investigate the hypothesis that excessive reassurance seeking may function as a vulnerability for depressive symptoms. Pothoff and colleagues (1995) used structural equation modeling to demonstrate that excessive reassurance seeking predicts depressive symptoms, with minor social stressors mediating the effect. The authors suggest that these findings support an integration of Coyne's model with Hammen's (1991, 1992) stress-generation model in which depressed individuals are posited to generate stress in their lives (which contributes to their depression). Reassurance seeking is thus posited to be one mechanism by which depressed individuals create interpersonal stress, and consequently maintain or exacerbate their depressive symptoms.

Another route to demonstrate evidence for bidirectional causality among the variables in the reassurance-seeking process involves investigating social rejection as a predictor of depression, with reassurance seeking as a moderator. This temporal sequence essentially mirrors the original sequence discussed in this chapter. Evidence in support of both sequences would provide strong support for reassurance seeking (and its antecedents and consequences) as a transactional process with bidirectional causality. Joiner and Metalsky (2001, Study 4), provide evidence that excessive reassurance seeking predicts the development of depressive symptoms among initially symptom-free individuals. Using a sample of college roommates, Joiner and Metalsky (2001, Study 5) also provide evidence that the interaction of rejection (as measured by the RSE-P) and reassurance seeking predicts *increases* in depressive symptoms. This is the mirror hypothesis needed to support bidirectional causality. The form of the interaction confirmed that it was individuals with the lowest partner esteem at time 2 (i.e., high levels of rejection) combined with high reassurance-seeking scores who were most likely to report increases in depressive symptoms from time 1 to time 2.

In a prospective test of the hypothesis that social rejection may predict increases in depressive symptoms over time in heterosexual dating couples, Katz and colleagues (1998) found support for this hypothesis as well as evidence that reassurance seeking and self-esteem moderate the relationship. The interaction between rejection (measured with the RSE-P) and reassurance seeking significantly predicted increases in depressive symptoms from time 1 to time 2, 6 weeks later. The same was true for the interaction between rejection and self-esteem. However, when all possible two-way interaction terms were entered as predictors of increases in depressive symptoms (i.e., rejection by reassurance seeking, rejection by self-esteem, and reassurance seeking by self-esteem), only the interaction between rejection and reassurance seeking accounted for unique variance. Thus the authors conclude that the moderating effect of self-esteem on increases in depressive symptoms could be fully accounted for by the effects of reassurance seeking. Furthermore, they suggest that in this case the interpersonal variables were stronger moderators of the relationship between rejection and depression than were the intrapersonal variables. The authors concede that generalizing this finding to other intrapersonal and interpersonal variables would be premature, but they also suggest that at least regarding the increase of depressive symptoms following rejection, interpersonal variables that directly influence interaction partners may more strongly bring out the negative effects of rejection than intrapersonal variables that only influence interaction partners indirectly.

Support for bidirectional causality among the depression–rejection link, with reassurance seeking as moderator, can also be found in studies investigating contagious depression. Joiner (1994) investigated the hypothesis that an individual's level of depressive symptoms can predict a partner's future level of depressive symptoms among a sample of college roommates. The hypothesis was supported such that the target's BDI scores at time 1 predicted the partner's BDI scores at time 2 (after controlling for the partner's BDI scores at time 1 and level of negative life events at time 2). In addition, the interaction between the target's time 1 BDI scores and the partner's reassurance-seeking score at time 1 predicted increases in the partner's BDI scores. The form of this interaction revealed that target time 1 BDI only predicted increases in partner BDI for partners with high levels of reassurance seeking. Thus, reassurance seeking acted as a vulnerability for contagious depression. The author suggested that if a relationship partner has a greater tendency to seek reassurance, if his or her roommate gets depressed, the roommate will be less emotionally available to provide the needed reassurance. Thus the high reassurance-seeking roommate may not receive the reassurance he or she wants and will be more likely to experience increases in depressive symptoms.

Excessively seeking reassurance from others about self-worth seems to function as a behavior that links together intrapersonal and interpersonal experiences. Intrapersonal vulnerabilities like low self-esteem and depression can make it more likely that an individual will excessively seek reassurance from others, which will in turn increase that individual's risk for social rejection. Unfortunately, social rejection can in turn make it more likely that an individual will seek reassurance (possibly because he or she just received information that activates the sociometer), and as a result maintain his or her depression or become even more depressed. The reciprocal influences among the variables in the reassurance-seeking process if left unchecked may lead to a downward spiral. However, since there are so many links in the chain, this suggests that there are even more targets for intervention to prevent this downward cycle.

IMPLICATIONS FOR OUR UNDERSTANDING
OF THE SELF AND REJECTION

We have discussed intrapersonal antecedents as well as interpersonal consequences of reassurance seeking. We have also discussed how a component of
the reassurance-seeking process (e.g., depression) can function as both a vulnerability and a consequence of the process. The transactional quality of the
reassurance-seeking process suggests that changes may be occurring at both
the intrapersonal and the interpersonal levels to perpetuate the cycle. Self-
esteem is arguably the primary self-component involved in reassurance
seeking—without drops in self-esteem, individuals might never engage in
reassurance seeking. If changes occur at the intrapersonal level as a result of
engaging in the reassurance-seeking process, an understanding of reassurance
seeking may help elucidate our understanding of self-esteem.

Researchers of the self-concept commonly contend that the self is socially
constructed (e.g., Baldwin & Sinclair, 1996). In addition, self-esteem, as a construct in the self system, is influenced by the interpersonal environment,
including explicit and implicit feedback (Kernis & Goldman, 2003). Coyne
(1976) contends that the feedback individuals receive as a result of reassurance seeking is likely to be inconsistent and conflicting. Whereas partners
may initially provide convincing reassurance (which is nonetheless doubted),
over time, as they become annoyed, partners may begin to provide confusing,
conflicting feedback: they may say in words that they care about the individual, but do so in a disgusted or dismissive tone, or with body language that
conveys a meaning opposite to the explicit one they provide verbally. Individuals engaging in excessive reassurance seeking may on some level pick up on
the rejecting atmosphere in their interactions. These perceptions are likely to
fuel further self-doubts after nonsatisfying interactions. This process suggests
one example of how interpersonal feedback may influence self-esteem, particularly the stability of self-feelings. Kernis and his colleagues have asserted that
in addition to the level of self-esteem (i.e., high or low), an important dimension of self-feelings is their stability—how much self-esteem fluctuates across
contexts and over time (e.g., Kernis, Cornell, Sun, Berry, & Harlow, 1993).
Kernis, Paradise, Whitaker, Wheatman, and Goldman (2000) suggest that
unstable self-esteem involves fragile, easily shaken feelings of self-worth that
are dependent on self-evaluative events, such as self-perceptions of goal
achievement or interpersonal feedback. In contrast, stable self-esteem is not
so contextually dependent: having stable self-esteem "means that one's feelings of self-worth are stable and secure, that is, they do not need continual validation stroking" (Kernis et al., 2000, p. 1297). From this description of stable
self-esteem, we feel confident suggesting that individuals who engage in
excessive reassurance seeking probably do not possess stable self-esteem.
Furthermore, it is possible that reassurance seeking could be one mechanism

by which (1) unstable self-esteem develops after an initial blow to self-esteem or (2) unstable self-esteem that developed early in childhood (as suggested by Kernis & Goldman, 2003) may be maintained or exacerbated. The feedback individuals receive from reassurance seeking is likely to be highly variant (Coyne, 1976), thus representing a potential vulnerability for the development of unstable self-esteem.

An examination of reassurance seeking may also aid our understanding of interpersonal processes, especially rejection. Two of the proposed intra-personal vulnerabilities for reassurance seeking, depressive symptoms and trait level of self-esteem, have been found to moderate individuals' sensitivity to rejection (Nezlek, Kowalski, Leary, Blevins, & Holgate, 1997). Nezlek and colleagues (1997) found that both depressive symptoms and low self-esteem were associated with stronger reactions to an experimental rejection manipulation and that individuals with higher levels of depressive symptoms or lower self-esteem were more attuned to the information given to them in the form of interpersonal feedback. The sociometer theory of self-esteem mentioned briefly above (e.g., Leary & Baumeister, 2000) posits that individuals' self systems contain an internal interpersonal exclusion/inclusion monitor that signals individuals when exclusion or inclusion occurs. This monitor is termed the "sociometer." This interpersonal monitor signals individuals through fluctuations in state self-esteem, such that individuals feel good (i.e., higher state self-esteem) when they perceive inclusion and feel bad (i.e., lower state self-esteem) when they perceive exclusion. In this way, again relying on the "pleasure principle," individuals are motivated to pursue inclusion (because they feel good) and to avoid exclusion (so they will not feel bad). The sociometer functions much like a fuel gauge in a car: just as the goal in a car is not to have a fuel gauge that registers full, but rather to have a tank that is full of gas, the goal for humans in social interactions is not to have high self-esteem (which is merely a gauge), but rather to have experiences "full of" inclusion. In turn, these inclusionary experiences fulfill individuals' fundamental needs to belong (Baumeister & Leary, 1995).

Since the sociometer is sensitive to perceived inclusion and exclusion, and individuals with depressive symptoms and low self-esteem seem to be more sensitive to rejection in the lab (Nezlek et al., 1997), it is possible that individuals with those intrapersonal vulnerabilities of depression and low self-esteem might engage in reassurance seeking in part because they have overly sensitive sociometers. These individuals might be more likely to experiences drops in self-esteem and increases in anxiety following negative life events because they perceive interpersonal rejection where none may exist. In "true" instances of interpersonal rejections, others may recognize the pain the individual is most likely experiencing and provide unsolicited reassurance. However, in circumstances in which only an overly sensitive sociometer picks up on rejection (i.e., others do not perceive rejection), reassurance from others will not be forthcoming, and thus must be sought out. Individuals who engage in excessive reassurance seeking may have overly sensitive sociometers and unstable self-esteem, and consequently may respond to rejection differently than individuals without these intrapersonal vulnerabilities. Consequently, including reassurance seeking as a variable in studies of rejection and ego threat could help researchers more precisely predict reactions to these interpersonal events.

Vohs and Heatherton (2001) found that following an ego threat, individuals with high esteem sought competency feedback, whereas individuals with low self-esteem sought interpersonal feedback. This finding is consistent with our description of the process of reassurance seeking in which individuals with self-doubts seek reassurances from others about their self-worth. However, Vohs and Heatherton also found that after threats to self-esteem, individuals with high trait self-esteem were seen as *less* likeable by others, whereas individuals with low trait self-esteem were seen as *more* likeable by others. A naturalistic study that examined drops in self-esteem over 9 months in college freshman as they experienced the transition to a competitive college also found that among men, high self-esteem was related to lower likeability (when combined with the operationalization of ego threat; see Vohs & Heatherton, 2003). This raises the question of why low self-esteem seems to operate as a protective factor against rejection in studies investigating ego threat, yet operates as a vulnerability factor in studies investigating reassurance seeking. Vohs and Heatherton (2003) suggest that one moderator may be length of relationship. Thus they conducted their naturalistic study over 9 months. However, although all analyses done in the Vohs and Heatherton study controlled for length of acquaintance by the raters, this study did not focus on the same type of relationships as those studied in the reassurance-seeking literature (i.e., roommates and dating partners). Low self-esteem may function differentially as a protective or vulnerability factor for rejection depending on the type of relationship involved—and the type of interpersonal behaviors, such as reassurance seeking—used to combat the feelings of low self-esteem. Individuals are not likely to reassurance-seek with their classmates or in newly formed relationships. Boyfriends, girlfriends, spouses, and roommates are much more likely targets of reassurance seeking.

A FINAL NOTE OF REASSURANCE

We have described the interpersonally toxic process of excessive reassurance seeking that may result in rejection and even exacerbation of the intrapersonal vulnerabilities that started the process (i.e., depression and doubts about the self and the future). We have suggested that all of the intrapersonal and interpersonal components in this process interact to produce a self-perpetuating, interpersonally damaging cycle. But do not despair! Each one of these interactions is also a possible point of intervention: without all of the components in the process, the downward cycle cannot continue. Studying processes such as reassurance seeking that explicitly focus on the links between intrapersonal and interpersonal processes suggests that it is research that examines this crucial link that will allow us to predict when components of the self system as well as interpersonal behaviors will result in negative consequences. As mentioned above, low self-esteem seems to function as both a vulnerability and a protective factor: placing this intrapersonal component in a broader context, including the behaviors of both interaction partners as well as the type of relationship in question, might well elucidate the most psychologically healthy formulations of this variable.

The downward cycle of excessive reassurance seeking would never be initiated without the entrance of an intrapersonal vulnerability: increases in self-doubts. Yet these self-doubts would likely not be a problem and would not result in rejection if individuals did not engage in excessive reassurance seeking. Our need to belong conflicts with these self-doubts, and individuals may choose to place a Band-Aid on the self-doubts by seeking reassurance. Further delineating when and why individuals choose quick-fix self-soothing strategies like reassurance seeking, which unfortunately are ineffective, represents an exciting and hopeful avenue for future research. If conflicting and confusing feedback given to self-doubting individuals can maintain such a deleterious process, we suggest and hope that the effect of consistent and clear feedback might somehow stop the reassurance-seeking cycle in its tracks.

NOTES

1. Negative feedback seeking is often measured with the Feedback-Seeking Inventory (FSQ; Swann et al., 1992), which taps interest in receiving feedback about the self. Participants are given a list of 10 questions from multiple domains (e.g., intellectual ability, social competence), the answers to which have self-relevance. Half of the questions are framed positively and half negatively. The participant is asked to choose five questions he or she would most like to have his or her partner answer about him or her. Thus scores for negative feedback-seeking are derived by summing the number of negative feedback questions participants select.

2. Regarding the gender differences found in Joiner, Alfano, and Metalsky (1992) and Joiner and Metalsky (1995), but *not* in Joiner, Alfano, and Metalsky (1993), the authors of the latter paper suggest that females may need to "go to greater lengths" by seeking *both* reassurance and negative feedback in order to elicit rejection from their roommates (p. 128). However, both of these variables were included in the 1995 study. Thus those authors suggest that perhaps women participants were reluctant to provide responses indicative of rejection. Perhaps a more satisfying explanation is provided by Katz and Beach (1997) who suggest that responses to

reassurance seeking and negative feedback seeking may depend on the type of relationship (i.e., roommate vs. romantic). It may be that for women, rejection effects more often occur in romantic, not roommate, relationships; Katz and Beach provide support (discussed later) that this may be the case.

3. Kowalski asserts additional factors that relate to the obnoxious quality of the behavior; we discuss only those relevant to reassurance seeking. For a full discussion, see Kowalski (2003).

4. The correlation between depressive symptoms has not yet been supported in children (e.g., Joiner, 1999) or married couples (e.g., Benazon, 2000). See Joiner, Metalsky, Katz, and Beach (1999) for a discussion of this relationship across diverse samples, as well as a table listing correlation magnitudes.

REFERENCES

Baldwin, M. W., & Sinclair, L. (1996). Self-esteem and "if . . . then" contingencies of interpersonal acceptance. *Journal of Personality and Social Psychology, 71,* 1130–1141.

Baumeister, R. F., & Leary, M. R. (1995). The need to belong: Desire for interpersonal attachments as a fundamental human motivation. *Psychological Bulletin, 117,* 497–529.

Beck, A. T., Epstein, N., Brown, G., & Steer, R. (1988). An inventory for measuring clinical anxiety: Psychometric properties. *Journal of Consulting and Clinical Psychology, 56,* 893–897.

Beck, A. T., Rush, A. J., Shaw, B. F., & Emery, G. (1979). *Cognitive therapy of depression.* New York: Guilford Press.

Beck, A. T., & Steer, R. A. (1987). *Manual for the Revised Beck Depression Inventory.* San Antonio, TX: Psychological Corporation.

Benazon, N. R. (2000). Predicting negative spousal attitudes toward depressed persons: A test of Coyne's interpersonal model. *Journal of Abnormal Psychology, 109,* 550–554.

Coyne, J. C. (1976). Toward an interactional description of depression. *Psychiatry, 39,* 28–40.

Coyne, J. C. (1999). Thinking interactionally about depression: A radical restatement. In T. E. Joiner & J. C. Coyne (Eds.), *The interactional nature of depression: Advances in interpersonal approaches* (pp. 365–392). Washington, DC: American Psychological Association.

Davila, J. (2001). Refining the association between excessive reassurance seeking and depressive symptoms: The role of related interpersonal constructs. *Journal of Social and Clinical Psychology, 20,* 538–559.

Freud, S. (1920/1950). *Beyond the pleasure principle.* New York: Liveright.

Garber, J., & Hollon, S. D. (1991). What can specificity designs say about causality in psychopathology research? *Psychological Bulletin, 110,* 129–136.

Hamilton, J. C., & Deemer, H. N. (1999). Excessive reassurance-seeking as self-regulatory perseveration: Implications for explaining the relation between depression and illness behavior. *Psychological Inquiry, 10,* 293–297.

Hammen, C. (1991). Generation of stress in the course of unipolar depression. *Journal of Abnormal Psychology, 100,* 555–561.

Hammen, C. (1992). Life events and depression: The plot thickens. *American Journal of Community Psychology, 20,* 179–193.

Hollowell, E. M. (1997). *Worry: Hope and help for a common condition.* New York: Ballantine Books.

Joiner, T. E. Jr. (1994). Contagious depression: Existence, specificity to depressed symptoms, and the role of reassurance seeking. *Journal of Personality and Social Psychology, 67,* 287–296.

Joiner, T. E. Jr. (1999). A test of interpersonal theory of depression in youth psychiatric inpatients. *Journal of Abnormal Child Psychology, 27,* 77–85.

Joiner, T. E. Jr. (2000). Depression's vicious scree: Self-propagating and erosive processes in depression chronicity. *Clinical Psychology: Science and Practice, 7,* 203–218.

Joiner, T. E. Jr. (2002). Depression in its interpersonal context. In I. H. Gotlib & C. L. Hammen (Eds.), *Handbook of depression* (pp. 295–313). New York: Guilford Press.

Joiner, T. E. Jr., Alfano, M. S., & Metalsky, G. I. (1992). When depression breeds contempt. *Journal of Abnormal Psychology, 101,* 165–173.

Joiner, T. E. Jr., Alfano, M. S., & Metalsky, G. I. (1993). Caught in the crossfire: Depression, self-consistency, self-enhancement, and the response of others. *Journal of Social and Clinical Psychology, 12,* 113–134.

Joiner, T. E. Jr., Katz, J., & Lew, A. (1999). Harbingers of depressotypic reassurance seeking: Negative life events, increased anxiety, and decreased self-esteem. *Personality and Social Psychology Bulletin, 25,* 632–639.

Joiner, T. E. Jr., & Metalsky, G. I. (1995). A prospective test of an integrative interpersonal theory of depression: A naturalistic study of college roommates. *Journal of Personality and Social Psychology, 69,* 778–788.

Joiner, T. E. Jr., & Metalsky, G. I. (2001). Excessive reassurance seeking: Delineating a risk factor involved in the development of depressive symptoms. *Psychological Science, 12,* 371–378.

Joiner, T. E. Jr., Metalsky, G. I., Katz, J., & Beach, S. R. H. (1999). Depression and excessive reassurance-seeking. *Psychological Inquiry, 10,* 269–278.

Joiner, T. E. Jr., & Schmidt, N. B. (1998). Excessive reassurance-seeking predicts depressive but not anxious reactions to acute stress. *Journal of Abnormal Psychology, 107,* 533–537.

Katz, J., & Beach, S. R. H. (1997). Romance in the crossfire: When do women's depressive symptoms predict partner relationship dissatisfaction? *Journal of Social and Clinical Psychology, 16,* 243–258.

Katz, J., Beach, S. R. H., & Joiner, T. E. Jr. (1998). When does partner devaluation predict emotional distress?: Prospective moderating effects of reassurance-seeking and self-esteem. *Personal Relationships, 5,* 409–421.

Katz, J., & Joiner, T. E. Jr. (2001). The aversive interpersonal context of depression: Emerging perspectives on depressotypic behavior. In R. M. Kowalski (Ed.), *Behaving badly: Aversive behaviors in interpersonal relationships* (pp. 117–147). Washington, DC: American Psychological Association.

Kernis, M. H., Cornell, D. P., Sun, C., Berry, A., & Harlow, T. (1993). There's more to self-esteem than whether it's high or low: The importance of stability of self-esteem. *Journal of Personality and Social Psychology, 65,* 1190–1204.

Kernis, M. H., & Goldman, B. M. (2003). Stability and variability in self-concept and self-esteem. In M. R. Leary & J. P. Tangney (Eds.), *Handbook of self and identity* (pp. 106–127). New York: Guilford Press.

Kernis, M. H., Paradise, A. W., Whitaker, D. J., Wheatman, S. R., & Goldman, B. N. (2000). Master of one's psychological domain: Not likely if one's self-esteem is unstable. *Personality and Social Psychology Bulletin, 26,* 1297–1305.

Kovacs, M. (1992). *Children's Depression Inventory manual.* Los Angeles: Western Psychological Services.

Kowalski, R. M. (2003). *Complaining, teasing, and other annoying behaviors.* New Haven, CT: Yale University Press.

Leary, M. R. (2001). Toward a conceptualization of interpersonal rejection. In M. R. Leary (Ed.), *Interpersonal rejection* (pp. 3–20). Oxford, UK: Oxford University Press.

Leary, M. R., & Baumeister, R. F. (2000). The nature and function of self-esteem: Sociometer theory. *Advances in Experimental Social Psychology, 32,* 1–62.

Metalsky, G. I., & Joiner, T. E. Jr. (1992). Vulnerability to depressive symptomatology: A prospective test of the distress–stress and causal mediation components of the hopelessness theory of depression. *Journal of Personality and Social Psychology, 63,* 667–675.

Mischel, W., & Shoda, Y. (1995). A cognitive-affective system theory of personality: Reconceptualizing situations, dispositions, dynamics, and invariance in personality structure. *Psychological Review, 102,* 246–268.

Nezlek, J. B., Kowalski, R. M., Leary, M. R., Blevins, T., & Holgate, S. (1997). Personality moderators of reactions to interpersonal rejection: Depression and trait self-esteem. *Personality and Social Psychology Bulletin, 23,* 1235–1244.

Norton, R. (1983). Measuring marital quality: A critical look at the dependent variable. *Journal of Marriage and the Family, 45,* 141–151.

Pelham, B. W., & Swann, W. B. Jr. (1989). From self-conceptions to self-worth: On the sources and structure of global self-esteem. *Journal of Personality and Social Psychology, 57,* 672–679.

Pothoff, J. G., Holahan, C. J., & Joiner, T. E. Jr. (1995). Reassurance seeking, stress generation, and depressive symptoms: An integrative model. *Journal of Personality and Social Psychology, 68,* 664–670.

Rosenberg, M. (1965). *Society and the adolescent self-image.* Princeton, NJ: Princeton University Press.

Sacco, W. P., & Dunn, V. K. (1990). Effect of actor depression on observer attributions: Existence and impact of negative attributions toward the depressed. *Journal of Personality and Social Psychology, 59,* 517–524.

Sacco, W. P., & Nicholson, K. J. (1999). A social-cognitive perspective on reassurance-seeking and depression. *Psychological Inquiry, 10,* 298–302.

Segrin, C., & Dillard, J. P. (1992). The interactional theory of depression: A meta-analysis of the research literature. *Journal of Social and Clinical Psychology, 11,* 43–70.

Swann, W. B. Jr. (1990). To be known or to be adored: The interplay of self-enhancement and self-verification. In E. T. Higgins & R. M. Sorrentino (Eds.), *Handbook of motivation and cognition: Volume 2* (pp. 408–448). New York: Guilford.

Swann, W. B. Jr., & Bosson, J. K. (1999). The flip side of the reassurance-seeking coin: The partner's perspective. *Psychological Inquiry, 10,* 302–304.

Swann, W. B. Jr., Griffin, J. J., Predmore, S. C., & Gaines, B. (1987). The cognitive-affective crossfire: When self-consistency confronts self-enhancement. *Journal of Personality and Social Psychology, 52,* 881–889.

Swann, W. B. Jr., Wenzlaff, R. A., Krull, D. S., & Pelham, B. W. (1992). Allure of negative feedback: Self-verification strivings among depressed persons. *Journal of Abnormal Psychology, 101,* 293–306.

Van Orden, K., Wingate, L. R., Gordon, K. H., & Joiner, T. E. (2005). Interpersonal factors as vulnerability to psychopathology over the life course. In B. L. Hankin & J. R. Z. Abela (Eds.), *Development of psychopathology: A vulnerability–stress perspective* (pp. 136–160). Thousand Oaks, CA: Sage.

Vohs, K. D., & Heatherton, T. D. (2001). Self-esteem and threats to self: Implications for self-construals and interpersonal perceptions. *Journal of Personality and Social Psychology, 81,* 1103–1118.

Vohs, K. D., & Heatherton, T. D. (2003). The effects of self-esteem and ego threat on interpersonal appraisals of men and women: A naturalistic study. *Personality and Social Psychology Bulletin, 29,* 1407–1420.

INTERPERSONAL SCHEMAS AND ORIENTATIONS

CHAPTER 7

An Attachment Theory Perspective on the Interplay between Intrapersonal and Interpersonal Processes

BROOKE C. FEENEY

Attachment theory provides a useful perspective from which to consider the interplay between personal and interpersonal processes because it stipulates that, from the cradle to the grave, very specific *interpersonal* processes are important in shaping specific *intrapersonal* characteristics (i.e., individual differences in personality)—and these *intrapersonal* characteristics exert an important influence on subsequent *interpersonal* processes. This chapter discusses attachment theory's stipulations regarding the interplay between intrapersonal and interpersonal processes, as well as research supporting these theoretical propositions.

IN THE BEGINNING: INTERPERSONAL PROCESSES INFLUENCING INTRAPERSONAL CHARACTERISTICS

Attachment theory centers on the idea that the interpersonal dynamics that occur in specific relationship contexts play an important role in shaping personality (Bowlby, 1969/1982, 1973, 1980, 1988). Important propositions of attachment theory are:

1. Individuals come into the world genetically predisposed to form strong emotional bonds with particular individuals who care for them (generally referred to as "attachment figures"). During childhood, bonds are formed typically with parents, who are looked to for protection, comfort, and support; during adolescence and adulthood, these important bonds persist but are supplemented by new bonds, primarily romantic ones.

2. These bonds exist and are important because they reduce the risk of the individual coming to harm. In times of adversity, individuals seek proximity to known and trusted others, and they derive a sense of protection, safety, and security by doing so. Therefore, individuals are genetically biased to develop a set of behavioral patterns that enable them to keep attachment figures within certain limits of accessibility.

3. The way in which attachment figures respond to the individual's need for close contact in times of adversity is presumed to play an important role in shaping facets of the individual's personality. An attachment figure who is available and responsive when needed serves a protective function with regard to any number of threats that an individual may encounter (e.g., illness, fear, pain).

Thus an important aspect of attachment theory is its assertion that a healthy dependence on a reliably sensitive and responsive "attachment figure" is important for optimal functioning and well-being from the cradle to the grave (Bowlby, 1988).

John Bowlby, the pioneer of attachment theory, describes personality development from a very interpersonal perspective (Bowlby, 1969/1982, 1973, 1988). He argues that relationships are critically important throughout the lifespan, in infancy and in adulthood, and he asserts that we must genuinely respect the need for affection and intimacy that everyone shares. An important proposition of attachment theory is that attachment behavior (or a reliance on significant others) in certain circumstances is not something to be discouraged and looked down upon. Instead, it is something that should be accepted as an intrinsic part of human nature and acknowledged for the role it plays in promoting optimal human functioning. Bowlby emphasizes the important function of attachment figures in this regard: attachment figures promote healthy functioning by providing a *safe haven* to which a relationship partner can come for comfort, support, reassurance, assistance, and protection, and by providing a *secure base* from which a relationship partner can explore the world and strive to meet his or her full potential. In the most healthy, stable partnerships, this can be viewed as a cyclical process in which individuals are able to move out from the attachment figure to learn, explore, and discover when feeling secure and content, and in which individuals are able to move in toward the attachment figure to derive comfort and security when threatened in any way (Bowlby, 1988; Feeney, 2004; Marvin, Cooper, Hoffman, &

Powell, 2002). Bowlby (1988) states that "this concept of the secure personal base, from which a child, an adolescent, or an adult goes out to explore and to which he returns from time to time, is one [that is] crucial for an understanding of how an emotionally stable person develops and functions *all through his life*" (p. 60).

Evidence for this process has been shown particularly with regard to parent–child relationships (Ainsworth, 1982; Ainsworth, Blehar, Waters, & Wall, 1978; Bowlby, 1988). Children who are brought up in an affectionate home and have attachment figures who are responsive to their needs (e.g., tuned in to the child's signals, likely to interpret them correctly and to respond promptly and appropriately, accepting of the child and cooperative in dealing with him or her) are confident and clear about whom to seek out in times of need (e.g., when they are tired, frightened, or sick). This type of attachment figure is usually able, by his or her presence or ready accessibility, to create the conditions that enable the child to feel secure and to resume exploration in a confident way (Bowlby, 1988). Thus children raised in this type of caregiving environment can be seen to make a series of excursions away from the attachment figure, often returning to "check in" and engage in mutually enjoyable contact before making the next excursion. When any type of threat arises (e.g., when frightened, tired, ill, injured, or worried about being separated from the attachment figure), the child's top priority is to regain the presence of the attachment figure, and the child's explorations and organized excursions cease. Thus, according to attachment theory, exploratory behavior is incompatible with attachment behavior and has a lower priority; it is only when conditions are favorable and attachment behavior is inactive that true exploration can occur (Ainsworth, 1982; Bowlby, 1988).

In contrast, children who are raised in homes where attachment figures are less sensitive and responsive to their needs (e.g., fail to notice the child's signals, often misinterpret signals when they are noticed, and then respond tardily, inappropriately, or not at all; ignore or reject the child; interfere with the child's activities in an arbitrary way) are less confident about receiving care in times of need (Ainsworth, 1982; Ainsworth et al., 1978; Bowlby, 1988). The conditions created by unresponsive attachment figures restrict the child's ability to explore the world in a confident way. Thus children raised in this type of caregiving environment either tend to be anxious about their attachment figure's whereabouts and availability even in the presence of the attachment figure (crying a lot and difficult to soothe) or they tend to be independent and ignoring of the attachment figure altogether (seeming not to need the attachment figure or to enjoy contact with him or her). According to the theory, consistent experiences of unresponsiveness may lead people to hide desires for love and support, and to refuse to ask for help or ever acknowledge a need for it (Bowlby, 1988). Avoidance (refusing to express or feel the natural desire for a close, trusting relationship and for care/comfort) may help the individual avoid being rejected or treated in a hostile way, whereas anxious preoccupation with the attachment figure may enable the individual to obtain occasional support.

Attachment theory states that as an individual grows older, his or her life continues to be organized as a series of excursions away from a close relationship partner; however, the excursions become steadily longer in time and space, and the threshold for activation of attachment behavior is raised because adolescents and adults have more complex representational models of themselves, the environment, and the people who are important to them (Bowlby, 1969/1982, 1973, 1988). However, a major proposition of attachment theory is that throughout adult life the availability of a responsive attachment figure remains the source of a person's feeling secure. In fact, Bowlby (1988) states that "all of us, from the cradle to the grave, are happiest when life is organized as a series of excursions, long or short, from the secure base provided by our attachment figures" (p. 62), and he argues that a secure home base is necessary for optimal functioning and mental health.

Attachment behavior is presumed to be organized by means of a control system within the central nervous system, analogous to the physiological control systems that maintain physiological measures like blood pressure and body temperature within certain limits (Bowlby, 1969/1982, 1988). An important postulate of attachment theory is that the attachment system will become activated in stressful or threatening situations and lead an individual of any age to desire proximity to a known and trusted other. In support of this postulate, Mikulincer, Gillath, and Shaver (2002) examined attachment system activation in adulthood and provided the first empirical evidence that when threatened, even unconsciously through the use of threat primes, the adult mind turns automatically to representations of attachment figures. According to the theory, the attachment system maintains a person's relation to his or her attachment figure within certain limits of distance and accessibility, and, as individuals grow older, they tend to use increasingly sophisticated methods for maintaining comfortable levels of proximity to important relationship partners.

Bowlby (1988) claims that in order for the attachment system to operate efficiently, it must have at its disposal as much information as possible about the self and others (particularly attachment figures) with regard to how each is likely to respond to the other in particular relationship contexts (particularly in attachment-relevant situations in which the individual's psychological sense of security is threatened). This information includes knowledge of others' intentions, dependability, accessibility, and responsiveness, as well as knowledge of the self (e.g., one's own goals and intentions, the degree to which the self is perceived to be the type of person who is likely to receive affection and support from others) and patterns of interaction that have developed between the self and attachment figures. According to the theory, knowledge of the self and the social world becomes organized in the form of "internal working models" of the self and others. These working models can be thought of as relationship schema that function to simulate relationship events and that enable individuals to plan their own behavior and predict the behavior of others (Baldwin, 1992; Baldwin, Keelan, Fehr, Enns, & Koh-Rangarajoo, 1996). Of course, the more accurate and adequate the representations, the better adapted behavior based on them is likely to be. These working models are presumed to be in constant use; therefore, their influence on thought, feeling, and behavior is likely to become routine and to operate outside of awareness. Thus an important proposition of attachment theory is that working models are based on actual, real-life interactions with attachment figures. The influences of these interpersonal experiences on personality development is described by Bowlby (1988) as follows:

> A principle means by which such experiences influence personality development is held to be through their effects on how a person construes the world about him and on how he expects persons to whom he might become attached to behave, both of which are derivatives of the representational models of his parents that he has built up during his childhood. (p. 65)

Researchers have identified specific patterns of attachment (presumed to reflect the specific content of working models) and the family conditions that promote them. *Secure individuals* are confident that attachment figures will be available, responsive, and helpful in stressful situations, and with this assurance, they are bold in their explorations of the world. *Anxious individuals* are uncertain of their attachment figures' availability and responsiveness when called upon; thus they tend to be clinging and anxious about exploring the world. *Avoidant individuals* have no confidence that they will be responded to helpfully when they seek care from others; therefore, they attempt to be emotionally self-sufficient and live without the support of others. These working models (and resulting patterns of attachment) are considered to be central features of personality throughout life. Although they are amenable to change, they tend to become increasingly a property of the individual and to be self-perpetuating because they become established as influential cognitive structures that may operate at an unconscious level, and because the individual tends to impose them on new relationships (Collins & Read, 1994; Main, Kaplan, & Cassidy, 1985). The important point with regard to the theme of this book is that these personality characteristics (including views of the self and expectations of the availability and responsiveness of others) are based on the individual's actual interactions with significant others and they influence feelings, social behaviors, social perceptions, and relationship functioning across the lifespan. Working models and resulting attachment patterns are thought to be central components of personality that guide interactions with others.

THE INFLUENCE OF WORKING MODELS: INTRAPERSONAL CHARACTERISTICS INFLUENCING INTERPERSONAL PROCESSES

Working models of attachment are presumed to operate "as part of a broader system of cognitive, affective, and behavioral processes that enable people to make sense of their experiences and to function in a way that serves their personal needs" (Collins & Read, 1994, p. 69). They are considered to be "highly accessible cognitive constructs" that become activated automatically whenever attachment-relevant events occur. Once these models are activated in memory, they are predicted to have a direct impact on the cognitive processing of social information (including attention, memory, and inference) and on emotional response patterns. Moreover, because most individuals have developed (based on past relationship experiences) a behavioral repertoire consisting of well-learned responses to attachment-relevant events, working models of attachment should also have a direct impact on behavior (Collins & Read, 1990; Collins, Guichard, Ford, & Feeney, 2004). It is a major postulate of attachment theory that much of this system will operate automatically (i.e., spontaneously, with little effort, and outside of awareness); therefore, it is not necessary to assume that people are consciously directing these processes, or even that they are aware of them.

The different patterns of attachment also can be understood in terms of rules that guide individuals' responses to emotionally distressing situations (Kobak & Sceery, 1988). These rules may organize strategies for regulating distress in situations that normatively elicit attachment behavior. For example, secure attachment is organized by rules that allow acknowledgment of distress and turning to others for support. Avoidant attachment is organized by rules that restrict acknowledgment of distress, as well as any attempts to seek comfort and support from others. Anxious attachment is organized by rules that direct attention toward distress and attachment figures in a hypervigilant manner that inhibits the development of autonomy and self-confidence.

One specific attachment-relevant domain in which working models of attachment are presumed to influence interpersonal processes involves the interactive social support process. According to the theory, individual differences in attachment patterns should be most evident when an individual is distressed and in need of support—that is, when the attachment system is activated and a safe haven is needed. Individual differences in attachment patterns should also be evident in the individual's use of attachment figures as a secure base for exploration. The next part of this chapter reviews the existing literature examining the influence of working models of attachment (or attachment styles) on the interactive social support process in adulthood. Evidence regarding the influence of attachment style on support-seeking behavior is reviewed first, followed by evidence for attachment style differences in support-giving behavior and interpersonal perception.

Support-Seeking Behaviors

Attachment theory states that the need for security is a fundamental human need; therefore, adults as well as children will have developed characteristic strategies for terminating the activation of the attachment system (i.e., strategies for seeking support, reducing feelings of distress, and increasing feelings of security) when they are feeling distressed or threatened. The specific strategies used to achieve this goal are contingent on an individual's history of regulating distress with attachment figures. If attachment figures have been available and responsive to distress signals, then distress can be successfully regulated with strategies that involve active seeking of comfort and support from others. However, in less optimal circumstances, such as when attachment figures have rejected attempts to gain comfort or have been inconsistently available and/or inept at providing comfort, distress may come to be associated with negative outcomes; therefore, alternative methods of coping with distress and regulating the attachment system must evolve.

Consistent with these propositions, a number of studies have found links between attachment style and self-reported support-seeking behaviors (Armsden & Greenberg, 1987; DeFronzo, Panzarella, & Butler, 2001; Florian, Mikulincer, & Bucholtz, 1995; Greenberger & McLaughlin, 1998; Mikulincer & Florian, 1995; Mikulincer, Florian, & Weller, 1993; Ognibene & Collins, 1998; Pierce & Lydon, 1998). Armsden and Greenberg (1987) were the first to document a link between a secure attachment style and the self-reported use of support-seeking as a coping strategy. However, two other studies are particularly noteworthy because they examined the association between attachment style and coping during two different real-life stressful situations. First, Mikulincer and colleagues (1993) examined the association between adult attachment style and the way people coped with the Iraqi missile attack on Israel during the Gulf War. Secure individuals reported using more support-seeking strategies (turning to others for both emotional and instrumental support) than both anxious and avoidant individuals, and anxious individuals reported using more emotion-focused strategies (trying to change one's feelings about the situation) than both secure and avoidant individuals. Next, Mikulincer and Florian (1995) assessed the effects of attachment style on the ways that young Israeli soldiers coped with a 4-month combat training period—a different real-life stressful situation to which most of Israel's young adults are regularly exposed. In this study, both secure and anxious individuals reported more support seeking than did avoidant individuals.

Two other self-report studies assessed the extent to which people with different attachment styles generally (1) seek emotional and instrumental support from various sources: mothers, fathers, same-sex friends, opposite-sex friends, and romantic partners (Florian et al., 1995) and (2) seek support from others when they are experiencing specific types of stressors: an interpersonal versus an academic stressor (Ognibene & Collins, 1998). In both of these studies, individuals with a secure attachment style reported seeking social support (e.g., talking to someone about one's feelings) in dealing with life problems, whereas avoidant individuals reported an unwillingness to do so (see also DeFronzo et al., 2001, and Pierce & Lydon, 1998). However, the results for anxious individuals were mixed in the two studies. In one study (Florian et al., 1995), anxious individuals did not differ from avoidant individuals in the degree to which they reported seeking support from others; in the other (Ognibene & Collins, 1998), anxious individuals were similar to secure individuals in their seeking of support.

Researchers have also found that attachment style is predictive of directly observable support-seeking behavior (Collins & Feeney, 2000; Larose, Boivin, & Doyle, 2001; Simpson, Rholes, & Nelligan, 1992). Simpson and colleagues (1992) provided the first empirical demonstration of the effects of attachment styles on support-seeking behavior. They designed a methodology to induce anxiety in the female member of dating couples so that (1) the attachment system would be strongly activated and (2) behaviors associated with different attachment styles would be directly elicited. The female member of each couple was told that she would be exposed to a situation and a set of experimental procedures that arouse considerable anxiety and distress in most people. Participants were then escorted to a private room where they waited for 5 minutes with their male partners, during which time the couple's spontaneous interaction was unobtrusively videotaped. At the beginning of this interaction period, the male partner knew nothing about his partner's impending stressful situation.

Results indicated that among secure and avoidant women, levels of observer-rated anxiety were related to levels of observer-rated support seeking. Specifically, more secure women sought more support (emotional and physical comfort) from their partners as their level of anxiety increased, whereas more avoidant women sought less support as their anxiety increased. More securely attached women used their partners as a source of comfort and reassurance as their anxiety increased, whereas more avoidant women retracted from their partners both emotionally and physically. It is interesting to note, however, that at lower levels of anxiety, more avoidant women sought *more* support from their partners than did secure women. Because the proximity needs of avoidant individuals are often frustrated and rarely satisfied, it is believed that these individuals may overcompensate with proximity seeking under less threatening conditions. It is also interesting to note that 16 of the 83 women in this study did not even mention the anxiety-provoking situation to their partners; exploratory analyses revealed that these 16 were the more avoidant women (Simpson et al., 1992).

These results were corroborated in two other observational studies: one in which dating couples were videotaped as one member of the couple discussed a current problem or stressor with his or her partner (Collins & Feeney, 2000), and another in which couples were observed as they were separating from each other at an airport (Fraley & Shaver, 1998). Individuals with more secure working models of attachment were less likely to use indirect (e.g., hinting and sulking) and somewhat more likely to use direct (e.g., asking for advice) support-seeking strategies when discussing a current stressor in their lives (Collins & Feeney, 2000). Avoidant attachment, however, was associated with the use of ineffective support-seeking strategies. Individuals who were higher in avoidance tended to seek relatively low levels of support regardless of how stressful they perceived their problem to be, and when they did seek support they were more likely to use indirect strategies. Consistent with these results, avoidant attachment was associated with less contact seeking in couples who were separating at an airport (Fraley & Shaver, 1998).

Taken together, the results of these studies reveal that attachment security is associated with both a greater willingness to seek social support in response to stress and a more direct support-seeking style. Adults with secure attachment characteristics seek support from others as a primary method of coping with distress, whereas avoidant individuals use more distancing strategies in order to cope with stress. Under conditions of stress (when the attachment system is likely to be activated) adults who are higher in attachment-related avoidance tend to direct their attention away from attachment figures. However, the support-seeking behavior exhibited by individuals who are higher in attachment-related anxiety is less clear. The self-report studies have yielded mixed results. Moreover, an anxious attachment style was not predictive of support-seeking behavior in the observational studies reviewed above. However, anxious attachment was associated with both more support-seeking behavior and more negative/hostile affect in a recent study examining the interaction dynamics of adolescents as they discussed current life concerns with a same-age, same-sex peer they were meeting for the first time (Feeney, Ramos-Marcuse, & Cassidy, 2005). It is possible that the support-seeking behavior of these individuals may depend on particular circumstantial and contextual factors to be identified in future research (Mikulincer et al., 1993) or that the samples for the existing observational studies have not included an adequate representation of the insecure attachment types (Collins & Feeney, 2000).

It is interesting to note that the results of these studies indicate that avoidant individuals do not distance themselves from others when they are not experiencing high degrees of stress—that is, when their attachment systems are not activated (Ognibene & Collins, 1998; Simpson et al., 1992). When avoidant individuals reported their support-seeking behavior in response to hypothetical social stressors, avoidant attachment was negatively related to support seeking under high-stress conditions, but was not related to support-seeking under low-stress conditions (Ognibene & Collins, 1998). Moreover, secure attachment was not related to support seeking under low-stress conditions, but was strongly related to support seeking under high-stress conditions. However, the association between anxious attachment and support seeking did not differ under conditions of high and low stress, suggesting that anxious individuals may be less discriminating in their need for support. These findings are consistent with the major tenets of attachment theory, which state that the intensity of the stressor is important with regard to attachment system activation such that the behavioral propensities associated with the various attachment styles should be most evident in highly stressful situations—that is, when the attachment system is activated.

Support-Giving Behaviors

According to attachment theory, behaviors that support a relationship partner's attachment and exploration needs should also be predictable from one's working models of attachment. Because working models include information about the likelihood of *receiving* care from others, it is likely that they encompass personal beliefs about *providing* care to others as well (Kunce & Shaver, 1994). Thus working models of attachment should consist not only of rules that guide support-seeking behaviors and the regulation of personal distress, but also rules that guide support/caregiving behaviors and the regulation of a significant other's distress.

Based on an extensive review of the literature describing caregiving behaviors associated with infant attachment styles, Kunce and Shaver (1994) identified four major caregiving dimensions, which include *proximity* (the ability to provide a distressed partner with physical and psychological accessibility), *sensitivity* (the ability to notice and accurately interpret a partner's needs, feelings, and nonverbal as well as verbal signals), *cooperation* (the ability to support a partner's own efforts and attempts to solve problems as opposed to taking control of the situation), and *compulsive caregiving* (the tendency to get overinvolved in a partner's problems). In a series of studies, these researchers found that each attachment style is associated with a unique pattern of caregiving. Individuals with a secure attachment style report relatively low levels of compulsive caregiving, and relatively high levels of cooperation, proximity, and sensitivity. In contrast, anxious–preoccupied individuals report relatively high levels of proximity and compulsive caregiving, but relatively low levels of sensitivity and cooperation, suggesting that although these individuals are capable of providing affectionate care, their support behaviors may be somewhat intrusive and out of synch with their partner's needs. Dismissing avoidant individuals report the lowest levels of compulsive caregiving and provision of proximity, as well as relatively low levels of sensitivity, whereas fearful avoidant individuals report relatively low levels of proximity and sensitivity and relatively high levels of compulsive caregiving. The patterns for the two avoidant types (dismissing and fearful) are consistent with the hypothesis that the two styles are similar in their avoidance of intimacy, but differ in their need for others' acceptance and approval (Bartholomew & Horowitz, 1991).

Other studies examining associations between attachment characteristics and self-reported support/caregiving within the relationship corroborated these findings (Carnelley, Pietromonaco, & Jaffe, 1996; Feeney, 1996; Feeney & Collins, 2001). Taken together, the results of these studies indicate that secure individuals have the most favorable caregiving style (high responsiveness and lack of compulsive caregiving), whereas fearful individuals have the least favorable style (low responsiveness and high compulsive caregiving). Anxious–preoccupied individuals seem to have a mixed caregiving style to the extent that they provide warm physical contact (although in the absence of sensitivity and cooperation) but also engage in compulsive caregiving. It seems that despite their desire for intimacy and closeness, anxious–preoccupied individuals may be too wrapped up in their own relationship concerns to provide their partners with consistently sensitive and responsive care. It is also likely that anxiety over possible relationship loss (characteristic of preoccupied and fearful individuals) may lead to self-sacrifice and feelings of underappreciation—a compulsive caregiving style (Feeney, 1996; Hazan & Shaver, 1990). Dismissing avoidant individuals appear to be unresponsive, controlling, and the least engaged in any sort of caregiving activity.

Attachment style has also been predictive of support-giving behavior exhibited during observational studies. Results of the Simpson and colleagues (1992) study described earlier (in which the female members of romantic couples were told that they would be participating in an activity known to elicit anxiety in people) indicated that among more secure men, higher levels of partner anxiety were associated with greater support efforts. In contrast, among more avoidant men, higher levels of partner anxiety were associated with lower levels of support. In other words, more secure men offered more support (comfort and reassurance) as their partners displayed greater anxiety, and avoidant men offered less support as their partners displayed greater anxiety. Similar results were obtained in the study involving observations of couples separating at an airport: Avoidant individuals exhibited less caregiving behavior (e.g., reassurance, embracing) toward their partner during the separations (Fraley & Shaver, 1998). In both of these studies, no significant effects emerged for individuals who had a more anxious attachment style.

It is important to note that, similar to the results for support-seeking behavior, avoidance was associated with lower levels of support only when the potential recipient of support was distressed. Simpson and colleagues (1992) found that when their female partners displayed lower levels of stress, avoidant men actually provided *more* support than did secure men. However, as their partner's level of distress increased, securely attached men offered greater reassurance and emotional support, and they made more supportive comments. An observational study in which partner distress was experimentally manipulated confirmed this behavioral pattern (Feeney & Collins, 2001). In this study, couple members were given an opportunity to write a note to a partner they believed to be experiencing either a great deal of distress about giving a speech (high need condition) or very little distress about giving the speech (low need condition). Results indicated that avoidant individuals provided the least support when their partner needed it the most: In the high need condition, when support providers were clearly aware that their partners were distressed, higher levels of avoidance were associated with less support provision. However, in the low need condition, when support providers were led to believe that their partner was not distressed, avoidance was associated with increased support provision. Thus avoidant individuals cannot be characterized as uniformly neglecting, cold, distant, or aloof. They seem to behave in this manner primarily when their partner experiences higher levels of distress. Expressions of distress appear to impede the establishment of proximity in dyadic interactions involving avoidant individuals, both when distress is experienced directly (as experienced by the female participants in this study) and when it is experienced vicariously (as experienced by the male partners in this study). Simpson et al. concluded that distressed adult partners, as well as distressed infants (Belsky, Rovine, & Taylor, 1984; cited in Simpson et al., 1992), present significant relationship problems for avoidant individuals. These results are consistent with literature showing that mothers of avoidant infants, who tend to be avoidant themselves, withdraw from interaction when their infant is distressed but engage in interaction when their infant is content (Escher-Graub & Grossman, 1983, cited in Cassidy, 2001), and with research indicating that avoidant individuals appear to actively dismiss or devalue attachment needs and expressions of distress—an affect regulation strategy that may function to deactivate one's own attachment/caregiving system (Cassidy, 1994; Feeney & Collins, 2001; Fraley, Davis, & Shaver, 1998; Fraley, Garner, & Shaver, 2000; George & Solomon, 1999; Simpson et al., 1992).

Anxious attachment has also been predictive of support behavior in observational studies. Results of the observational study in which couples were videotaped as they discussed a current stressor showed that attachment anxiety was associated with less instrumental support provision, less responsiveness, and more negative support behaviors such as blaming the partner and dismissing the problem (Collins & Feeney, 2000). Interestingly, anxious individuals were able to provide relatively high levels of support when their partner's needs were clear and direct, but they provided much lower levels of support when their partner's needs were less clear. In contrast, secure individuals provided relatively high levels of support regardless of the clarity and directness of their partner's support-seeking efforts. The fact that anxious adults were able to provide effective support when their partner's needs were clear suggests that they have the skills needed to be responsive support providers, but they may lack the motivational or attentional resources to do so consistently (Collins & Feeney, 2000).

A study in which recipient distress and thus need for support was experimentally manipulated also indicated that anxious individuals are not uniformly poor support providers. Attachment-related anxiety was associated with (1) high levels of emotional support provision in both high- and low-need conditions and (2) higher levels of instrumental support provision in the high-need condition, the condition in which the partner presumably needed support the most, than in the low-need condition (Feeney & Collins, 2001). The fact that anxious individuals provided emotional support regardless of their partner's degree of distress reflects their tendency to be overinvolved caregivers. However, the fact that they provided more instrumental support in the high-need condition and less in the low-need condition suggests that at least some aspects of their support behavior were appropriately contingent on their partner's needs. These results are compatible with work in the infant attachment literature indicating that mothers of anxious children (who are often classified as preoccupied with attachment) tend to interfere with infant exploration in an effort to keep their children close to them (see Cassidy & Berlin, 1994, for a review) and they tend to overinterpret attachment cues and engage in caregiving behaviors that promote dependency (George & Solomon, 1996, 1999).

Studies conducted with the goal of identifying the underlying mechanisms that explain attachment style differences in support behavior provide additional insight into the associations reviewed above (Feeney & Collins, 2001, 2003). The purpose of these investigations was to go beyond the mere documentation of patterns of support behavior to identify the mechanisms that may help explain these patterns. Because effective support provision (i.e., sensitively responding to needs as they arise) is likely to require a variety of skills, motives, and resources that individuals are likely to possess to varying degrees, these variables were examined as potential mediators of the links between attachment and support provision. Results of this research suggest that avoidant adults may be unresponsive and controlling support providers at least partly because they lack knowledge about how to support others, they lack a prosocial orientation toward others (i.e., they lack empathic abilities and a communal orientation toward their relationship partner), and they fail to develop the deep sense of relationship closeness, commitment, interdependence, and trust that appears to be critical for the motivation of responsive support (Feeney & Collins, 2001). Avoidant adults also seem to be poor support providers because their underlying motives for helping their partners are relatives egoistic ones: Avoidant attachment is positively associated with selfish and obligation motives for helping one's partner (e.g., helping to get something in return, helping to avoid negative consequences) and negatively associated with motives involving feelings of love and concern for one's partner and feelings of enjoyment from helping (Feeney & Collins, 2003). Avoidant individuals also report motivations for *not* supporting their relationship partners including lack of skills, dislike of distress, lack of concern for the partner, dislike of helping a difficult partner, and dislike of partner dependence. Thus avoidant individuals appear to lack both the requisite skills and the motivation to be responsive and effective support providers.

Anxious individuals, on the other hand, appear to be compulsive, controlling, and inconsistently responsive support providers at least partly because they feel close, committed, and interdependent with their partners while simultaneously distrusting their partners and being selfishly motivated in their support attempts (Feeney & Collins, 2001). Anxious attachment is positively associated both with relatively altruistic motives for supporting one's partner including feelings of love/concern for one's partner and enjoyment of helping, and with relatively egoistic motives for supporting one's partner including a desire for self-benefit, a desire to achieve one's own relationship goals, and feelings of obligation (Feeney & Collins, 2003). This suggests that the lack of a consistent link between anxious attachment and responsive support provision may be due to the particular mediating force (selfish motives or feelings of concern for the partner's well-being) that takes precedence in a given situation. Anxious individuals do appear to possess some of the requisite skills and motives for being effective support providers; however, other conflicting motives may cause them to care for their partners in a compulsive, controlling, and inconsistent manner.

Taken together, the studies reviewed above provide evidence that responsive support provision is facilitated by attachment security and hindered by attachment insecurity. Recent work by Mikulincer and Shaver (2005) has provided impressive evidence that even experimentally induced attachment security (in addition to dispositional attachment security) produces compassionate feelings, values, and behavior as manifested in a greater willingness to volunteer and help others. These findings suggest that knowledge of attachment dynamics may be useful in promoting responsive support/helping behavior not only among close relationship partners, but also in a number of other real-world contexts.

Interpersonal Perception

Previous research in social cognition suggests that people are not simply passive recipients of environmental stimuli; instead, they are active participants in the construction of their own reality (Fiske & Taylor, 1991). Because social perception is heavily influenced by top-down, theory-driven processes in which existing goals, schemas, and expectations shape the way people view new information, working models of attachment (which include relationship schemas and expectations) should have a significant influence on perceptions of interpersonal behaviors. In fact, working models of attachment relationships could be thought of as social support schemas because they include information about the self and about significant others with regard to the giving and receipt of social support in stressful situations. Therefore, these models should guide interpretation of, and memory for, support-relevant behaviors and events (Lakey & Cassady, 1990).

Several studies have been conducted in an effort to examine distressed individuals' perceptions of specific support behaviors. Researchers (e.g., Fincham & Bradbury, 1990; Pierce, Baldwin, & Lydon, 1997) have proposed that the evaluation of an individual's supportiveness is likely to be influenced both by characteristics of the perceiver (e.g., the attachment style of the distressed individual) and by that which is available to be perceived (i.e., objective features of the situation, such as actual support behavior). Internal working models are likely to influence the interpretation of significant others' potentially supportive behaviors because people tend to interpret behaviors in ways consistent with their expectations (e.g., Collins & Feeney, 2000, 2004; Feeney & Cassidy, 2003; Lakey, Moineau, & Drew, 1992; Lakey, Tardiff, & Drew, 1994; Pierce, Sarason, & Sarason, 1992). Therefore, social support expectancies may be maintained through attributional patterns (Bradbury & Fincham, 1990; Fletcher & Fincham, 1991; Murray & Holmes, 1993; Murray, Holmes, & Griffin, 1996). For example, if a distressed individual expects that support is generally available from a significant other, then any positive behavior from that person is likely to be attributed to internal, global, and stable factors, and seen as helpful and supportive. However, if the distressed individual does not expect his or her partner to be supportive, then any supportive attempts by the partner might be discredited by attributions to external, unstable, and specific factors (Pierce et al., 1997). Therefore, working models of attachment may foster an attributional style that confirms and strengthens these preexisting models.

Drawing on the cognition in marriage literature, Fincham and Bradbury (1990) have emphasized the importance of attributions or explanations for understanding perceptions of support. They argue that understanding why a particular support behavior occurred is a critical determinant not only of its immediate impact, but also of expectations concerning future support. In particular, they argue that whether a partner's support behavior is viewed as voluntary and selflessly motivated is a critical determinant of whether the behavior is perceived as supportive. These researchers propose that supportive acts are maximally supportive when they are viewed as voluntary behaviors intended solely to benefit the person in need of support. Therefore, support behaviors will be viewed as less supportive to the extent that attributional processing results in the suspicion that the behavior is not entirely voluntary or reflects an ulterior motive. It is also important to remember that individuals in close relationships are *expected* to be responsive to one another's needs (e.g., Mills & Clark, 1994; Williamson, Clark, Pegalis, & Behan, 1996). Therefore, support seekers who are forced to expressly request support (as opposed to receiving instinctive support from the partner) may interpret their partner's support behavior more negatively than if it had been offered spontaneously (Cutrona, Cohen, & Igram, 1990; Dunkel-Schetter, Folkman, & Lazarus, 1987; Pierce et al., 1997).

Fincham and Bradbury (1990) further propose that relevant information most accessible in memory, or most salient at the time the judgment of social support is made, is likely to influence judgments of support. Increased accessibility of a concept can result from external primes, as well as from internal stimuli that are not prompted by external events, such as negative thoughts or beliefs. Such internal stimuli can make a concept "chronically accessible" and serve to maintain perceptions of lack of support despite the occurrence of supportive behaviors by the partner. Working models of attachment relationships are chronically accessible internal primes that may serve to maintain preexisting perceptions of support such that all support behaviors may be viewed in a predetermined positive or negative light.

Individual Differences in General Perceptions of Support

Several recent studies have revealed links between attachment style and general perceptions of available social support (e.g., Blain, Thompson, & Whiffen, 1993; Florian et al., 1995; Kobak & Sceery, 1988; Ognibene & Collins, 1998; Priel & Shamai, 1995; Wallace & Vaux, 1993). Using self-report questionnaire measures, these studies have generally shown that individuals with secure attachment characteristics perceive that more social support is available to them (i.e., they are more likely to hold positive support appraisals) than individuals with insecure attachment characteristics. For example, Wallace and Vaux (1993) found that secure individuals were less negatively oriented toward their support networks than were either avoidant or anxious individuals. In contrast, adults with an insecure attachment style were more likely to endorse beliefs and expectations reflecting the risks, costs, and futility of seeking help from network members. Other researchers have shown that the attachment groups differ in their perceptions of support availability regardless of the particular type of support being considered (e.g., emotional vs. instrumental) and regardless of the identity of the support provider (e.g., mother, father, romantic partner, same-sex friend, opposite-sex friend; Florian et al., 1995). Secure individuals report having more social support available to them in all the categories assessed than insecure people.

Individual Differences in Perceptions of Specific Support Behaviors

Several researchers have examined the ways in which general perceptions of social support influence the evaluation and recall of ambiguous and non-ambiguous support behaviors (Lakey & Cassady, 1990; Lakey et al., 1992; Mankowski & Wyer, 1996; Pierce et al., 1992). In one study, individuals high and low in perceived social support imagined describing a personal or academic problem to a friend or relative (Lakey & Cassady, 1990). Each scenario was accompanied by descriptions of hypothetical supportive behaviors provided by the friend or relative; these behaviors were ambiguous (they were neither clearly supportive nor clearly nonsupportive) to allow for greater latitude in individual interpretation. After reading each scenario, participants rated the degree to which they viewed each supportive behavior as helpful; then, after they completed a distractor task, they were given the paragraph describing the hypothetical stressful situation again, and were asked to recall as many of the previously rated supportive behaviors as they could. Results revealed that individuals low in perceived available support (which is most characteristic of insecure individuals) exhibited a bias toward perceiving supportive attempts as unhelpful, as well as a bias toward recalling fewer instances of helpful/supportive behavior.

A similar study that presented all participants with exactly the same support stimuli (standardized support behaviors) yielded similar results (Lakey et al., 1992). Specifically, participants watched a videotape on which several problem situations were presented. Each problem scenario was followed by a scene in which an ambiguous support behavior was provided by a stranger in response to the problem. Consistent with the findings of Lakey and Cassady (1990), individuals high in perceived available support interpreted the ambiguously supportive behaviors as more helpful than did individuals low in perceived available support. However, in contrast to prior findings, individuals high in perceived available support demonstrated better memory for negatively perceived, but not for positively perceived, support behaviors. The speculation is that these individuals may have better memory for support-*relevant* behaviors, regardless of whether the behaviors are schema-consistent or schema-inconsistent. However, the fact that these individuals did not demonstrate superior recall for both positive and negative support-related behaviors in the same study points to a need for future research that explores the precise conditions under which individuals will be most likely to recall schema-consistent versus schema-inconsistent information.

A study examining the effects of general perceptions of available support on judgments and recall of both ambiguous and unambiguous support behaviors revealed that (1) when considering *ambiguous* support behavior from the perspective of the recipient, participants judged the specific support behavior as being less supportive if their standard of comparison was high (if they had high perceptions of available support) than if it was low (if they had low perceptions of available support), and (2) when considering *unambiguous* behaviors from the recipient's perspective, participants' general perceptions of support availability were unrelated to their judgments (Mankowski & Wyer, 1996). In addition, participants taking the recipient's perspective recalled more rejecting than supportive behaviors overall; however, consistent with the recall findings of Lakey and colleagues (1992), this difference was more pronounced when their level of perceived support availability was high than when it was low. Although this study did not resolve the discrepant findings reported above, it did reveal another interesting piece of information: participants' judgments of the support provider were *not* related to their recall of the support provider's specific support behaviors. This finding suggests that participants based their judgments on some more general concept around which they organized the behaviors—which could be their working models of attachment relationships or social support schemas.

Pierce and colleagues (1992) also conducted a study in order to investigate the effects of (1) general expectations for support, (2) relationship-specific expectations for support and conflict, and (3) situational stress on the extent to which standardized support notes from a close other are perceived to be supportive. Students were assigned to either a high-stress speech condition or a low-stress speech condition, during which their mothers provided a standardized amount of social support through the use of handwritten notes. Before the speech, mothers were asked to copy a note that read "Don't worry—just say how you feel and what you think and you'll do just fine." Then, after the speech, mothers copied a note that read "I liked your speech. That's a tricky topic to spend a whole lot of time on, and you covered it well." Although these notes were clearly supportive, students who expected high levels of social support from their mothers (relationship-specific expectations for support) perceived the prespeech note and postspeech note (in the high-stress condition) as more supportive than did other students. Contrary to predictions, however, general expectations for support appeared to have no impact on perceived supportiveness of the notes after controlling for relationship-specific expectations.

Taken together, the results of these studies suggest that individuals' a priori beliefs about the social support available to them affect their evaluation and recall of new support information. However, future research is needed to determine the mechanisms that underlie the maintenance of these beliefs in light of that information. It is likely that relatively stable internal working models of attachment relationships are responsible for guiding the judgments and recall of the support behaviors reported here; however, we still know very little about the specific conditions under which these working models will be modified in light of contradictory information. Next, research examining the ways in which working models of attachment influence perceptions of specific support behaviors is reviewed.

Attachment Differences in Perceptions of Specific Support Behaviors

Before describing research specific to perceptions of support behaviors, it is important to note that attachment researchers also have examined the ways in which working models of attachment bias the construal of relationship events more generally. One recent investigation provided empirical support for attachment theory's proposition that working models of attachment influence the processing of new social information (Feeney & Cassidy, 2003). In this study, adolescents participated in laboratory conflict interactions with each of their parents and rated their perceptions of the interactions both immediately after the discussions and 6 weeks later. Consistent with theory, results indicated that adolescents' immediate perceptions of the interactions were influenced by their attachment-related representations of their parents (secure representations predicted more positive perceptions), and adolescents' perceptions, over the 6-week period, shifted such that their later perceptions were even more congruent with their attachment-related representations than were their immediate perceptions.

Researchers also have shown that adults with different attachment styles explain and interpret potentially negative attachment-relevant events (e.g., your partner didn't respond when you tried to cuddle; your partner didn't comfort you when you were feeling down) in ways consistent with their beliefs and expectations about themselves and others (Collins, 1996; Collins, Ford, Guichard, & Allard, in press). In these studies, young adults were presented with a series of hypothetical relationship events and asked to provide attributions for their partner's behavior. Individuals high in attachment-related anxiety provided more negative interpretations for their partner's behavior—explanations reflecting a low sense of perceived self-worth and a view of the partner as being generally unresponsive to their needs. They responded to hypothetical partner transgressions by endorsing relationship-threatening attributions, experiencing emotional distress, and endorsing behavioral intentions that were likely to result in conflict. Secure adults, however, provided more positive explanations for the potentially negative relationship events—construing events in ways that minimized their negative impact on the relationship. Individuals high in attachment-related avoidance endorsed pessimistic attributions for their partner's positive behavior, but they were less pessimistic in their explanations for their partner's transgressions and did not report emotional distress.

In a recent experimental study using a design similar to that of Pierce and colleagues (1992), Collins and Feeney (2004) experimentally induced stress in one member of a romantic couple by having him or her perform a speech task that would be videotaped and watched by his or her partner. Immediately after giving couples the speech instructions (which were designed to induce stress), the experimenter left the room and unobtrusively videotaped the couple's spontaneous interaction. Then, in order to examine individual differences in perceptions of support behaviors, romantic partners copied in their own handwriting standardized support notes that were delivered to the speech giver both before and after the speech. Partners were randomly assigned to either a high-support condition in which they copied two objectively supportive notes (e.g., "Don't worry—just say what you think and how you feel and you'll do great." and "I liked your speech. That was a hard thing to do and you did a really good job.") or a low-support condition in which they copied two relatively unsupportive notes ("Try not to say anything too embarrassing—especially since so many people will be watching your speech." and "Your speech was a little hard to follow, but I guess you did the best you could under the circumstances."). The recipients rated their perceptions of the supportiveness of these notes, as well as their perceptions of the prior interaction with their partner. Results indicated that insecure participants (anxious and avoidant) who received low-support messages appraised these messages more negatively, misremembered a prior behavioral interaction with their partner as having been less supportive, and performed significantly worse at their task compared with secure participants. A follow-up study in which partners were permitted to send genuine support messages confirmed the finding that insecure participants perceived their partners' messages as less supportive, even after controlling for independent ratings of the messages.

Taken together, these studies indicate that working models of attachment influence social construal processes in general and predict differences in perceptions of social support in particular. Relative to secure adults, insecure adults appear to be predisposed to perceive their partners as less helpful and less well intentioned. However, these biased construal effects appear to occur primarily when the behavior being interpreted is ambiguous, negative, or open to subjective interpretation. Thus insecure working models appear to be a cognitive liability when ambiguous or negative relational events activate doubts or vulnerabilities.

It is important to mention, however, that the studies reviewed above do not definitively answer the question of whether insecure individuals and individuals with low perceived support underestimate the actual level of support that is available to them—or whether secure individuals and individuals with high perceived support are overly optimistic about their social resources. Sarason and colleagues (1991) have shown that low perceived support students (compared to high perceived support students) reported less positive estimates of the perceived support of the "typical" student, but that high perceived support students' estimates more closely matched the actual mean scores of students—suggesting that low perceived support individuals tend to underestimate the level of support available to them. In addition, Collins and

Feeney (2004) showed that insecure participants misremembered an earlier interaction as being unsupportive after experiencing an intervening negative event when it really had not been (based on the ratings of objective observers). Nonetheless, additional research is needed in this regard because there is also ample evidence indicating that people exhibit positive biases/illusions when evaluating their relationship partners (Murray & Holmes, 1993; Murray et al., 1996).

COMING FULL CIRCLE: INTERPERSONAL PROCESSES INFLUENCING INTRAPERSONAL CHARACTERISTICS

In this chapter, attachment theory's propositions regarding the influence of interpersonal processes on the development of working models of attachment were reviewed, as well as research showing that these personality characteristics influence subsequent interpersonal processes. The interpersonal processes highlighted in this chapter were interpersonal social support processes. Taken as a whole, the existing research provides compelling evidence that individual differences in attachment characteristics play an important role in shaping interpersonal behaviors and perceptions.

It is important to at least briefly mention, however, that these interpersonal processes, which are shaped to some extent by attachment models as reviewed above, are presumed to subsequently influence intrapersonal functioning. One example involves the influence of interpersonal dynamics centering on the support of relationship partners' goal strivings and exploration (secure base support provision) on a variety of personal outcomes (Feeney, 2004; Feeney & Collins, 2004; Ruehlman & Wolchik, 1988). A study examining the influence of support dynamics both during couples' discussions of personal goal strivings and during a laboratory exploration activity indicated that the responsive (nonintrusive) support of a relationship partner's goal strivings and explorations have important implications for the recipient's happiness, self-esteem, and perceived likelihood of achieving specific goals (Feeney, 2004). Other related work has provided evidence for the influence of interpersonal support and hindrance of personal goals on an individual's psychological distress and well-being (Ruehlman & Wolchik, 1988).

In addition, although it is beyond the scope of this chapter to review, a massive literature indicates that social support is associated with better mental and physical health outcomes (e.g., Cohen, 1988; Cohen & Syme, 1985; Cohen & Wills, 1985; Reis & Franks, 1994; Vaux, 1988). This literature generally indicates that people with satisfying levels of support are healthier both psychologically and physically, they recover from illness more quickly, and they seem to be better adjusted both personally and socially (see Sarason,

Sarason, & Gurung, 1997, for a review). Although the perceived availability of social support (as opposed to actual support received) has been most consistently and strongly associated with various health outcomes (Cohen & Wills, 1985; Wethington & Kessler, 1986), both support perceptions and support behaviors have been shown to be influenced to some extent by working models of attachment.

It is also interesting to note that attachment characteristics have been associated with a variety of personal adjustment variables, and these links are likely to be mediated by important interpersonal dynamics. For example, individuals with secure attachment characteristics are better adjusted than individuals with insecure attachment characteristics both personally and socially (Kobak & Sceery, 1988; Priel & Shamai, 1995). Specifically, secure individuals report fewer symptoms of psychological distress and higher social competence than insecure individuals. Based on the literature reviewed above, it is likely that secure individuals are so well adjusted because they are involved in intimate relationships that engender the social support behaviors and perceptions that have been shown to be predictive of personal and relationship well-being.

CONCLUDING STATEMENT

As the above review indicates, attachment theory provides an important theoretical framework for considering the dynamic interplay between personal and interpersonal processes. Attachment theory is unique in its ability to provide a lifespan perspective on the ways in which complex personal and interpersonal processes are likely to influence one another. The richness of this theory is evident in both the breadth and depth of its postulates regarding (1) the role that relationships play in certain aspects of personality development, (2) the influence of these specific personality characteristics (attachment styles) on subsequent relationship functioning, and (3) the continual influence of relationships on various aspects of personal functioning throughout the lifespan. Although an abundance of evidence for attachment theory's postulates has already accumulated, many other important propositions remain untested, and much remains to be discovered about the interplay between personal and relationship processes in adulthood. It is inevitable that attachment theory will continue to play a major role in illuminating the importance of relationships for optimal human functioning.

ACKNOWLEDGMENTS

Preparation of this chapter was supported by National Institute of Mental Health Grant No. MH-066119 and National Science Foundation Grant No. BCS-0424579.

REFERENCES

Ainsworth, M. D. (1982). Attachment: Retrospect and prospect. In C. M. Parkes & J. Stevenson-Hinde (Eds.), *The place of attachment in human behavior* (pp. 3–30). New York: Basic Books.

Ainsworth, M. D., Blehar, M. C., Waters, E., & Wall, S. (1978). *Patterns of attachment: Psychological study of the Strange Situation*. Hillsdale, NJ: Erlbaum.

Armsden, G. C., & Greenberg, M. T. (1987). The Inventory of Parent and Peer Attachment: Individual differences and their relationship to psychological well-being in adolescence. *Journal of Youth and Adolescence, 16*, 427–455.

Baldwin, M. W. (1992). Relational schemas and the processing of social information. *Journal of Personality and Social Psychology, 112*, 461–484.

Baldwin, M. W., Keelan, J. P., Fehr, B., Enns, V., & Koh-Rangarajoo, E. (1996). Social-cognitive conceptualization of attachment working models: Availability and accessibility effects. *Journal of Personality and Social Psychology, 71*, 94–109.

Bartholomew, K., & Horowitz, L. M. (1991). Attachment styles among young adults: A test of a four-category model. *Journal of Personality and Social Psychology, 61*, 226–244.

Belsky, J., Rovine, M., & Taylor, D. G. (1984). The Pennsylvania Infant and Family Development Project: III. The origins of individual differences in infant–mother attachment: Maternal and infant contributions. *Child Development, 55*, 718–728.

Blain, M. D., Thompson, J. M., & Whiffen, V. E. (1993). Attachment and perceived social support in late adolescence: The interaction between working models of self and others. *Journal of Adolescent Research, 8*, 226–241.

Bowlby, J. (1969/1982). *Attachment and loss: Vol. 1. Attachment*. New York: Basic Books.

Bowlby, J. (1973). *Attachment and loss: Vol. 2. Separation, anxiety and anger*. New York: Basic Books.

Bowlby, J. (1980). *Attachment and loss: Vol. 3. Sadness and depression*. New York: Basic Books.

Bowlby, J. (1988). *A secure base*. New York: Basic Books.

Bradbury, T. N., & Fincham, F. D. (1990). Attribution in marriage: Review and critique. *Psychological Bulletin, 107*, 3–33.

Bradbury, T. N., & Fincham, F. D. (1992). Attributions and behavior in marital interaction. *Journal of Personality and Social Psychology, 63*, 613–628.

Bretherton, I. (1985). Attachment theory: Retrospect and prospect. *Monographs of the Society for Research in Child Development, 50*(1–2), 3–35.

Carnelley, K. B., Pietromonaco, P. R., & Jaffe, K. (1996). Attachment, caregiving, and relationship functioning in couples: Effects of self and partner. *Personal Relationships, 3*, 257–278.

Cassidy, J. (1994). Emotion regulation: Influences of attachment relationships. *Monographs of the Society for Research in Child Development, 59*(2–3), 228–283.

Cassidy, J. (2001). Truth, lies, and intimacy: An attachment perspective. *Attachment and Human Development, 3*, 121–155.

Cassidy, J., & Berlin, L. J. (1994). The insecure/ambivalent pattern of attachment: Theory and research. *Child Development, 65*, 971–991.

Cohen, S. (1988). Psychosocial models of the role of social support in the etiology of physical disease. *Health Psychology, 7,* 269–297.

Cohen, S., & Syme, S. L. (1985). *Social support and health.* San Diego, CA: Academic Press.

Cohen, S., & Wills, T. A. (1985). Stress, social support, and the buffering hypothesis. *Psychological Bulletin, 98,* 310–357.

Collins, N. L. (1996). Working models of attachment: Implications for explanation, emotion, and behavior. *Journal of Personality and Social Psychology, 71,* 810–832.

Collins, N. L., & Feeney, B. C. (2000). A safe haven: An attachment theory perspective on support-seeking and caregiving in adult romantic relationships. *Journal of Personality and Social Psychology, 78,* 1053–1073.

Collins, N. L., & Feeney, B. C. (2004). Working models of attachment shape perceptions of social support: Evidence from experimental and observational studies. *Journal of Personality and Social Psychology, 87,* 363–383.

Collins, N. L., Ford, M. B., Guichard, A. C., & Allard, L. M. (in press). Working models of attachment and attribution processes in intimate relationships. *Personality and Social Psychology Bulletin.*

Collins, N. L., Guichard, A. C., Ford, M. B., & Feeney, B. C. (2004). Working models of attachment: New developments and emerging themes. In W. S. Rholes & J. A. Simpson (Eds.), *Adult attachment: Theory, research, and clinical implications* (pp. 196–239). New York: Guilford Press.

Collins, N. L., & Read, S. J. (1990). Adult attachment, working models, and relationship quality in dating couples. *Journal of Personality and Social Psychology, 58,* 644–663.

Collins, N. L., & Read, S. J. (1994). Cognitive representations of adult attachment: The structure and function of working models. In K. Bartholomew & D. Perlman (Eds.), *Advances in personal relationships: Vol. 5. Attachment processes in adulthood* (pp. 53–90). London: Jessica Kingsley.

Cutrona, C. E., Cohen, B. B., & Igram, S. (1990). Contextual determinants of the perceived supportiveness of helping behaviors. *Journal of Social and Personal Relationships, 7,* 553–562.

DeFronzo, R., Panzarella, C., & Butler, A. C. (2001). Attachment, support seeking, and adaptive inferential feedback: Implications for psychological health. *Cognitive and Behavioral Practice, 8,* 48–52.

Dunkel-Schetter, C., Folkman, S., & Lazarus, R. (1987). Correlates of social support receipt. *Journal of Personality and Social Psychology, 53,* 71–80.

Feeney, B. C. (2004). A secure base: Responsive support of goal strivings and exploration in adult intimate relationships. *Journal of Personality and Social Psychology, 87,* 631–648.

Feeney, B. C., & Cassidy, J. A. (2003). Reconstructive memory related to adolescent–parent conflict interactions: The influence of attachment-related representations on immediate perceptions and changes in perceptions over time. *Journal of Personality and Social Psychology, 85,* 945–955.

Feeney, B. C., & Collins, N. L. (2001). Predictors of caregiving in adult intimate relationships: An attachment theoretical perspective. *Journal of Personality and Social Psychology, 80,* 972–994.

Feeney, B. C., & Collins, N. C. (2003). Motivations for caregiving in adult intimate relationships: Influences on caregiving behavior and relationship functioning. *Personality and Social Psychology Bulletin, 29*, 950–968.

Feeney, B. C., & Collins, N. L. (2004). Interpersonal safe haven and secure base caregiving processes in adulthood. In W. S. Rholes & J. A. Simpson (Eds.), *Adult attachment: Theory, research, and clinical implications* (pp. 300–338). New York: Guilford Press.

Feeney, B. C., Ramos-Marcuse, F., & Cassidy, J. (2005). *Support-seeking and support-provision in adolescence: Interactional dynamics and individual differences.* Unpublished manuscript.

Feeney, J. A. (1996). Attachment, caregiving, and marital satisfaction. *Personal Relationships, 3*, 401–416.

Fincham, F. D., & Bradbury, T. N. (1990). Social support in marriage: The role of social cognition. *Journal of Social and Clinical Psychology, 9*, 31–42.

Fiske, S. T., & Taylor, S. E. (1991). *Social cognition.* New York: McGraw-Hill.

Fletcher, G., & Fincham, F. D. (1991). Attribution processes in close relationships. In G. J. O. Fletcher & F. D. Fincham (Eds.), *Cognition in close relationships* (pp. 7–35). Hillsdale, NJ: Erlbaum.

Florian, V., Mikulincer, M., & Bucholtz, I. (1995). Effects of adult attachment style on the perception and search for social support. *Journal of Psychology, 129*, 665–676.

Fraley, R. C., Davis, K. E., & Shaver, P. R. (1998). Dismissing-avoidance and the defensive organization of emotion, cognition, and behavior. In J. A. Simpson & W. S. Rholes (Eds.), *Attachment theory and close relationships* (pp. 249–279). New York: Guilford Press.

Fraley, R. C., Garner, J. P., & Shaver, P. R. (2000). Adult attachment and the defensive regulation of attention and memory: Examining the role of preemptive and postemptive defensive processes. *Journal of Personality and Social Psychology, 79*, 816–826.

Fraley, R. C., & Shaver, P. R. (1998). Airport separations: A naturalistic study of adult attachment dynamics in separating couples. *Journal of Personality and Social Psychology, 75*, 1198–1212.

George, C., & Solomon, J. (1996). Representational models of relationships: Links between caregiving and attachment. *Infant Mental Health Journal, 17*, 198–216.

George, C., & Solomon, J. (1999). Attachment and caregiving: The caregiving behavioral system. In J. Cassidy & P. R. Shaver (Eds.), *Handbook of attachment: Theory, research, and clinical applications* (pp. 649–670). New York: Guilford Press.

Greenberger, E., & McLaughlin, C. S. (1998). Attachment, coping, and explanatory style in late adolescence. *Journal of Youth and Adolescence, 27*, 121–139.

Hazan, C., & Shaver, P. R. (1990). Love and work: An attachment-theoretical perspective. *Journal of Personality and Social Psychology, 59*, 270–280.

Kobak, R. R., & Sceery, A. (1988). Attachment in late adolescence: Working models, affect regulation, and perception of self and others. *Child Development, 59*, 135–146.

Kunce, L. J., & Shaver, P. R. (1994). An attachment-theoretical approach to caregiving in romantic relationships. In K. Bartholomew & D. Perlman (Eds.), *Advances in personal relationships* (Vol. 5, pp. 205–237). London: Jessica Kingsley.

Lakey, B., & Cassady, P. (1990). Cognitive processes in perceived social support. *Journal of Personality and Social Psychology, 59*, 337–343.

Lakey, B., Moineau, S., & Drew, J. B. (1992). Perceived social support and individual differences in the interpretation and recall of supportive behaviors. *Journal of Social and Clinical Psychology, 11*, 336–348.

Lakey, B., Tardiff, T. A., & Drew, J. B. (1994). Negative social interactions: Assessment and relations to social support, cognition, and psychological distress. *Journal of Social and Clinical Psychology, 13*, 42–62.

Larose, S., Boivin, M., & Doyle, A. B. (2001). Parental representations and attachment style as predictors of support-seeking behaviors and perceptions of support in an academic counseling relationship. *Personal Relationships, 8*, 93–113.

Main, M., Kaplan, N., & Cassidy, J. (1985). Security in infancy, childhood, and adulthood: A move to the level of representation. *Monographs of the Society for Research in Child Development, 50*(1–2), 66–104.

Mankowski, E. S., & Wyer, R. S. Jr. (1996). Cognitive processes in perceptions of social support. *Personality and Social Psychology Bulletin, 22*, 894–905.

Marvin, R., Cooper, G., Hoffman, K., & Powell, B. (2002). The Circle of Security Project: Attachment-based intervention with caregiver–preschool child dyads. *Attachment and Human Development, 4*, 107–124.

Mikulincer, M., & Florian, V. (1995). Appraisal of and coping with a real-life stressful situation: The contribution of attachment styles. *Personality and Social Psychology Bulletin, 21*, 406–414.

Mikulincer, M., Florian, V., & Weller, A. (1993). Attachment styles, coping strategies, and posttraumatic psychological distress: The impact of the Gulf War in Israel. *Journal of Personality and Social Psychology, 64*, 817–826.

Mikulincer, M., Gillath, O., & Shaver, P. R. (2002). Activation of the attachment system in adulthood: Threat-related primes increase the accessibility of mental representations of attachment figures. *Journal of Personality and Social Psychology, 83*, 881–895.

Mikulincer, M., & Shaver, P. R. (2005). Attachment security, compassion, and altruism. *Current Directions in Psychological Science, 14*, 34–38.

Mills, J., & Clark, M. S. (1994). Communal and exchange relationships: Controversies and research. In R. Eber & R. Gilmour (Eds.), *Theoretical frameworks for personal relationships* (pp. 29–42). Hillsdale, NJ: Erlbaum.

Murray, S. L., & Holmes, J. G. (1993). Seeing virtues in faults: Negativity and the transformation of interpersonal narratives in close relationships. *Journal of Personality and Social Psychology, 65*, 707–722.

Murray, S. L., Holmes, J. G., & Griffin, D. W. (1996). The benefits of positive illusions: Idealization and the construction of satisfaction in close relationships. *Journal of Personality and Social Psychology, 70*, 79–98.

Ognibene, T. C., & Collins, N. L. (1998). Adult attachment styles, perceived social support and coping strategies. *Journal of Social and Personal Relationships, 15*, 323–345.

Pierce, G. R., Baldwin, M. W., & Lydon, J. E. (1997). A relational schema approach to social support. In G. R. Pierce, B. Lakey, I. G. Sarason, & B. R. Sarason (Eds.), *Sourcebook of social support and personality* (pp. 19–47). New York: Plenum Press.

Pierce, G. R., Sarason, B. R., & Sarason, I. G. (1992). General and specific support expectations and stress as predictors of perceived supportiveness: An experimental study. *Journal of Personality and Social Psychology, 63*, 297–307.

Pierce, T., & Lydon, J. (1998). Priming relational schemas: Effects of contextually activated and chronically accessible interpersonal expectations on responses to a stressful event. *Journal of Personality and Social Psychology, 75*, 1441–1448.

Priel, B., & Shamai, D. (1995). Attachment style and perceived social support: Effects on affect regulation. *Personality and Individual Differences, 19*, 235–241.

Reis, H. T., & Franks, P. (1994). The role of intimacy and social support in health outcomes: Two processes or one? *Personal Relationships, 1*, 185–197.

Ruehlman, L. S., & Wolchik, S. A. (1988). Personal goals and interpersonal support and hindrance as factors in psychological distress and well-being. *Journal of Personality and Social Psychology, 55*, 293–301.

Sarason, B. R., Pierce, G. R., Shearin, E. N., Sarason, I. G., Waltz, J. A., & Poppe, L. (1991). Perceived social support and working models of self and actual others. *Journal of Personality and Social Psychology, 60*, 273–287.

Sarason, B. R., Sarason, I. G., & Gurung, R. A. R. (1997). Close personal relationships and health outcomes: A key to the role of social support. In S. Duck (Ed.), *Handbook of personal relationships* (pp. 547–573). New York: Plenum Press.

Simpson, J. A., Rholes, W. S., & Nelligan, J. S. (1992). Support seeking and support giving within couples in an anxiety-provoking situation: The role of attachment styles. *Journal of Personality and Social Psychology, 62*, 434–446.

Vaux, A. (1988). *Social support.* New York: Praeger.

Wallace, J. L., & Vaux, A. (1993). Social support network orientation: The role of adult attachment style. *Journal of Social and Clinical Psychology, 12*, 354–365.

Wethington, E., & Kessler, R. C. (1986). Perceived social support, received support and adjustment to stressful life events. *Journal of Health and Social Behavior, 27*, 78–89.

Williamson, G. M., Clark, M. S., Pegalis, L. J., & Behan, A. (1996). Affective consequences of refusing to help in communal and exchange relationships. *Personality and Social Psychology Bulletin, 22*, 34–47.

CHAPTER 8

Implicit Theories of Relationships and Coping in Romantic Relationships

C. RAYMOND KNEE

AMY CANEVELLO

People often bring assumptions with them when they enter a romantic relationship. Among these assumptions are certain beliefs and expectations about how romantic relationships typically function. Two particular beliefs, or "implicit theories," that have been shown to be important in predicting and understanding how people attempt to negotiate their romantic lives are belief in romantic destiny and belief in relationship growth (Knee, 1998). Recent findings suggest that assumptions people hold about the stability of their perceptions of both partner compatibility and the nature of problems in romantic relationships guide how meaning is assigned to particular relationship events and situations (Knee, Patrick, & Lonsbary, 2003).

Destiny belief concerns the stability of one's *impressions* about relationships. For example, Ben and Jennifer have recently begun dating. Jennifer is very attracted to Ben but feels that they have a difficult time relating to each other (e.g., they do not seem to have much in common). Jennifer may begin to think about their budding relationship in terms of the long-term stability of this impression about their compatibility. If Jennifer was high in destiny belief, she might conclude that since she and Ben are unable to relate now, they probably never will relate in the manner she would like. This scenario could lead Jennifer, guided by her belief about the stability of her impressions about romantic relationships, to end their relationship in its early stages. Conversely, if Jennifer were low in destiny belief, she might conclude that although she and Ben do not seem to have much in common right now, that does not mean that they will continue to have little in common in the future. In this case, guided by her belief that the future potential of a relationship can change and is not immediately or easily evident, Jennifer would be more likely to stay in the relationship for the time being. Destiny belief, the conviction that one's impressions of relationships are generally fixed and stable (and accurate), sets up an emphasis on determining the compatibility of a potential romantic partner and the future success of the relationship from whatever information is immediately available.

Independently, *growth belief* concerns the stability of *problems* in relationships. For example, Ben is worried about his relationship with Jennifer because he often feels neglected by her. On the one hand, Ben is high (relative to low) in growth belief, he might begin to think about his relationship in terms of the stability of this particular problem, guided by his belief that problems in relationships are unstable and can change. Ben may think that he and Jennifer can work through their problem, and that this might lead to a stronger relationship. On the other hand, if Ben is low (relative to high) in growth belief, he might believe that even if he and Jennifer tried to work things out, Jennifer's neglect of him will always remain an issue in the relationship. Growth belief is characterized by an emphasis on relationship development and the belief that relationships grow not despite obstacles but in part because of them.

In this chapter, we discuss a model hypothesizing that implicit theories of relationships (ITRs) contribute to the meaning assigned to relationship events, thus impacting not only relationship outcomes, but how one attempts to cope with relationship events.

THE CONSTRUCT OF IMPLICIT THEORIES

The concept of implicit, or naive, theories about the self and others is rooted in Heider's (1958) field theory of social perception and Kelly's (1955) theory of personality. Implicit theories refer to personal constructs or naive assumptions about the self and the social world that help guide how people perceive and interpret events. Ross (1989) defined *implicit theories* as schematic knowledge structures that involve specific beliefs about the stability of an attribute and the conditions that are likely to promote change. Along these lines, Dweck and her colleagues (Dweck, Chiu, & Hong, 1995) examined implicit theories along the dimension of stability. For example, an entity theory reflected the assumption that a particular attribute (e.g., intelligence) was stable and immutable, whereas an incremental theory reflected the assumption that a particular attribute was capable of changing. These naive assumptions were shown to have considerable influence on the meaning that people assign to failure and how people respond to such challenging experiences—for example, whether they persist in learning a particular task or instead give up. When one assumes that one's standing on a particular attribute (e.g., intelligence) is stable, then even minor setbacks may suggest that one cannot do the task and that one will never be able to do the task. In contrast, when one assumes that one's standing on the attribute is unstable, then setbacks are regarded as learning experiences that may eventually improve one's standing on later attempts.

A key aspect of the assumptions that people hold about themselves and the world is that such assumptions guide the way people assign meaning to events and situations, and also the way they draw inferences about themselves and others in those situations. When one assumes that attributes are stable, then behaviors that are thought to reflect those attributes will take on great meaning when one is making inferences about a person. For example, if one assumes that honesty is stable—that people are fundamentally either honest or dishonest—then learning that one's romantic partner has been unfaithful would suggest that unfaithful behavior will occur again. Furthermore, when attempting to determine the cause of the infidelity, one will likely make stronger dispositional inferences and thus blame the partner, because the behavior is assumed to reflect an underlying stable trait (in this case, dishonesty) in the partner. The tendency to make stronger trait inferences about others from ambiguous situations has long been recognized by social psychologists as the "fundamental attribution error." Many models of how this occurs cognitively have been put forth (Gilbert & Malone, 1995; Quattrone, 1982; Trope, 1986). Interestingly, implicit theories can, in part, determine the extent to which people will make such trait inferences in the first place, based on the assumptions they bring with them when witnessing the experience.

People also bring fundamental assumptions with them to their romantic relationships. In the domain of relationships, the dimension of stability can be further broken down into two independent dimensions. ITRs consist of a belief in romantic destiny and an independent belief in relationship growth (see Knee et al., 2003, for a review). Destiny belief involves assuming that relationships are either meant to be or they are not meant to be. This dimension concerns the stability of one's impressions about relationships. When one believes strongly (relative to weakly) in romantic destiny, one assumes that one's impression of the match between partners is relatively accurate and that one can forecast the future of the relationship. Growth belief involves the conviction that relationships can be maintained and problems in relationships can be overcome. This dimension concerns the assumption of stability of problems in the relationship. When one believes strongly (relative to weakly) in relationship growth, one assumes that problems and disagreements are unstable and can be managed as they occur and fluctuate over the course of the relationship. These beliefs about relationships operate as fundamental assumptions about the nature of romantic relationships, and, as such, they guide inferences and attributions about relationship experiences. For example, those who believe in romantic destiny (relative to those who do not) tend to be especially sensitive to their initial impressions of the relationship and tend to make stronger inferences about cues that might suggest that the relationship is not "meant to be." Specifically, relationship survival is more strongly linked to initial feelings of satisfaction and closeness among those who believe strongly in romantic destiny. Among those who do not endorse a destiny belief, early impressions of satisfaction and closeness do not significantly predict how long the relationship will last (Knee, 1998). Those who strongly endorse a destiny belief also tend to cope with negative relationship events in a predictable manner. Specifically, belief in destiny is associated with denying the negative event, disengaging from the relationship, and restraining oneself from maintenance attempts.

Returning to Jennifer's initial negative impression of her relationship with Ben, if she is higher (relative to lower) in destiny belief, she may pay particular attention to this information and interpret it as a cue or sign that their relationship is not meant to be. As a result, she is likely to report lower initial satisfaction with the relationship, and may conclude that if she and Ben do not relate now, there is little chance that they will ever really relate to each other. Consequently, it is more likely that Jennifer will break off the relationship in response to these early cues. However, if Jennifer were lower (relative to higher) in destiny belief, it is likely that she will put less stock in her initial feelings, believing that just because the two are having difficulty now does not mean that they will not have a good relationship in the future.

Endorsing a growth belief is also related to how one approaches and makes sense of relationships. Higher (relative to lower) growth belief is associated with the notion that relationship problems are solvable and that it is through this process that partners grow closer and the relationship becomes stronger. For example, college freshmen who more strongly endorse a growth belief tend to have fewer one-night stands during their first month of college and tend to date a specific person for a longer period of time (Knee, 1998). When it comes to coping with negative relationship events, growth belief is associated with relationship-maintenance strategies, including more active coping, more planning, and more suppression of competing activities, as well as more positive and optimistic reinterpretation of the situation. Returning to Ben and Jennifer's relationship problems (Ben's belief that Jennifer neglects him), if Ben is higher (relative to lower) in growth belief, he will be more likely to conclude that they will be able to work through this issue, and become even closer in the process. He will also likely have a more optimistic interpretation of the situation, taking a relatively more positive perspective on the event. Thus he is also more likely to make a conscious effort to talk with

Jennifer about the issue and actively work on fixing the problem. If Ben is lower (relative to higher) in growth belief, he is more likely to believe that there is nothing he can do to fix the situation and either hope that Jennifer is aware of the problem and fixes it herself or conclude that Jennifer's neglect will always be a problem in the relationship.

The assumptions people hold about the stability of their perceptions of partners and the nature of problems in their romantic relationships guide how meaning is assigned to particular relationship events and situations. For example, a specific relationship event may or may not actually predict the future course of the relationship. What really matters is the meaning that the person assigns to the event. On the dimension of one's impressions of the relationship, perceiving a discrepancy between one's partner and one's ideal may be interpreted as a serious limitation that will forever plague one's satisfaction with the relationship. With a high destiny belief, Jennifer views her less-than-ideal impression of the relationship as holding great meaning for the future of the relationship. Her initial dissatisfaction with her relationship is a sign that she will always be dissatisfied. Conversely, with a low destiny belief, Jennifer sees this impression as less central to the success of the relationship. Her initial impressions are not necessarily a good indicator of future satisfaction. On the dimension of the stability of problems, having an argument with one's partner may be interpreted as a stable and threatening event that would need to be overcome to achieve a successful relationship. With a low growth belief, Ben views his feelings of being neglected as meaningful for the future of the relationship in that this problem is stable and is likely to continue. He believes that this will always be an issue in the relationship. With a high growth belief, Ben would assign less meaning to this problem by viewing it as something that says little about the future of the relationship. Instead, he would believe that working through the issue will lead to resolution, possibly allowing the couple to become closer. The assumptions that people bring with them to their relationships, in part, guide how this type of meaning is assigned to specific relationship events such as these.

IMPLICIT THEORIES OF RELATIONSHIPS AS MODERATORS OF HOW RELATIONSHIP EVENTS PREDICT RELATIONSHIP OUTCOMES

ITRs are thought to guide the meaning that is given to relationship events and perceptions in a relatively direct manner, as described above. However, the meaning that is assigned to the events and perceptions can moderate how the events and perceptions affect outcomes. This is essentially one way that ITRs are linked to coping with relationship challenges. While ITRs have often been found to moderate how relationship events and perceptions predict relationship outcomes, it is really the meaning that is assigned, because of the ITRs, that is key. In this way, the ascribed meaning theoretically mediates how ITRs buffer coping responses. For example, ITRs have been shown to moderate the association between wanting a better partner and feeling satisfied in the relationship (Knee, Nanayakkara, Vietor, Neighbors, & Patrick, 2001). In their Study 1, Knee and colleagues (2001) defined "wanting more" as perceiving a discrepancy between the qualities of an ideal partner and the qualities of one's current partner. In this design, believing that problems and impressions are unstable (rather than fixed) buffered the association between the perception that one's partner falls short and feeling less satisfied with the relationship. Generally, wanting more in one's partner was strongly related to feeling less happy with the relationship. However, this association was buffered by ITRs such that, when higher in growth and lower in destiny beliefs, how one viewed one's partner did not predict how happy (or unhappy) one was with the relationship.

In Study 2, Knee and colleagues (2001) examined the *projected illusions hypothesis* (Murray, Holmes, & Griffin, 1996), which postulates that those in satisfying relationships generally tend to view their partner more favorably than the partner views him- or herself. Conversely, those in less satisfying relationships generally tend to view their partner less favorably than the partner views him- or herself. In this study, believing that problems are unstable (higher growth belief) reduced the extent to which viewing one's partner in a less favorable manner was associated with feeling dissatisfied with the relationship. This result means that even though one viewed one's partner unfavorably, if one believed that these traits were unstable, then they no longer predicted satisfaction with the relationship.

In an independent line of research, Franiuk, Cohen, and Pomerantz (2002) found similar support for how ITRs moderate the link between perceptions and outcomes. They found that among "soul-mate theorists," the degree to which participants felt they were currently with their soul mate predicted how satisfied they were with the relationship. Furthermore, soul-mate and "work-it-out" beliefs interacted such that when *not* with one's soul mate (relative to when with one's soul mate), it was most beneficial to be lower in a soul-mate theory and higher in a work-it-out theory. This combination of beliefs has been described elsewhere as a "cultivation orientation," and has been shown to buffer the extent to which viewing one's partner as less than ideal predicts current satisfaction with the relationship (Knee et al., 2001, Study 1).

While ITRs were shown in these studies to buffer how perceptions predict outcomes, we expect that the key mediating variable is the meaning that is assigned to the perceptions as a function of one's assumptions about the stability of relationship problems and the stability of one's impressions of the relationship. In another study, believing that one's impressions of relationships are stable moderated the degree to which initial evaluations of the relationship predicted how long it would last (Knee, 1998). That is, early feelings of satisfaction with one's relationship and closeness to the partner generally predicted how long relationships would last. However, this was moderated by destiny belief, or the belief that one's impressions are stable and fixed such that early impressions predicted later relationship survival only when one believed in destiny. Again, while one's ITR was shown to be the moderator in this study, we expect that the key intervening variable was the meaning assigned to impressions and evaluations of the relationship, as a function of assuming that one's impressions are stable and fixed (or unstable and changing).

IMPLICIT THEORIES OF RELATIONSHIPS: FROM INTRAPERSONAL TO INTERPERSONAL PROCESSES

Figure 8.1 presents a conceptual model of how ITRs moderate the way relationship events predict outcomes. As shown, a key aspect of this inferential process is the meaning that is assigned to the event as a function of one's ITRs. As Figure 8.1 shows, on the left, with the innermost box, some initiating event relevant to the relationship occurs. We define *initiating events* broadly as those experiences that may or may not actually impact the relationship, but that potentially provoke inferences about the relationship in one way or another. Initiating events include, but are not limited to, a disagreement or conflict between partners, and feedback or information about how well the relationship is going or how well one is "achieving" a successful relationship. Initiating events also include other events in the relationship that may seem relevant to the current or future quality of the relationship—for example, comments about the relationship from friends or family or even events that may make salient potential alternative partners, as well as one's own feelings of discontent (Vangelisti & Alexander, 2002). While initiating events, by themselves, may not logically imply anything in particular about the quality of the relationship, it is our assertion that they certainly may be perceived differently depending on the assumptions one brings to the relationship.

Most of the analysis of Figure 8.1 assumes that such feedback and events tend to be negative. Indeed, the theoretical process seems clearer about how ITRs operate with potentially negative events. Bad events generally tend to be more influential than good events (e.g., Baumeister, Bratslavsky, Finkenauer, & Vohs, 2001). However, that is not to say that the inferential process discussed here is limited to negative events. To the contrary, positive feedback and events may be interpreted through similar mechanisms, albeit more or less strongly. Indeed, future research needs to examine the extent to which ITRs operate on positive events in a manner similar to negative events whereby greater inferential validity and processing is given to both positive

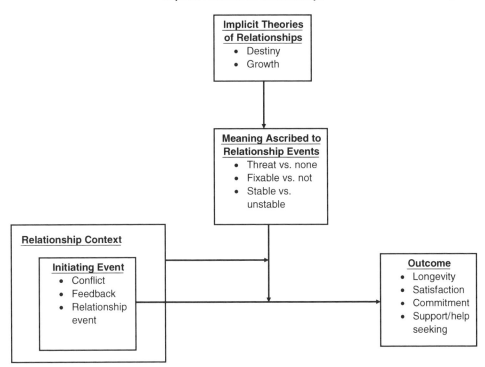

FIGURE 8.1. ITRs and coping processes in romantic relationships. These processes have been studied more extensively with respect to negative rather than positive events.

and negative events. It is likely that when one assumes that one's impressions of relationships are fixed and determined, both positive and negative events can take on greater meaning.

Once an initiating event occurs, or several such events occur over time, it or they may lead to changes (both momentary and long-term changes) in relationship outcomes including satisfaction with and commitment to the relationship. However, the key point of the model is that the assumptions one brings to the relationship in part determine the extent to which momentary and long-term changes in such outcomes emerge as a function of those initiating events. Thus the path between initiating events and relationship outcomes is intersected by the meaning ascribed to relationship events, which is in turn driven by the ITRs one holds. As we mentioned earlier, ITRs moderate how initiating events predict relationship outcomes. However, the intervening variable in this moderation is thought to be the meaning ascribed to these events or the degree to which the initiating event is interpreted as something that is stable versus unstable, something that is unchangeable versus changeable, and something that threatens the potential of the relationship or not. These inter-pretations, in turn, rest largely on one's underlying assumptions about how relationships operate. For example, when one believes in destiny, one tends to interpret negative relationship events as relatively fixed, stable, and unchang-ing, and thus as threatening to the potential of the relationship. Interpreting relationship events in this way will in turn affect one's feelings about the rela-tionship more strongly. This moderation is, once again, largely based on the assumption that one's impressions of a relationship are relatively stable. Inde-pendently, when one believes in growth, one tends to assume and expect that problems can be resolved and that relationships can improve. This assumption leads to an interpretation of immediate relationship events (both positive and negative) as relatively unimportant in what they may imply about the quality of the relationship or its future course. Negative events are not viewed as a threat because such events are expected and regarded as changeable because it is assumed that relationships require maintenance and coping with issues as they arise. This interpretation of initiating events as relatively expected and irrelevant to the success of the relationship leaves one's feelings about the relationship relatively unaffected by those events. This moderation is largely based on the assumption that problems and differences in relationships are typical and that, with effort, they can be resolved as they arise.

In the case of Ben and Jennifer's relationship problem, the initiating event would be Ben's worries about Jennifer's apparent neglect of him. In terms of the initial meaning or importance of the event, if Ben brings a stron-ger growth belief to the relationship, he is more likely to interpret this prob-lem as being less influential or meaningful for his overall satisfaction with the relationship. It is this assigned meaning that determines how the initiating event leads to relationship outcomes. In this case, there would be little change in satisfaction based on this single relationship event because those who are high (relative to low) in growth belief tend to view problems as less stable and threatening. Therefore, outcomes in this scenario might include little inter-ruption in the longevity of the relationship and unchanged satisfaction or com-mitment. However, if Ben holds a weaker growth belief, it is easier to see how the problem may have substantially different meaning for his relationship sat-isfaction. Again, the path from the initiating event to relationship outcomes is moderated by ITRs. In this case, a weaker growth belief would change the meaning assigned to Jennifer's neglect. The problem would be viewed as a potential threat to the continued success of the relationship because it would be interpreted as being relatively stable and irreparable. The meaning ascribed to this event may lead Ben to report less satisfaction with and com-mitment to the relationship and may even impact the relationship's longevity.

Finally, Figure 8.1 also portrays the importance of the context of the rela-tionship in this process. By *relationship context*, we mean the preexisting tone, impression, limiting conditions, or other factor that surrounds the relationship and varies between relationships. For example, some relationships may already have preexisting challenges—for example, long-distance relationships. Partners in long-distance relationships are thought to have greater challenges in remaining together, although research on this is somewhat mixed (e.g., Guldner & Swensen, 1995; Helgeson, 1994; Rohlfing, 1995). Another example might be interracial relationships in which the partners feel pressure from themselves or others against the relationship. Finally, another contextual factor may be relationships in which conflict is more frequent than usual, such that intense conflict has become either expected or has become so extreme that another argument would set in motion attempts to terminate the relationship, regardless of one's underlying assumptions. These contextual factors, and others, are thought to mitigate the extent to which ITRs and the inferential processes they engender moderate how initiating events can predict outcomes. For example, Knee, Patrick, Vietor, and Neighbors (2004, Study 2) found that an initiating event—in this case, having a conflict in a controlled setting—was generally followed by lower relationship commitment. However, the degree to which this occurred depended on one's growth belief (and presumably the meaning assigned to conflict because of it) and on the context of the relationship. In this case, the context variable was operationalized as having a more negative view of one's partner to begin with. Under this condition of viewing one's partner more negatively at baseline, growth belief was an especially strong buffer of the general association between having a conflict and feeling less committed. When one held the assumption that problems are to be expected in the course of a relationship and can be resolved, having a disagreement in a laboratory setting was not followed by less commitment nearly as much as when one assumed that problems are relatively unexpected and cannot be resolved.

In the case of Ben and Jennifer, it is easy to see how the context of the relationship may further moderate how the meaning ascribed to the relationship affects outcomes. If Ben and Jennifer's relationship is a long-distance one, the meaning of this event may be amplified (relative to the absence of this contextual variable). Feedback regarding the success of the relationship may be at a minimum in this context, so Ben automatically may be receiving less information than normal from his partner. Additionally, the value of that feedback may increase solely because of its scarcity. If Ben has a weaker (relative to stronger) growth belief, then the meaning he assigns to the relationship problem may be magnified because of the scarcity and increased value of the information. This may potentially enhance the threatening nature of the problem and lead to decreased satisfaction and commitment, and even to early dissolution of the relationship (compared to if the relationship were not a long-distance one).

CAUSAL DIRECTION

The majority of available evidence suggests that ITRs operate primarily in a single causal direction from theories to inferences to behaviors (Franiuk, Pomerantz, & Cohen, 2004; Knee et al., 2003). Theoretically, in the relationships literature and elsewhere, it is posited that these underlying cognitive assumptions guide how events are interpreted and lead to subsequent emotions and behaviors, or buffer the degree to which particular perceptions lead to specific classes of emotions and behaviors. Indeed, in the achievement and social cognition literatures, causal manipulation of ITRs has repeatedly been shown to result in the predicted response patterns of persistence versus helplessness (see Dweck et al., 1995, for a review). In the relationships literature, only recently has evidence emerged from momentary experimental manipulation of one's ITRs (Franiuk et al., 2004). Franiuk and her colleagues (2004) induced participants to hold soul-mate or work-it-out theories, and replicated previously demonstrated moderation of the association between perceptions of one's partner and feelings of satisfaction with the relationship. Analogous to studies that have employed questionnaire measures of one's ITRs, there was a stronger association between perceiving one's partner as ideal and feeling satisfied with the relationship among those who were momentarily induced to hold a soul-mate theory of relationships. In Study 2, experimentally manipulated ITRs led to biased cognitive processing, especially when the relationship was threatened. Specifically, inducing participants to hold a soul-mate theory (relative to a work-it-out theory) resulted in more relationship-enhancing cognitions if they believed they were with the "right" partner, but more relationship-detracting cognitions if they did not believe they were with the right partner. Furthermore, these biases in processing were enhanced when participants were told that the chances of success for their relationship were very low.

Generally, ITRs tend to be relatively persistent over time, with respectable test–retest reliabilities (Franiuk et al., 2002; Knee et al., 2003). However, as the research above attests to, this persistence may have more to do with the methods of studying the construct than with the nature of the construct itself. Clearly, as with implicit theories in other literatures, they can be experimentally manipulated as well. Indeed, it may be important to distinguish between "chronic" ITRs that are assessed as general beliefs about relationships and "induced," or primed, ITRs that are momentarily enhanced or primed. Further research is needed, to be sure, but if similar findings emerge at both "trait" and "state" levels of the construct, it can be argued that this testifies to the power of the ITRs construct. It is also important to note that, although preliminary studies suggest that ITRs can be manipulated experimentally, this does not preclude the possibility that cause also runs in the opposite direction, such that if relationship events were manipulated strongly enough, then ITRs may be amenable to revision. It also does not rule out the possibility that other naturally occurring factors may alter or modify the ITRs one holds. For example, Knee (1998) had participants report the most stressful event (regardless of whether it was a relationship event or not) that occurred during the semester. Interestingly, the correlation between destiny beliefs measured a few months apart (test–retest) was half as large in magnitude among those who reported a relationship event as the most stressful event they experienced during that time, compared to those who reported a nonrelationship event as the most stressful event. Thus, while ITRs are thought to guide how meaning is assigned to events, and in turn lead to particular inferences and coping behaviors, that is not to say that salient relationship experiences do not sometimes shape one's ITRs. For example, if Jennifer has a strong growth belief and is in an abusive relationship and leaves her partner, her growth belief may weaken as a function of being in a relationship where early indicators of potential abuse were once considered unstable and changeable. A possible scenario involving change in destiny belief may be a weakening of Ben's destiny belief as a function of the dissolution of a relationship he once believed was destined to continue. Further research is needed to examine potential influences on one's ITRs, including longitudinal research on the process of breakup and research on transitions between relationships.

IMPLICIT THEORIES OF RELATIONSHIPS
AND COPING WITH RELATIONSHIP EVENTS

There are many perspectives on how people attempt to cope with stressful events. One of the more popular approaches views coping as a transactional process that involves cognitions and behaviors directed at altering the situation in the form of problem-focused coping, or regulating one's emotions in the form of emotion-focused coping (Lazarus & Folkman, 1984). More recently, this approach and others have been adapted for the study of coping in relationships (e.g., Badr, 2004; Bodenmann, 1995; Coyne & Smith, 1991). Relationship-focused coping is thought to have two main components, active engagement and protective buffering, which roughly parallel the distinction between problem-focused and emotion-focused coping in the mainstream literature (Badr, 2004; Coyne & Smith, 1991). Active engagement occurs when partners are actively involved in making decisions and other problem-solving strategies. Protective buffering occurs when partners deny problems and concerns, present a brave front, or defer to their partner to avoid disagreement.

Individuals' ITRs not only guide how meaning is assigned to relationship events and perceptions, they also predict how people will attempt to cope with relationship challenges. When one believes that one's impressions of the relationship are stable, then perceptions of the limitations of the relationship become something to deny, avoid, or abandon, because they imply that they will remain limitations and raise questions about better alternatives. This may also differ early on when one is trying to evaluate whether a relationship is worth pursuing, compared to once one is convinced that the relationship is a good match. When the investment is relatively limited, then limitations may suggest that one should bail out and abandon the relationship for a potentially better match. When the investment is relatively profound, in the sense of feeling that one has found the right partner, then limitations may become threats to the relationship's future success, a success that the person has committed considerable mental and emotional energy toward ensuring. Thus, once established, a destiny belief would guide one to deny or avoid awareness of problems and limitations. However, before that time, one would be especially sensitive to cues that could suggest something about the status and potential of the relationship.

Knee (1998) also found that destiny belief was independently associated with particular coping strategies, primarily those of the avoidant or disengagement variety. Participants described the most upsetting event during a semester, and completed the COPE (Carver, Scheier, & Weintraub, 1989) with regard to that specific event. For example, denial was operationalized as refusing to believe that a problem exists or trying to behave as though the problem is not real (Carver et al., 1989). The extent to which denial may be adaptive or maladaptive, like many coping strategies, probably depends on many factors including the potential for actually resolving the problem, whether the criterion is short-term or long-term benefit, and the context of the relationship. However, denial seems more likely to occur when it is believed that the situation or problem cannot be resolved. Indeed, Knee found that destiny belief was associated with denying a relationship problem when it arose. Denying that a problem exists is one way to avoid working on the problem. Another method of avoiding the problem involves reducing one's effort to deal with the problem, and even giving up the attempt to attain goals with which the problem is interfering (Carver et al., 1989). This behavioral disengagement is related to the notion of helplessness, in which one gives up trying to succeed and abandons the task. In other literatures, this behavioral syndrome in response to challenging situations has been linked strongly to the belief that attributes (such as intelligence) are fixed and stable (see Dweck et al., 1995, for a review). Indeed, this association carries over to the relationships literature in that destiny belief is associated with behavioral disengagement when problems arise (Knee, 1998). Part of a destiny belief is assuming that one's impressions of the relationship are stable and that how one views the relationship now is how one will view the relationship later. Events that challenge an established impression are likely to be ignored or defended against because these tend to violate a strongly held underlying assumption about the nature of relationships. Similarly, disengaging from the relationship is also more likely when one assumes that one's impressions are stable and that negative events can be interpreted as cues that the relationship will not succeed. Finally, another way of coping with a relationship involves restraining oneself from doing anything about it immediately. While this form of restraint coping has been considered a problem-focused strategy, it is also considered to be a passive strategy in that it implies not acting to deal with the problem (Carver et al., 1989). Consistent with the tendency for those who believe in destiny to deny or disengage from a relationship problem, Knee also found that destiny belief is associated with restraining oneself from doing anything about the problem.

Denying a relationship problem, disengaging from dealing with an acknowledged problem, and restraining oneself from doing anything immediately all appear to be relatively avoidant methods of dealing with a relationship event. Such avoidance of potential problems makes sense when one assumes that impressions of the relationship are stable and unchanging. It is possible that if one's impression of the relationship is relatively established, denial and restraint may be more likely, whereas one's impression is still developing, then strategies that involve disengaging from the relationship may be more likely. However, additional research is needed to examine these processes more carefully. Theoretically, cues that may suggest that the relationship is not "the one" can take on greater meaning with destiny belief. Whether such cues play an equally important role once a strong impression has been established is not clear. However, those who fundamentally assume that relationship potential can be determined easily probably never finish evaluating the relationship and inferring relatively grand meaning from relationship events. One would expect that the tendency to make stronger inferences about such events would set up a relatively evaluative and vigilant mindset that carries throughout the course of the relationship. Although their sample was limited to relatively brief college student relationships, Franiuk and colleagues (2002) independently tested whether holding a soul-mate theory of relationships was correlated with reported reactions to arguments. They found that, indeed, those who believed that partners are destined to be together tended to report giving in when having an argument with their partner. In addition, these soul-mate believers also tended to generally perceive more agreement with their partner.

Independently of belief in destiny, one's belief in growth also predicts how one will attempt to cope with relationship limitations. When one believes that relationship problems are relatively unstable, these issues are interpreted as opportunities to come to know one's partner better and improve the relationship. Thus, when growth belief is high (relative to low), problems are approached in ways that are likely to foster resolution and relationship development. As mentioned earlier, Knee (1998) examined associations between one's implicit theories of relationships and several coping strategies when dealing with relationship experiences. Associations emerged for both the growth and destiny dimensions. Specifically, growth belief was associated with several problem-focused strategies that seem geared toward maintaining the relationship, including more active coping, planning, and suppression of competing activities, as well as more positive and optimistic reinterpretation of the situation.

Active coping involves actively attempting to do something about the stressful relationship event, including initiating direct action, increasing one's efforts, and trying to cope with the problem in a head-on fashion (Carver et al., 1989). When one believes in growth, one assumes that problems can be resolved and that maintaining the relationship is a typical and required behavior. Attempting to deal directly and openly with problems as they arise exemplifies the assumption that underlies the belief that relationship problems and events can be altered and managed. Planning is another problem-focused strategy in which one thinks about how to cope with the stressor and plans a course of action for addressing and dealing with the problem. Again, this is more likely to occur when one believes that relationship problems are unstable and changeable. If one assumes that problems are fixed and that relationships do not require much maintenance, then one would be less likely to attempt to actively plan and cope with the situation.

Also included in the category of problem-focused coping is the strategy of suppressing competing activities. Sometimes one puts other projects aside when necessary in order to deal with a relationship problem, essentially trying to "clear one's plate" to facilitate dealing with the event at hand. The association between growth belief and suppression of competing activities when relationship problems arise makes considerable sense. If one assumed that relationship problems were incapable of remedy, one would not likely bother to focus all one's resources on the immediate problem. Finally, growth belief was associated with making a more optimistic reinterpretation of the relationship event. This kind of positive reappraisal is typically considered as a type of emotion-focused coping (Lazarus & Folkman, 1984). However, Carver and colleagues (1989) pointed out that the value of seeing the best in a situation is not limited to merely reducing one's distress, but rather should promote continued problem-focused coping attempts.

While not necessarily an active, problem-focused approach, an optimistic perspective on stressful events has been found to be linked to positive health outcomes and other benefits (e.g., Salovey, Rothman, Detweiler, & Steward, 2000). Seeing the best in a particular relationship situation makes sense when one assumes that relationships grow and change over time, and may facilitate continued efforts to deal with the problem in a more active fashion rather than viewing the problem as immutable and giving up on attempts to change it. More research needs to examine how destiny and growth beliefs (and similar constructs) operate in long-term committed relationships and whether the inferential process that is set up early on carries through for a longer time.

In conclusion, the ITRs framework has much to say about the beliefs and assumptions that people bring with them into their relationships. We feel that this framework helps explain how the same events within a relationship can be interpreted in rather different ways. These different interpretations, or assignments of meaning, in turn guide how the events are appraised and the coping responses that tend to follow. Whether studied as relatively chronic and stable beliefs or as primed and relatively temporary constructs, ITRs tend to consistently buffer the degree to which events in one's relationship predict one's satisfaction, one's coping responses, and even the survival or demise of the relationship. While ITRs are only one conceptual vehicle for understanding how intrapersonal processes can influence interpersonal processes, they offer a rich theoretical foundation that parallels literatures outside the relationships domain. At the same time, the framework and research in the relationships domain is relatively young and sparse, with many potential avenues for further study.

ACKNOWLEDGMENTS

We thank Cynthia Lonsbary for her help in commenting on previous drafts of this chapter.

REFERENCES

Badr, H. (2004). Coping in marital dyads: A contextual perspective on the role of gender and health. *Personal Relationships, 11*, 197–211.

Baumeister, R. F., Bratslavsky, E., Finkenauer, C., & Vohs, K. D. (2001). Bad is stronger than good. *Review of General Psychology, 5*, 323–370.

Bodenmann, G. (1995). A systemic-transactional view of stress and coping among couples. *Swiss Journal of Psychology, 54*, 34–49.

Carver, C. S., Scheier, M. F., & Weintraub, J. K. (1989). Assessing coping strategies: A theoretically based approach. *Journal of Personality and Social Psychology, 56*(2), 267–283.

Coyne, J. C., & Smith, D. A. F. (1991). Couples coping with myocardial infarction: A contextual perspective on wives' distress. *Journal of Personality and Social Psychology, 61*, 404–412.

Dweck, C. S., Chiu, C., & Hong, Y. (1995). Implicit theories: Elaboration and extension of the model. *Psychological Inquiry, 6*, 322–333.

Franiuk, R., Cohen, D., & Pomerantz, E. M. (2002). Implicit theories of relationships: Implications for relationship satisfaction and longevity. *Personal Relationships, 9*(4), 345–367.

Franiuk, R., Pomerantz, E. M., & Cohen, D. (2004). The causal role of theories of relationships: Consequences for satisfaction and cognitive strategies. *Personality and Social Psychology Bulletin, 30,* 1494–1507.

Gilbert, D. T., & Malone, P. S. (1985). The correspondence bias. *Psychological Bulletin, 117,* 21–38.

Guldner, G. T., & Swensen, C. H. (1995). Time spent together and relationship quality: Long- distance relationships as a test case. *Journal of Social and Personal Relationships, 12*(2), 313–320.

Heider, F. (1958). *The psychology of interpersonal relations.* New York: Wiley.

Helgeson, V. S. (1994). The effects of self-beliefs and relationship beliefs on adjustment to a relationship stressor. *Personal Relationships, 1*(3), 241–258.

Kelly, G. A. (1955). *The psychology of personal constructs.* New York: Norton.

Knee, C. R. (1998). Implicit theories of relationships: Assessment and prediction of romantic relationship initiation, coping, and longevity. *Journal of Personality and Social Psychology, 74,* 360–370.

Knee, C. R., Nanayakkara, A., Vietor, N., Neighbors, C., & Patrick, H. (2001). Implicit theories of relationships: Who cares if romantic partners are less than ideal? *Personality and Social Psychology Bulletin, 27,* 808–819.

Knee, C. R., Patrick, H., & Lonsbary, C. (2003). Implicit theories of relationships: Orientations toward evaluation and cultivation. *Personality and Social Psychology Review, 7*(1), 41–55.

Knee, C. R., Patrick, H., Vietor, N., & Neighbors, C. (2004). Implicit theories of relationships: Moderators of the link between conflict and commitment. *Personality and Social Psychology Bulletin, 30*(5), 617–628.

Lazarus, R. S., & Folkman, S. (1984). *Stress appraisal and coping.* New York: Springer.

Murray, S. L., Holmes, J. G., & Griffin, D. W. (1996). The benefits of positive illusions: Idealization and the construction of satisfaction in close relationships. *Journal of Personality and Social Psychology, 70,* 79–98.

Quattrone, G. A. (1982). Behavioral consequences of attributional bias. *Social Cognition, 1,* 358–378.

Rohlfing, M. E. (1995). "Doesn't anybody stay in one place anymore?": An exploration of the under-studied phenomenon of long-distance relationships. In J. T. Wood & S. Duck (Eds.), *Understanding relationship processes series: Vol. 6. Understudied relationships: Off the beaten track* (pp. 173–196). Thousand Oaks, CA: Sage.

Ross, M. (1989). Relation of implicit theories to the construct of personal histories. *Psychological Review, 96,* 341–357.

Salovey, P., Rothman, A. J., Detweiler, J. B., & Steward, W. T. (2000). Emotional states and physical health. *American Psychologist, 55,* 110–121.

Trope, Y. (1986). Identification and inferential processes in dispositional attribution. *Psychological Review, 93,* 239–257.

Vangelisti, A. L., & Alexander, A. L. (2002). Coping with disappointment in marriage: When partner's standards are unmet. In P. Noller & B. Feeney (Eds.), *Understanding marriage* (pp. 201–227). Cambridge, UK: Cambridge University Press.

Organization of Partner Knowledge

Implications for Liking and Loving, Longevity, and Change

CAROLIN J. SHOWERS
ALICIA LIMKE

A wide range of literature on memory processes and knowledge structures (Kihlstrom, Beer, & Klein, 2003; Markus, 1977; Smith & Medin, 1981) would suggest that some intrapersonal processes that affect interpersonal relationships stem from the organization of relationship-relevant information in an individual's working or long-term memory. This chapter focuses on the way an individual organizes beliefs about a romantic partner (i.e., partner knowledge), with particular emphasis on positive or negative valence as an organizing dimension (cf. Niedenthal, Halberstadt, & Innes-Ker, 1999; Osgood, 1969) and the impact of this kind of organization on relationship quality. More specifically, the relationship variables of interest include the individual's attitudes or feelings for the partner, the overall quality of the relationship, and its eventual outcome (ongoing or ended status).

The term *organization* refers to the category structure of relevant partner knowledge. Although memory models often present knowledge structures as the cause of subsequent feelings, judgments, and behaviors, these structures may often be the consequence of particular styles or strategies of thinking about a partner or of certain types of interactions or behaviors (cf. Klein, Loftus, & Sherman, 1993). In either case, the organization of partner knowledge may reflect or correspond to the individual's cognitive strategies for regulating thoughts, feelings, and behaviors toward the partner (Cantor & Kihlstrom, 1987). In other words, a certain type of organization may be adopted because it serves a person's goals pertaining to the partner or the relationship. For example, some types of organization may help to maintain relationships despite a partner's salient flaws by minimizing the impact of negative attributes on subsequent feelings and behaviors. Other types of organization that do not cushion negative attributes may prevail when individuals are motivated to be cautious about continuing a problematic relationship or trusting an unstable partner. In a study of the organization of *self*-knowledge, Showers, Abramson, and Hogan (1998) suggested that the positive or negative content of beliefs may be a direct reflection of current positive or negative experiences (e.g., high conflict or external stresses), whereas organizational structure may correspond to the strategies an individual uses that ameliorate or exaggerate that experience. Similarly, then, the positive or negative content of beliefs about a partner may be a relatively direct reflection of an individual's experience of the partner, whereas the structure of partner knowledge may reflect motives to see a person in an especially positive or negative light. Thus the organization of partner knowledge may represent some of the intrapersonal processes that influence relationship outcomes.

EVALUATIVE ORGANIZATION OF PARTNER KNOWLEDGE

The existing model of the evaluative organization of self-knowledge (Showers, 1992a, 2002) can easily be applied to the case of partner knowledge. Positive and negative beliefs about a relationship partner can be described as *evaluatively compartmentalized* (i.e., positive and negative beliefs are segregated into separate categories of partner knowledge) or *evaluatively integrative* (i.e., positive and negative beliefs frequently appear within the same categories of partner knowledge). These two types of organization fall on a continuum from perfectly compartmentalized (all categories of partner knowledge are purely positive or purely negative) to perfectly integrated (positive and negative beliefs or attributes are equally distributed across all categories). Examples of each are presented in Table 9.1. According to the theoretical model, category structure determines which set of beliefs about a partner are activated in a particular situation. For example, the thought of going out with one's partner and a group of friends on Saturday night will likely activate very different beliefs for the individuals who generated the partner descriptions depicted in Panels A and B. For the individual in Panel A, activating the category "Around his friends" brings to mind purely positive attributes (happy, friendly, outgoing, energetic, fun). For the individual in Panel B, the relevant "Social" category brings to mind a mixed set of attributes (energetic and fun, but also indecisive and disorganized).

TABLE 9.1. Actual Card Sorts Illustrating Compartmentalized and Integrative Organization of Partner Knowledge

Panel A: Compartmentalized organization

Around his friends	Around me	At work	In a bad mood	General attitude	When I go out without him
Happy	Happy	Mature	-Disagreeing	Happy	-Self-centered
Friendly	Friendly	Intelligent	-Irritable	Independent	-Disagreeing
Outgoing	Comfortable	Friendly	-Self-centered	-Self-centered	-Irritable
Energetic	Organized	Comfortable	-Tense	Confident	-Tense
Fun and entertaining	-Lazy	Organized	-Isolated	Interested	-Uncomfortable
	Communicative	Communicative		Organized	-Insecure
	Independent	Independent		Communicative	-Immature
	Giving	Interested		Comfortable	
	Interested	Needed		Friendly	
	Lovable	Confident			
		Capable			
		Hardworking			

Panel B: Integrative organization

Love life	Social	School	Family	Friends	Work	Athletics
Lovable	Outgoing	-Irritable	-Unloved	Outgoing	Confident	-Like a failure
Giving	Confident	Successful	-Hopeless	Friendly	-Irritable	Hardworking
Needed	Energetic	Hardworking	Needed	Lovable	Successful	Capable
Fun and entertaining	Fun and entertaining	Intelligent	-Irritable	Confident	Hardworking	Energetic
Communicative	-Indecisive	-Tense	-Sad and blue	Energetic	Capable	
Happy	-Disorganized	Capable	-Insecure	Fun and entertaining	Maturer	
Mature	Lovable	Confident	-Tense	Happy		
-Irritable	Friendly		Communicative			
Friendly			Friendly			

Note. A minus sign indicates negative attributes. These card sorts, including the aspect labels, were generated by two participants in this study. From Showers and Zeigler-Hill (2004). Copyright 2004 by Sage Publications. Adapted by permission.

179

Current Feelings

The partner attributes activated by the category structure should influence an individual's feelings about upcoming events. Thus the individual in Panel A may be more optimistic about the evening and her feelings about her partner than the individual in Panel B. If the most important experiences for both of these couples were social ones, a simple prediction would be that the individual in Panel A would ultimately like her partner better and be more satisfied in her relationship than the individual in Panel B. However, as already implied, a critical moderator of this prediction is the importance of the activated categories. If, on this particular Saturday evening, the partner represented in Panel A is in a bad mood (activating attributes like disagreeing, irritable, self-centered, and tense), the likely outcome of the evening would favor the individual represented in Panel B. Thus an individual's experience of a partner represented by a compartmentalized structure is likely to be either extremely positive or extremely negative, depending on whether positive or negative compartments are activated most frequently. Moreover, the individual's feelings about this partner may fluctuate widely if both positive and negative compartments are relatively important and are activated frequently, but at different times (Zeigler-Hill, 2004).

In contrast, individuals' experience of partners who are represented by integrative structures should be more moderate, given the proportions of positive and negative attributes perceived. For a partner with many positive attributes, an integrative structure may actually water down positive impressions by bringing to mind at least a few negative attributes in any context. The advantage of integrative structures should emerge when a partner is perceived to have important negative attributes, in which case the integrative structure helps to balance salient negative characteristics with relevant positive beliefs, and is preferable to a compartmentalized structure that has many important negative attribute categories (Showers, 1992a, 1992b).

Long-Term Outcomes

A basic prediction of this theoretical causal model is that the structure determines the set of positive and/or negative beliefs that are activated in a given situation, and therefore influences the content of working knowledge about the partner as well as current feelings. However, the consequences of adopting compartmentalized or integrative structures over the long term may be different from their implications for current feelings. For example, successful integration (which creates links between salient negative attributes and ameliorating positive ones) may be difficult to maintain over the long term. People may be unwilling or unable to sustain the effort and cognitive resources necessary to maintain associations between oppositely valenced beliefs over long periods of time (Showers & Kling, 1996; Showers & Zeigler-Hill, 2003). Thus integration as a strategy for minimizing the impact of a partner's negative attributes may wear itself out over time. It is also the case that individuals with compartmentalized perceptions of their partners may experience shifts in the relative importance of positive versus negative beliefs, consequently changing feelings about the partner from one extreme to another. Thus the structures that predict relatively positive feelings about a partner in the short term may not predict long-term outcomes for a relationship.

Change in Partner Structure

When considering the long-term consequences of the structure of partner knowledge, another possibility to consider is that the structure itself will change. The dynamic model of self-organization suggests that people shift from easy and efficient compartmentalized self-structures to the more effortful integrative style when stressful events make negative attributes salient, thereby eliciting the individual's attention and interest in active coping (Showers, 2002). One possibility is that there is a tendency to start with a very simple evaluatively compartmentalized perception of a potential partner's strengths and weaknesses. However, as negative attributes emerge or conflict arises, an engaged partner may focus attention on these potential problem areas, resulting in integration. This effort may be continent on a growing sense of commitment to the relationship. However, the integrative process need not be successful: for some individuals, the extra effort to ameliorate or understand a partner's negative attributes may pay off; for others, this effort may fail.

EMPIRICAL EVIDENCE

To examine the association between partner structures, an individual's current feelings about a partner, potential long-term change in partner structures, and long-term outcomes, a sample of 99 college students in ongoing romantic relationships were followed for the course of 1 year. They provided assessments of self- and partner structure at the outset of the study. One year later, 94 of these individuals were contacted by phone and were questioned about the current (ongoing or ended). Sixty-seven of them also provided a second assessment of the structure of partner knowledge at that time.

Measures

Partner Structure (Card-Sorting Task)

To assess partner structure, participants generated a description of their partner by sorting a deck of 40 cards, each containing a personal attribute. There were 20 positive and 20 negative attributes. Participants were told, "Your task is to think of the different aspects of your partner or his or her life and then form groups of traits that go together, where each group of traits describes an aspect of your partner or his or her life." Participants could form as many groups as they needed, with as many or as few attributes as fit each one. They could use the same attribute in more than one group, and they did not have to use attributes that did not describe their partner. (See Showers & Kevlyn, 1999, for complete instructions.) Table 9.1 presents sample card sorts from this study.

Feelings for Partner

The measure of an individual's feelings for his or her partner was Rubin's (1970) Liking and Loving Scales.

Liking and Loving

The findings for a composite measure of liking and loving at time 1 were consistent with the predictions of the basic model of compartmentalization for current feelings (Showers & Kevlyn, 1999). These findings are presented in the line graphs shown in Figure 9.1. The association between the structure of partner knowledge and the individual's feelings of liking and loving differs depending on the proportion of negative attributes used in the partner descriptions. When the individual's characterization of the partner was basically positive, greater compartmentalization was correlated with greater liking and loving. However, when many negative attributes were used to describe the partner, those individuals who presented integrative partner structures reported more positive feelings. According to the model outlined above, compartmentalized structures for basically positive partners may enhance feelings because they keep any negative attributes out of mind. However, when negative attributes are already salient, integration is more likely to enhance feelings because it minimizes the impact of negative attributes that are already salient by linking them to the partner's positive attributes.

Relationship Status

Interestingly, although these findings for current feelings at time 1 were replicated in an analysis of liking and loving for individuals in ongoing relationships at time 2, current feelings at time 1 did not predict relationship status (ongoing or ended) at time 2 (Showers & Zeigler-Hill, 2004). The results of the ongoing/ended analysis are shown in italics in Figure 9.1. The individuals who had the highest rate of breakup at time 2 were those who reported the most positive feelings at time 1, that is, those who had described their partners in positive and compartmentalized terms. This is consistent with the suggestion

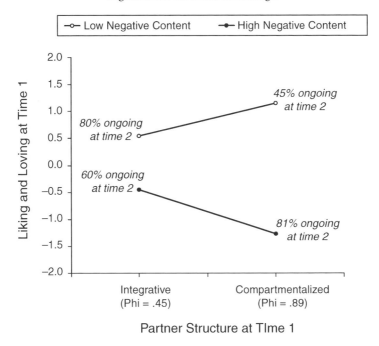

FIGURE 9.1. Associations of partner structure at time 1 with both current feelings and relationship status (ongoing or ended) at time 2. The line graphs represent current feelings as assessed by a composite measure of Rubin's (1977) Liking and Loving Scales, shown on the *y*-axis. Relationship status (proportion ongoing) at time 2 (1 year later) is shown in italics. From Showers and Zeigler-Hill (2004). Copyright 2004 by Sage Publications. Reprinted by permission.

that compartmentalized structures are vulnerable to shifts in the perceived importance or salience of the positive or negative categories, which may cause extreme variation in feelings, depending on which categories are activated at the time (Zeigler-Hill, 2004). Ironically, the individuals who reported the most negative feelings at time 1 were highly likely to stay together. We have suggested that these individuals may use compartmentalization as a way of managing important negative aspects of the partner that are unlikely to change (e.g., "My partner when he is out with his bowling buddies"), and that they may have extrinsic reasons (e.g., finances or family ties) for staying with a partner whom they do not especially like. Generally speaking, integrative individuals (who reported relatively moderate feelings at time 1) tended to stay together. The moderate feelings of those with positive partners may reflect a kind of realism about the partner's attributes that contributes to relationship longevity and helps to inoculate individuals against the emergence of new negative beliefs. Individuals who were integrating negative partner descriptions reported feeling relatively good about them in the short term, but had no advantage in terms of relationship longevity. This is consistent with our view that integrative processes require effort to maintain over time and may not always be successful in the long term.

Change in Partner Structure

The third major finding from these data had to do with change in the structure of partner knowledge over 1 year's time (Showers & Zeigler-Hill, 2004). We predicted that individuals might become more integrative in their partner structures either as they learned new negative beliefs about the partner or as a means of coping with relationship stresses that emerged. Interestingly, there was a tendency toward increased integration over 1 year in individuals who had *either* relatively negative partners *or* relatively high relationship conflict, *but not both*. Individuals whose partner negativity and relationship conflict were consistent (i.e., either low-low or high-high) tended to become more compartmentalized. Certainly, it makes sense that those whose perceptions (in terms of partner negativity) and experience (in terms of relationship conflict) were inconsistent would be those most likely to engage in the integrative struggle to resolve negative thoughts and feelings. Interestingly, only those who became integrative under conditions of low relationship conflict seem to have succeeded in their struggle. Increased integration under conditions of high conflict was associated with a high likelihood of the relationship ending. Those who experienced high partner negativity and high conflict may have felt that further effort and attention to problems and issues would be fruitless; their increased compartmentalization should have either isolated or accentuated negative attributes (depending on which compartments were perceived to be important). Conflict per se was less strongly associated with breakup in individuals who increased compartmentalization over time.

COGNITIVE MECHANISMS AND OUTCOME VARIABLES

The compartmentalization model illustrates how intrapersonal processes (here, the individual's knowledge structure for beliefs about the partner) affect interpersonal outcomes. The interpersonal outcome variables emphasized in the present research included feelings of liking and loving, as well as relationship status (ongoing or ended). The underlying mechanisms are presumed to be the fundamental cognitive processes of category activation and accessibility. Although associative network models increasingly seem out of date, they work well to explain the processing effects of these cognitive structures (e.g., Bower, 1981). Presumably, attributes that appear within the same conceptual category are more closely associated with each other than they are with attributes in other partner categories. When an everyday event activates either a category of the partner structure or an attribute within a category, all other closely linked attributes should come to mind. Thus, in integrative structures, positive and negative beliefs should frequently be activated together, and the salience of a negative attribute would not necessarily reduce the accessibility of relevant positive attributes. Moreover, it seems plausible that compartmentalized structures may not only reduce the accessibility of unwanted negative attributes, but may also ultimately make them unavailable, essentially excluding them from the partner concept. When an individual is motivated to see a partner's negative attributes as unimportant, compartmentalization should make them less accessible in the short term; if the compartmentalization succeeds, these negative attributes may be activated so infrequently that they are no longer part of the partner concept. However, this possible process has not yet been tested.

Because the present model focuses on the activation and accessibility of an individual's beliefs about the partner, the strongest predictions of this model should be for outcomes that are largely in the head of the perceiver, that is, the individual's feelings of liking or loving for his or her partner or, more generally, the individual's attitudes toward his or her partner. Although one would certainly expect the partner's feelings and behaviors or the partner's role in the relationship to influence an individual's liking and loving for the partner, it is also entirely plausible that an individual could have strong feelings of liking or loving for someone who did not reciprocate or encourage those feelings in any way. Other relationship variables, such as relationship status, or even measures of relationship quality or satisfaction or closeness, would seem to be more heavily influenced by the partner's attitudes and behaviors (i.e., by the relationship itself). Thus the way an individual organizes beliefs about the partner could potentially maintain feelings of liking and loving even after the partner has ended the relationship.

Another important outcome in the head of the perceiver is the attributions made for partner behavior. Showers and Kevlyn (1999) found that in older relationships, integrative organization for relatively negative partners was associated with more benign attributions for hypothetical bad behaviors. In contrast, when relationships were newer or "older" partners were perceived positively, compartmentalization of partner beliefs was associated with more positive attributions. The latter results fit well with findings that, under conditions of high trust, communication about negative "noise" in a relationship is not necessary to avoid detrimental effects (see Van Lange, Chapter 10, this volume); in the case of "older" negative partners, the integrative style may reflect an internal dialogue whose function parallels that of overt communication with the partner about negative noise.

Despite strong effects for intrapersonal outcome variables, the fact that the intrapersonal variable of partner structure does predict an interpersonal outcome like relationship status suggests that an individual's partner structure reflects more than just the individual's perceptions of the partner and the individual's strategies for dealing with the relationship. To some extent, these structures must reflect characteristics of the relationship as well as the partner's behaviors and feelings.

OTHER INTRAPERSONAL PROCESSES: SELF-STRUCTURE

In the present chapter, we have emphasized the structure of partner knowledge and change in that structure as the intrapersonal processes of interest. But there are other closely related intrapersonal process variables that should be considered in future research. For example, it is important to consider how the organization of *self-knowledge* is associated with interpersonal outcomes. In the present studies, effects related to partner structure persisted even when self-structure was taken into account (Showers & Kevlyn, 1999). However, the links between self-structure and partner structure are not well understood. One possibility is that individuals tend to apply the organizational framework they use for the self-concept to the organization of partner knowledge. For example, an individual who is not willing to make the effort to integrate self-knowledge is not likely to employ an integrative approach for relationship partners. Alternatively, if specific structures are selected because they serve important goals, there is every reason to believe that goals pertaining to the self (e.g., to self-enhance) may be quite independent of goals related to a partner (e.g., to distance oneself from a problematic partner), and therefore the most appropriate structures would not be the same.

DIRECTIONS OF CAUSALITY

Although the discussion so far has largely assumed that the structure of partner knowledge has a causal impact on an individual's feelings or relationship outcomes, we indicated at the outset that these structures may simply reflect an individual's strategies for coping with a partner's negative attributes, and, if so, then these structures could in fact be epiphenomena. It is also possible that the current state of the relationship itself may determine the choice of strategy or the organizing structure. For example, an emotionally intimate and satisfying relationship may motivate the search for a positive interpretation of a partner's bad behavior, resulting in an associative link between the bad behavior and an ameliorating positive attribute, which in turn is available and accessible at the next activation of that category of behavior. That is, because the relationship is satisfying, the individual may be willing to make the effort to use an integrative structure to maintain the most positive view of his or her partner that is possible. The failure to integrate in times of relationship stress may sometimes reflect a lack of commitment. In less emotionally intimate relationships (e.g., casually dating couples) or chronically unhappy pairs, individuals may also be content to live with their partners' negative attributes, or they may try to deny the importance of these negative attributes altogether. Their modest relationship goals may lead them to choose easier (and perhaps more efficient) compartmentalized structures.

In the present study, partner structures assessed at time 1 predicted relationship status 1 year later, after controlling for relationship variables at time 1 (Showers & Zeigler-Hill, 2004). This suggests that these structures are stable enough to correspond to long-term outcomes. It also suggests that they are not constructed on the spot to reflect the outcome. In the case of self-knowledge, multiple studies have shown that initial assessments of self-structure predicted reactions to events that took place at least 1 week later (e.g., Showers & Kling, 1996; Showers, Niedenthal, & Nugier, 2002; Zeigler-Hill, 2004). However, this kind of evidence clearly does not preclude the possibility that the organizational structure primarily reflects behavior, feelings, or coping strategies rather than serving as an instrumental cause of them via mechanisms of activation and accessibility.

IMPLICATIONS AND FUTURE DIRECTIONS

Increasingly, it is evident that the valence of beliefs alone may not be adequate to predict an individual's feelings about a partner or subsequent relationship outcomes. A focus on the structure of partner knowledge takes us beyond the mere perception of the *content* of an individual's experience to a perspective that emphasizes the *active construction* of that experience (Cantor, 1990; Mischel, 1973). The content of beliefs about a partner are surely sometimes biased. However, considering the role of structure allows for the possibility that the content of beliefs may often be a relatively accurate reflection of one's experience of a partner, and that it is often organizational factors that introduce an individual's own interpretations and perspectives.

More specifically, a focus on partner structure highlights motivational influences, especially if the type of organization is chosen because it serves an individual's relationship goals. An individual's partner structure likely corresponds to a cognitive strategy for achieving those goals. Thus compartmentalized structures may serve goals of simplifying judgments and decisions about a partner, or enhancing attitudes toward the partner without regard for accuracy. In contrast, integrative structures may serve goals of accuracy in representing aspects of the partner, in which it is more important to the individual that the partner is predictable and well understood instead of merely seen as positive. Integrative structures may also be employed by individuals who would rather be constantly aware of a partner's negative characteristics than be "surprised" by them in times of stress. Other structural features that have been identified in the self literature such as self-complexity (Linville, 1985, 1987), self-clarity (Campbell, 1990), and differential importance (Pelham & Swann, 1989) may also correspond to ways of thinking (cognitive strategies) that can be applied to interpersonal contexts (cf. Showers & Zeigler-Hill, 2003).

The focus on structure of partner knowledge also highlights the choices that individuals have in responding to the content of the experiences that present themselves. The same experiential content, organized differently, can map onto very distinct outcomes. For example, when a partner engages in negative behaviors (e.g., failing to show up for a date), compartmentalized individuals may suddenly be overwhelmed with negative feelings toward the partner. For these individuals, the partner's negative behavior activates only other negative feelings and memories of the partner. For some, this sudden fluctuation in feelings toward the partner may motivate them to end the relationship. In contrast, integrative individuals should have more stable feelings about their relationship partners (cf. Zeigler-Hill, 2004). Although they may be disappointed when their partner forgets a date, they may easily be able to recall other positive characteristics of the partner, thereby maintaining their optimism and trust in the relationship. The accessibility of these positive beliefs should influence reactions to the partner's negative behaviors (e.g., their willingness to discuss the incident or their commitment to staying together).

The present work also highlights the possibility that people have the flexibility to alter the type of organizational structure they use in response to stress or to serve an immediate goal. In particular, when faced with a partner's negative characteristics or behaviors, compartmentalized individuals who are motivated to maintain their relationship and their positive views of their partners may show the flexibility needed to switch to an integrative style (cf. McMahon, Showers, Rieder, Abramson, & Hogan, 2003; Showers & Zeigler-Hill, 2004). Such individuals may routinely rely on compartmentalized structures, but when faced with a partner's negative traits they begin to link these traits to positive ones.

Finally, by applying the model of evaluative organization of self-knowledge to interpersonal relationships, the cognitive processes of compartmentalization and integration can be examined in a broader context. Unlike self-descriptions, which may be heavy laden with motives to self-enhance (Sedikides, 1993), descriptions of relationship partners may be driven by a variety of goals including relationship maintenance, relationship enhancement, or relationship dissolution. Moreover, although partner descriptions generally tend to be more positive than self-descriptions (Showers & Kevlyn, 1999), some partners may be viewed as basically bad, providing an interesting challenge for structural strategies. The study of interpersonal relationships also offers an interesting array of outcomes beyond global feelings about a partner, such as relationship satus (ongoing or ended) or various dimensions of relationship quality (e.g., preferred level of intimacy or behavioral closeness).

Future research might apply the present structural model to an even wider range of interpersonal relationships, such as family or workplace relationships. Unlike romantic relationships, these relationships are often involuntary and may involve important status differences. They also often cannot be voluntarily dissolved. For example, compartmentalization and integration may be useful in understanding how adult children manage their relationships with abusive parents (cf. Showers, Zeigler-Hill, & Limke, in press). Relevant outcomes for these relationships might include variables such as a sense of interpersonal control, feelings of trust, or the emotional influence of the relationship partner. More generally, the examination of people's most important attachment relationships (e.g., with their early caregivers) may offer insight into the origins of preferred styles of organization and whether these partner structures correspond to attachment processes over the long term.

Future research could also apply the model of evaluative organization to an individual's beliefs about groups, especially groups that are vulnerable to stereotyping. Compartmentalization or integration of positive and negative beliefs about a stereotyped group may predict adherence to the stereotype and prejudicial attitudes. For example, it is possible that individuals who represent the characteristics of a stereotyped group in an integrative fashion would score lower on measures of explicit and implicit prejudice because they would be able to access both positive and negative characteristics of that group. In contrast, the process of subtyping (in which membership in a stereotyped group is acknowledged but not applied) may correspond to compartmentalization of the attributes associated with the negative stereotype.

Yet another direction for future research would focus on the importance of flexibility, especially structural flexibility, in perceptions of others. Showers and colleagues have suggested that the most adaptive strategy of self-organization is one that is flexible, and that developing structural flexibility may be an important component of psychological treatment and long-term well-being (Showers, Limke, & Zeigler-Hill, 2004; Showers & Zeigler-Hill, 2004). In the case of couples' relationships, flexibility in partner structure may be important for accommodating a partner's negative attributes in flexible ways, depending on the circumstances in which they arise. At times, compartmentalization of a partner's negative attributes may be advisable (e.g., so as not to confront relationship issues in times of external stress). However, appropriate and well-timed use of integrative thinking may be essential to a relationship's growth and long-term success.

CONCLUSIONS

Recent research on the structure of partner knowledge (Showers & Kevlyn, 1999; Showers & Zeigler-Hill, 2004) suggests that the model of evaluative organization of self-knowledge can be usefully applied to the study of interpersonal relationships. The structure of partner knowledge represents a set of intrapersonal processes that predict interpersonal outcomes. The present studies first examined current feelings about a relationship partner. When an individual's description of the partner was basically positive, compartmentalization was linked with greater liking and loving; when an individual's description was basically negative, integration was associated with more positive feelings toward the partner. However, after 1 year's time, positive compartmentalized individuals had the highest rate of breakup, suggesting that these individuals were vulnerable to shifts in the importance of the partner's negative characteristics. Interestingly, negative compartmentalized individuals seemed to have especially stable relationships, perhaps because compartmentalization allowed them to avoid a partner's important negative characteristics when there were extrinsic reasons for staying together. Integrative individuals generally tended to have ongoing relationships after 1 year's time, consistent with the view that this structure facilitates a realistic and resilient perspective on the partner and the relationship. Finally, change in partner structure was also observed. Integration increased under conditions of high relationship conflict or high partner negativity (but not both), a finding consistent with the view that integration reflects a struggle with negative attributes or events that are not well understood—a struggle that may or may not succeed.

In conclusion, a focus on the organization of partner knowledge offers new possibilities for research on interpersonal relationships. Future work might go on to explore the interrelatedness of self- and partner structures; the links between those intrapersonal processes and a broad range of interpersonal outcomes (e.g., trust, contact, closeness, or attachment); and, ultimately, whether structural flexibility is an important and desirable characteristic for individuals in close relationships.

REFERENCES

Bower, G. H. (1981). Mood and memory. *American Psychologist, 36,* 129–148.

Campbell, J. D. (1990). Self-esteem and clarity of the self-concept. *Journal of Personality and Social Psychology, 59,* 538–549.

Cantor, N. (1990). From thought to behavior: "Having" and "doing" in the study of personality and cognition. *American Psychologist, 45,* 735–750.

Cantor, N., & Kihlstrom, J. F. (1987). *Personality and social intelligence.* Englewood Cliffs, NJ: Prentice-Hall.

Kihlstrom, J. F., Beer, J. S., & Klein, S. B. (2003). Self and identity as memory. In M.

R. Leary & J. Tangney (Eds.), *Handbook of self and identity* (pp. 47–67). New York: Guilford Press.

Klein, S. B., Loftus, J., & Sherman, J. W. (1993). The role of summary and specific behavioral memories in trait judgments about the self. *Personality and Social Psychology Bulletin, 19,* 305–311.

Linville, P. W. (1985). Self-complexity and affective extremity: Don't put all of your eggs in one cognitive basket. *Social Cognition, 3,* 94–120.

Linville, P. W. (1987). Self-complexity as a cognitive buffer against stress-related illness and depression. *Journal of Personality and Social Psychology, 52,* 663–676.

Markus, H. (1977). Self-schemata and processing information about the self. *Journal of Personality and Social Psychology, 35,* 63–78.

McMahon, P. D., Showers, C. J., Rieder, S. L., Abramson, L. Y., & Hogan, M. E. (2003). Integrative thinking and flexibility in organization of self-knowledge. *Cognitive Therapy and Research, 27,* 167–184.

Mischel, W. (1973). Toward a cognitive social learning reconceptualization of personality. *Psychological Review, 80,* 252–253.

Niedenthal, P. M., Halberstadt, J. B., & Innes-Ker, A. H. (1999). Emotional response categorization. *Psychological Review, 106,* 337–361.

Osgood, C. E. (1969). On the whys and wherefores of E, P, and A. *Journal of Personality and Social Psychology, 12,* 194–199.

Pelham, B. W., & Swann, W. B. Jr. (1989). From self-conceptions to self-worth: On the sources and structure of global self-esteem. *Journal of Personality and Social Psychology, 57,* 672–680.

Rubin, Z. (1970). Measurement of romantic love. *Journal of Personality and Social Psychology, 16,* 265–273.

Sedikides, C. (1993). Assessment, enhancement, and verification determinants of the self-evaluation process. *Journal of Personality and Social Psychology, 65,* 317–338.

Showers, C. J. (1992a). Compartmentalization of positive and negative self-knowledge: Keeping bad apples out of the bunch. *Journal of Personality and Social Psychology, 62,* 1036–1049.

Showers, C. J. (1992b). Evaluatively integrative thinking about characteristics of the self. *Personality and Social Psychology Bulletin, 18,* 719–729.

Showers, C. J. (2002). Integration and compartmentalization: A model of self-structure and self-change. In D. Cervone & W. Mischel (Eds.), *Advances in personality science* (pp. 271–291). New York: Guilford Press.

Showers, C. J., Abramson, L. Y., & Hogan, M. E. (1998). The dynamic self: How the content and structure of the self-concept change with mood. *Journal of Personality and Social Psychology, 75,* 478–493.

Showers, C. J., & Kevlyn, S. B. (1999). Organization of knowledge about a relationship partner: Implications for liking and loving. *Journal of Personality and Social Psychology, 76,* 958–971.

Showers, C. J., & Kling, K. C. (1996). Organization of self-knowledge: Implications for recovery from sad mood. *Journal of Personality and Social Psychology, 70,* 578–590.

Showers, C. J., Limke, A., & Zeigler-Hill, V. (2004). Self-structure and self-change: Applications to psychological treatment. *Behavior Therapy, 35,* 167–184.

Showers, C. J., Niedenthal, P. M., & Nugier, A. (2002). Self-structure and the acquisition of self-knowledge. *Revue Internationale de Psychologie Sociale, 15*, 25–46.

Showers, C. J., & Zeigler-Hill, V. (2003). Organization of self-knowledge: Features, functions, and flexibility. In M. R. Leary & J. P. Tangney (Eds.), *Handbook of self and identity* (pp. 47–67). New York: Guilford Press.

Showers, C. J., & Zeigler-Hill, V. (2004). Organization of partner knowledge: Relationship outcomes and longitudinal change. *Personality and Social Psychology Bulletin, 30*, 1198–1207.

Showers, C. J., Zeigler-Hill, V., & Limke, A. (in press). Self-structure and childhood maltreatment: Successful compartmentalization and the struggle of integration. *Journal of Social and Clinical Psychology.*

Smith, E. E., & Medin, D. L. (1981). *Categories and concepts.* Cambridge, MA: MIT Press.

Zeigler-Hill, V. (2004). *Evaluative organization of self-knowledge: The hidden vulnerability of compartmentalization.* Unpublished doctoral dissertation, University of Oklahoma.

CHAPTER 10

From Altruism to Aggression

Understanding Social Interaction

PAUL A. M. VAN LANGE

What interpersonal orientations drive social interactions? Does selfishness underlie most of our behavior? Are we also inclined to benefit others? Are we naturally committed to sharing and pursuing equality? Do we tend to compete with others, even if we suffer from it by doing so? When and why do we aggress? Such questions are among the most fundamental to understanding interpersonal relations and group processes, which may explain why these topics have attracted the attention of so many scientists from so many fields and disciplines for so long. A complementary reason may be that the questions raised above touch upon the long-standing scientific debate about "human nature": Are people by nature good or bad?

Nothwithstanding the relevance of the debate about human nature, it took a long time before questions regarding human nature were studied empirically. In fact, it is only five to six decades ago that some influential books were written that systematically addressed such issues from a formal, mathematical perspective (Luce & Raiffa, 1957; Von Neuman & Morgenstern, 1944) and from a psychological perspective (Thibaut & Kelley, 1959). These books, and especially the empirical research that they inspired, have exerted an enormous influence on the science of interpersonal orientations. Two broad scientific benefits are especially important.

The first scientific benefit is that these analyses, and subsequent work, help us understand *situations*. That is, they helped us understand some basic features of situations and how they can be more or less "objectively" defined. For example, in classic games research, scientists were able to logically deduce around 96 situations from 2 × 2 matrices (which represented two persons each having two behavioral options). This work has led to an understanding that there are many kinds of conflicts in everyday life: conflicts between self-interest and collective interest, conflicts between self-interest and equality, conflicts between equality and collective interest, and so on. More recently, in the *Atlas of Interpersonal Situations* (Kelley et al., 2003) around 20 situations have been identified as essential, based on their relevance to social interactions in relationships. One situation that has attracted the interests of scientists working in various disciplines are social dilemmas, or conflicts between self-interest and collective interest. This situation is arguably important to understanding dilemmas in close relationships (e.g., whether to preemptively do the dishes), in relationships with colleagues (e.g., whether or not to prepare very well for a meeting, when it takes costly time to do so), and in our links with organizations or society at large (e.g., whether or not to engage in citizenship or volunteering activities to help others).

A second benefit is that these analyses, especially through later work by Kelley and Thibaut (1978), and Messick and McClintock (1968), helped us understand *interpersonal orientations* that are relevant to social situations. Indeed, various typologies of interpersonal orientations have been developed. This chapter reviews past research on social dilemmas and complementary situations to illustrate the potential importance of five relatively independent orientations: altruism, prosocial orientation (egalitarianism and cooperation), individualism, competition, and aggression. These orientations are essential to understanding what people make of situations—that is, how they construe situations. This inherently psychological process is essential to understanding how and why people behave and interact as they do.

BEYOND IMMEDIATE SELF-INTEREST:
TRANSFORMATION OF SITUATIONS

The notion that people go beyond direct self-interest is explicated in interdependence theory (Kelley & Thibaut, 1978), which makes a distinction between the *given matrix* and the *effective matrix*. The given matrix is largely based on "objective" outcomes derived from hedonic, self-interested preferences. Examples are "nonsocial" preferences regarding a particular activity, such as the desire to listen to music at high volume, the preference to watch one particular movie, or the costs derived from investing time and energy in cleaning the kitchen. As such, the given matrix summarizes the consequences of the individual's own actions and the partner's actions on the individual's outcomes. Interdependence theory assumes that the pursuit of direct immediate outcomes often provides an incomplete understanding of interpersonal behavior. There is indeed increasing evidence, some of which is discussed later, that an individual's preferences is solely based on consideration of his or her own outcomes. That is why this theory introduces the concept of *transformation of situations*, defined as a movement away from preferences of direct self-interest by attaching importance to longer term outcomes or outcomes of another person (or other persons, or groups). As a result of such broader considerations, the given matrix is transformed into an effective matrix, which is assumed to be more strongly linked to actual behavior. As such, this transformation concept is important to understanding why many people do turn down the volume while listening to their favorite music, why one occasionally does attend a movie that is not the movie that he or she most preferred to watch, or why many or most people do clean the kitchen. In the present chapter, I focus on "outcome transformations," whereby individuals take account of both their own outcomes and the outcomes of interaction partners.

The concept of outcome transformation is based in part on the literature on social value orientation (McClintock, 1972), which distinguishes among eight distinct preferences or orientations, including altruism, cooperation, individualism, competition, aggression, nihilism, masochism, and inferiority (I do not discuss the latter three orientations because they are very infrequently adopted). In this typology, *cooperation* is defined as the tendency to emphasize positive outcomes for self and other ("doing well together"). In contrast, *competition* is defined as the tendency to emphasize relative advantage over others ("doing better than others"), thereby assigning positive weight to outcomes for self and negative weight to outcomes for other. *Individualism* is defined as the tendency to maximize outcomes for self, with little or no regard for outcomes for other; *altruism* is defined as the tendency to maximize outcomes for other, with no or very little regard for outcomes for self. *Aggression* is defined as the tendency to minimize outcomes for other. These outcome transformations can be schematically represented by two dimensions, including (1) the importance (or weight) attached to outcomes for self, and (2) the importance (or weight) attached to outcomes for other (McClintock, 1972).

THE MYTH OF SELF-INTEREST

The notion of self-interest, later extended and termed the assumption of *rational self-interest*, has dominated much of the traditional theories relevant to interpersonal and intergroup behavior, including early formulations of game theory (Luce & Raiffa, 1957; Von Neuman & Morgenstern, 1944) and of social exchange theory (Blau, 1964; Homans, 1961; Thibaut & Kelley, 1959). This seems especially true for economic theory. As Gordon Tullock (1976), an influential economist and theorist on public goods, once said, "The average human being is about 95 percent selfish in the narrow sense of the term" (quoted in Mansbridge, 1990, p. 12). But within psychology too the assumption of rational self-interest is embedded in several key constructs, such as reinforcement, the pursuit of pleasure, utility maximization, as developed in the context of behavioristic theory (including social learning theory), psychoanalytic theory, and theories of social decision making. Moreover, many of the "self-enhancement" phenomena documented in social psychology tend to assume that people seek out material- or esteem-related outcomes for the self, often neglecting the power of considerations aimed at benefiting others. Although there is little doubt that people seek to construct realities in ways that serve to maintain or enhance a positive self-imagine (i.e., self-enhancement), it is also likely that similar tendencies are at work in describing close partners, friends, and other members belonging to one's own group (e.g., Murray & Holmes, 1993).

In the current chapter, we do not wish to discard self-interest as a powerful motivation. We do, however, maintain that self-interest tells only part of the story, not all of it. Also, we suggest that Tullock's 95% should be regarded as an overestimation. But why are we so confident that self-interest tells only part of the story? Why do we think that the term "the myth of self-interest," coined by Miller (1999), is in many respects more accurate than the term "rational self-interest?"

First, several researchers have addressed the fundamental issue of whether people may be willing to make a cooperative choice, in the absence of several (although not all) self-serving goals such as reputational, self-presentational, or reciprocal concerns. Specifically, researchers have designed prisoner's dilemma situations in which participants are strangers, make a single and anonymous choice for relatively large amounts of money, and interaction among participants is prevented before and after the experiment. These studies have revealed that under such conditions a substantial number of people make a cooperative choice (for a review, see Caporeal, Dawes, Orbell, & Van de Kragt, 1989).

Second, in a different program of research, it has been demonstrated that feelings of empathy provide a powerful motivation to make a cooperative choice in single-trial prisoner's dilemmas, even if the other had just made a noncooperative choice (Batson & Ahmad, 2001). That is, people who are informed about the misfortune of another person (e.g., partner has ended a relationship) and instructed to put themselves in his or her position (i.e., empathy instruction), tend to act in ways that cannot be understood in terms of self-interest (for an overview of earlier evidence, see Batson, 1998).

Third, the long-standing research on justice and fairness reveals that (at least some) people are often inclined to favor fair outcomes over self-enriching outcomes that represent inequality. A more recent phenomenon is the notion of altruistic punishment, the well-supported tendency for people to punish others (at a cost to themselves) who fail to cooperate and thereby undermine the "cooperative atmosphere" in a small group (Fehr & Gächter, 2002). This phenomenon too clearly shows that people are strongly motivated to pursue equality and to "do justice" to those who tend to exploit others.

Fourth, what is impressive about the lines of research described above is that considerations other than selfishness can be observed with relative strangers, with whom the subjects of experiments interact in a fairly abstract social dilemma task, often under completely anonymous conditions. Clearly, in the context of ongoing relationships, people should be quite prepared to engage in self-sacrificial acts, to "nurture," or to accommodate in an attempt to promote the well-being of family members, close partners, and friends (see Rusbult & Van Lange, 2003). Although such tendencies are not easy to isolate from long-term selfish interest in ongoing relationships (because there is a history and a future to the relationship), research on communal relationships suggests that prosocial behavior often may occur in the absence of "record keeping," or reciprocity in favors. That is, people tend to respond to variation in the other's needs, and less so (or not at all) to whether the partner has engaged in similar acts in the past (Clark & Mills, 1993). And the fact that people harbor exceedingly favorable views of close others is certainly consistent with the notion that the partner's ego is quite important to themselves as well (Murray & Holmes, 1993).

Last but not least, the long-standing program of research on social value orientation, to be discussed later, is strongly at odds with the view of self-interest. In fact, this program of research was initiated in part because early research on the prisoner's dilemma and the like revealed pronounced intra-individual consistency in tendencies toward cooperation or selfishness.

Thus various lines of research provide support for the notion that selfishness is not the only orientation that people adopt in interaction situations with others, whether close others or complete strangers. In this respect, we agree with recent insights that suggest that the importance of self-interest may be overstated. In their research on "the myth of self-interest," Miller and Ratner (1998; see also Ratner & Miller, 2001) demonstrated that participants overestimate the impact of financial rewards on their peers' willingness to donate blood, as well as the power of social rewards (as assessed by group membership) on their peers' attitudes. Also, research has revealed that people tend to assume that most others adopt an individualistic orientation to a prisoner's dilemma, believing that most others are simply seeking to enhance their own outcomes with no or very little regard for other's outcomes (Iedema & Poppe, 1994; Maki & McClintock, 1983).

Several mechanisms may support the myth of self-interest. For example, people are more likely to reciprocate noncooperation than to reciprocate cooperation. The implication is that a belief in the selfishness of others is more easily confirmed than a belief in the cooperative nature of others (Kelley &

Stahelski, 1970). Moreover, there are several specific mechanisms that support selfishness rather than cooperativeness. One example is the strong tendency for people to assign greater weight and attention to negative behaviors than to positive behaviors (e.g., Fiske, 1980; Skowronski & Carlston, 1989). Another mechanism derives from availability of information. Often, in the context of groups, what we can observe (noncooperative interaction) may actually be due to a few or even only one person, in that the cooperative intentions are (often) not visible. In other words, observable noncooperative behavior in groups may be due to the noncooperative intentions of only a few group members. Finally, at the societal level, the myth of self-interest tends to be supported in the media, which tends to focus more on the bad parts of human nature than on the good parts.

To conclude, we suggest that self-interest is a powerful motivation, but one that is often overestimated in strength. Such overestimation often is accompanied by a neglect of other important interpersonal orientations, to which we direct our attention next.

INTERPERSONAL ORIENTATIONS

We suggest that there are six important orientations that can be meaningfully distinguished. These orientations include altruism (enhancement of other's outcomes), cooperation (enhancement of joint outcomes), egalitarianism (enhancement of equality in outcomes), individualism (enhancement of own outcomes), competition (enhancement of relative advantage over others), and aggression (minimization of other's outcomes). We discuss each of these orientations in turn.

Altruism

The claim that altruism should be considered an interpersonal orientation is rather controversial. Indeed, as most readers know, there has been considerable debate about the existence of altruism both within and beyond psychology. Much of the controversy, however, deals with definitions of altruism, ranging from behavioral definitions (i.e., acts of costly helping are considered altruistic) to definitions that seek to exclude any possible mechanism that may be activated in some way by self-interest. If we limit our discussion for parsimony's sake to research on cooperation and competition, and to allocation measures, then we see that altruism is not very prominent. For example, in assessments of interpersonal orientations in a specific resource allocation task, the percentage of people who should be classified as altruistic (i.e., assigning no weight to their own outcomes while assigning substantial weight to others' outcomes) is close to zero (Liebrand & Van Run, 1985). Similarly, when people playing a single-choice prisoner's dilemma game observe that the other makes a noncooperative choice, the percentage of cooperation drops to 5% or less (Van Lange, 1999).

But this evidence should not be interpreted to indicate that altruism does not exist. In fact, what is more likely is that it does not exist under the (interpersonal) circumstances that are common in this tradition of research. People usually face a decision-making task—a social dilemma task, a resource allocation task, or a negotiation task—in which they are interdependent with a "relative stranger" with whom they share no history of social interaction or any other form of relationship. Accordingly, the experimental subjects have no basis for feelings of interpersonal attachment, sympathy, or relational commitment. We suggest that when such feelings are activated (in real life), altruism may very well exist.

As alluded to earlier, recent research by Batson and Ahmad (2001) provides convincing evidence. Specifically, they had participants play a single-trial prisoner's dilemma in which the other made the first choice. Before the social dilemma task, the other shared some personal information: her partner had just ended his relationship with her, and she finds it hard to think about anything else. Batson and Ahmad compared three conditions, one of which was a high empathy condition in which participants were asked to imagine and adopt the other person's perspective. The other conditions were either a low empathy condition, in which participants were instructed to take an objective perspective on the information shared by the other, or a condition in which no personal information was shared. After these instructions, participants were informed that the other made a noncooperative choice. Batson and Ahmad found that nearly half of the participants (45%) in the high empathy condition made a cooperative choice, while the percentages in the low empathy and control conditions were very low, as shown in earlier research (less than 5%, as in Van Lange [1999]). Hence this study provides a powerful demonstration of the power of empathy in activating choices that can be understood in terms of altruism, in that high empathy participants presumably assigned substantial weight to the outcomes for the other at the expense of their own outcomes.

The existence of altruism is also supported by earlier research that was designed to test the hypothesis that feelings of empathy could promote choices that benefit one particular individual in a group rather than the collective as a whole (Batson et al., 1995). Specifically, participants could choose to benefit themselves, the group, or other group members as individuals, which extends the dichotomy of self versus collective-as-a-group that is so common in social dilemma research. Using experimental manipulations of empathy (Study 1) and naturally occurring variation in empathy (Study 2), Batson et al. found that feelings of empathy created or enhanced the desire to benefit one particular other person in the group (i.e., the one for whom strong empathy was felt), thereby reducing tendencies toward benefiting the collective. This study indicates that, just as tendencies toward individualism may form a threat to collective well-being, so may tendencies toward benefiting specific others, or altruism, form a threat to collective well-being. That is, feelings of empathy may lead one to provide tremendous support to one particular person, thereby neglecting the well-being of the collective. For example, as noted by Batson and colleagues (1995, p. 621), an executive may retain an ineffective employee for whom he or she feels compassion to the detriment of the organization. We suggest that such tendencies toward altruism are likely to be observed when individuals deal with others with whom they have developed attachment, closeness, or sympathy.

Cooperation

A fair amount of research shows that the enhancement of joint outcomes, or cooperation, is an important consideration. People have a pronounced tendency to consider not only outcomes for themselves but also outcomes for others. The enhancement of joint outcomes may sometimes take the form of self-interest and assigning positive weight to others' outcomes (or doing no harm to others). But perhaps just as often, or more often, the enhancement of joint outcomes takes the form of enhancing outcomes for the group as a whole (a tendency sometimes referred to as "collectivism"; see Batson, 1994). In terms of decision rules, in both cases individuals tend to enhance joint outcomes (even though they may assign greater weight to outcomes for self than to outcomes for other).

Psychologically, the two types of cooperation are substantially different. The tendency to assign some positive weight to others' outcomes may be accompanied by a variety of mechanisms, such as wanting to act in line with the "no harm" principle (Batson, 1994), or adopting a norm of social responsibility, which dictates helping. The tendency to enhance group outcomes may readily be activated (e.g., at the very beginning of group formation), and is powerfully activated by identification with the group (e.g., Brewer & Kramer, 1986; Kramer & Brewer, 1984). To the extent that a person feels more strongly part of the group, or valued by the group, or derives self-definition and esteem from the group, that person is more likely to behave cooperatively. A classic case in point is research by Brewer and Kramer (1986), in which participants were categorized as psychology students (i.e., the actual participants, hence strong group identity) or economics students (i.e., weak group identity). Using a specific resource dilemma, Brewer and Kramer showed that under conditions of strong identity individuals were more likely to behave cooperatively when it was essential to the group (i.e., when the resources were near depletion). Such cooperative efforts were not observed when group identity was low. It has been suggested that under conditions of strong identity, there may be a blurring of the distinction between personal outcomes and collective outcomes—that is, "me" and "mine" becomes "we" and "ours," just as "we" and "ours" becomes "me" and "mine" (e.g., Van Vugt & Hart, 2004).

Egalitarianism

The existence of egalitarianism or equality may be derived from various lines of research. To begin with, several experiments have been conducted within the realm of resource-sharing tasks to examine the factors that may determine different "rules of fairness." In these tasks, a group of people shares a resource. The problem that these decision makers are confronted with is how to optimally use the resource without overusing it. Research by Allison and Messick (1990) provided a powerful demonstration of what happens in such situations. Their results showed that when participants (in a group of six people) are asked to harvest first from the common resource, people almost without exception used the equal division rule. Individuals tend to favor equality in outcomes (rather than more complicated rules of fairness; for related evidence, see Van Dijk & Wilke, 2000). Allison and Messick suggested that equality represents a decision heuristic that has the advantages of being simple, efficient, and fair. As such, equality has great potential to promote the quality and effectiveness of interpersonal relationships, and therefore can be considered as a "decision rule" that is deeply rooted in people's orientations toward others (see also Deutsch, 1975; Grzelak, 1982; Knight & Dubro, 1984).

Another powerful illustration of equality in interdependence situations is when people have to negotiate allocations (e.g., how to allocate monetary outcomes). This problem is often addressed in research on ultimatum games, an exceedingly popular paradigm in experimental economics (see Güth, Schmittberger, & Schwarze, 1982). In this negotiation setting, two players have to decide on how to distribute a certain amount of money. One of the players, the allocator, offers a proportion of the money to the other player, the recipient. If the recipient accepts, the money will be distributed in agreement with the allocator's offer. If the recipient rejects the offer, both players get nothing. Some of the first studies using this research paradigm demonstrated that allocators generally proposed an equal distribution (i.e., a 50–50 split) of the money (for an overview, see Camerer & Thaler, 1995). Subsequent studies, however, wondered whether this was true fairness and argued that allocators may have acted out of fear that recipients would reject their offer. Recent evidence suggests that at least some people do persist in employing the equality rule in ultimatum games, even when recipients can be cheated or when recipients hardly have any power over the decision to reject the offer (see Van Dijk, De Cremer, & Handgraaf, 2004). Again, equality seems to be an orientation that people carry with them when engaging in social interactions.

Although equality is in the eye of many the prime example of fairness, we already noted that fairness might also take different forms independent of outcomes. More precisely, allocating outcomes is always accompanied by procedures guiding allocation decisions (Thibaut & Walker, 1975). People also wonder about how fair these procedures are, and these perceptions in turn also have strong effects on people's behaviors and experiences in social relationships (De Cremer & Tyler, 2005). The focus on procedural fairness was further inspired by research showing that when people are asked to talk about their personal experiences of injustice they are usually found to talk primarily about procedural issues, in particular about being treated with a lack of dignity and politeness when dealing with others (e.g., Messick, Bloom, Boldizar, & Samuelson, 1985; Mikula, Petri, & Tanzer, 1990).

Moreover, there is research revealing that the opportunity for "voice" (i.e., being asked to give your opinion) may convey strong surplus value, in that people feel more strongly valued and respected. Voice also means that people are given an opportunity to express their values (i.e., "value-expressive" worth). For example, research shows that people still rated a procedure to be fairer if they had voice than if they lacked voice, even if they estimated that what they said had little or no influence on the decisions made and, as such, on the outcomes that they would experience (Tyler, Rasinski, & Spodick, 1985).

An important field study by Tyler and Degoey (1995) examined people's perceptions of the fairness of the legal authorities in California and their sense of identification with their state. At the time of their study, California was plagued by a severe drought and as such people had to try to maintain water resources, a situation that resembles a social dilemma. Results revealed that perceptions of procedural fairness (i.e., how accurate, ethical, neutral, consistent, and participative they perceived the procedures enacted by the authorities to be) significantly influenced people's willingness to save and maintain water resources. This was especially true when they exhibited a strong sense of identification with the community. High identifiers particularly cared about the fairness of the procedures because this indicated to them that they were valued society members and as such were treated with respect (Tyler & Lind, 1992). More recent research supports the notion that procedural fairness (examined by the availability of voice or not) often is used as a cue or heuristic as to whether "authority" is to be trusted. In fact, Lind (2001, p. 65) notes that "people use overall impressions of fair treatment as a surrogate for interpersonal trust" (for empirical evidence, see Van den Bos, Wilke, & Lind, 1998).

To conclude, egalitarianism has received attention in distinct literatures, often supporting the notion that equality in outcomes and treatment is deeply rooted in our system, in that equality often serves as the norm as well as a heuristic for our own actions and our expectations regarding others' actions.

Competition

There is also strong evidence in support of competition as an orientation quite distinct from self-interest. As noted earlier, work by Messick and McClintock (1968) has inspired considerable research that reveals that not only cooperative orientations but also competitive orientations may underlie social interactions. For example, Kuhlman and Marshello (1975) have demonstrated that individuals with cooperative orientations do not tend to exploit others who exhibit cooperation at every interaction situation, irrespective of the individual's own behavior. They also showed that individuals with competitive orientations do not exhibit cooperation, even if cooperative behavior rather than noncooperative behavior best serves their own personal outcomes. This can be illustrated by research examining the effects of the partner pursuing Tit-for-Tat—a strictly reciprocal strategy that begins with a cooperative choice and subsequently makes the same choice as the other did in the previous interaction situation (Axelrod, 1984; Gallucci & Perugini, 2003; Van Lange, 1999). Even when one is interested in enhancing outcomes for themselves only, then it makes sense to cooperate with Tit-for-Tat. Cooperative choices yield mutual cooperation (good outcomes), whereas noncooperative choices yield mutual noncooperation (less good outcomes). Interestingly, unlike individualists who do respond cooperatively, competitors do not tend to behave cooperatively in response to a Tit-for-Tat strategy. The plausible reason is that competitors do not seek to enhance their own outcomes in an absolute sense—they seek to maximize the gain (or minimize the losses) *relative* to the other person.

The importance of competition is even more directly shown in research on a decision-making task that represents a conflict between cooperation and individualism (Option A) and competition (Option B). Hence, the only reason to choose Option B is to receive better outcomes (or less worse outcomes) than the other, even though one could do better for oneself by choosing Option A. Research using this Maximizing Difference Game has revealed that quite a few people choose the competitive alternative; it is also of some interest to note that among some (young) age groups competitive tendencies tend to be even more pronounced (McClintock & Moskowitz, 1976). Specifically, among very young children (3 years old) individualistic orientation dominates, after which competition becomes more pronounced (4–5 years), which is then followed by cooperative ortientation (6–7 years).

Finally, one might wonder whether it is aversion to "getting behind" or the temptation of "getting ahead" that underlies such competition. In a very nice study by Messick and Thorngate (1967), it was shown that the former tendency (aversive competition) is much more pronounced than the latter tendency (appetitive competition)—in other words, not losing seems to be a stronger motivation than winning. This early research was later extended and generalized by Kahneman and Tversky's (1979) gain-and-loss frames in their prospect theory, and by Higgins's (1998) distinction between prevention and promotion focus as two distinct self-regulatory systems. Recent research has also revealed that under conditions of uncertainty, competition may be especially pronounced, presumably because people really want to make sure that they do not get less than others (Poppe & Valkenberg, 2003). Thus there is little doubt that competition is an important orientation that needs to be carefully distinguished from self-interest.

Aggression

The orientation of aggression has received very little attention in research on social dilemmas. It is interesting to note that, especially in comparison to the orientation of altruism, much research on aggression focuses on genetic and biological factors. Examples include twin studies and studies focusing on the association of aggression with hormonal activity, such as variations in levels of testosterone. Generally, this body of research supports the view that aggressiveness, examined by self-report methodology, is substantially "influenced" by genetic factors and biological makeup. For example, there is research showing that manipulations of levels of testosterone, varied as part of a treatment for sexual transformations, influence the proclivity to anger. There is an increase in the tendencies toward anger among individuals who transform from woman to man, and a decrease in such tendencies among individuals who transform from man to woman (Van Goozen, Frijda, & Van de Poll, 1995).

Importantly, the correlation between aggressiveness and testosterone is especially pronounced for scale items assessing aggressiveness in response to provocation (Olweus, 1979), suggesting that aggression needs to be considered in terms of anger that is interpersonally activated. Indeed, the methods typically used to study aggression consist of examining aggressiveness in response to provocation by another person. Hence, anger and aggressiveness should be easily aroused by others who fail to exhibit cooperative behavior. The fact that there is little systematic research on aggression in social dilemmas does not indicate that aggression is an unimportant orientation or motivation in the context of social dilemmas. We suspect that many or most of the readers who have conducted social dilemma experiments will immediately recognize not only the involvement but also the hostility described by Dawes, McTavish, and Shaklee (1977):

> One of the most significant aspects of this study, however, did not show up in the data analysis. It is the extreme seriousness with which subjects take the problems. Comments such as, "If you defect on the rest of us, you're going to live with it the rest of your life," were not at all uncommon. Nor was it unusual for people to wish to leave the experimental building by the back door, to claim that they

did not wish to see the "sons of bitches" who double-crossed them, to become extremely angry at other subjects, or to become tearful. (p. 7)

Because it is unlikely that aggression is a self-activated phenomenon in social dilemmas, people are unlikely to approach one another aggressively with the primary goal in mind to reduce the outcomes for other(s). As noted earlier, aggression may be activated when others fail to cooperate. This interpersonal basis of aggression is important, and suggests several interesting phenomena. For example, it may well be that tendencies toward aggression are most pronounced among those who do not expect others to behave selfishly. Kelley and Stahelski (1970) provide some evidence for what they referred to as *overassimilation*, the tendency for cooperative individuals (at least, some cooperative individuals) to behave eventually even more noncooperatively than the fairly noncooperative partner with whom they interact (see also Liebrand, Jansen, Rijken, & Suhre, 1986).

But why might people respond so aggressively to noncooperative behavior by another person? Is it only because other's noncooperative behavior provides one with much less good outcomes than other's cooperative behavior? We think not. In fact, it may well be strongly linked to a violation in equality of outcomes that often is created (and often perceived as intentionally created) by the other's noncooperative behavior. But then the question becomes "Why would people respond so aggressively to a violation of equality in outcomes?" Speculatively, three reasons seem especially noteworthy.

First, a violation of equality is generally easily observed. When comparing two outcome situations, it seems easier to compare both situations in terms of equality in outcomes than it is to compare them in terms of quality of joint outcomes (cf. Allison & Messick, 1990). Second, people often use social standards for evaluating the quality of their own outcomes (cf. Comparison Level; Kelley & Thibaut, 1978). In the context of a social dilemma, the social standard (or social comparison) is also salient (1) because typically people can "explain" any given outcome directly in terms of the other's behavior, and to some degree, the other's intentions; and (2) because individuals' own behavior, at least in part, may be guided by expectations regarding other's behavior (e.g., Kelley & Stahelski, 1970). Third, people are generally aversive to receiving less good outcomes than others. One is reminded here of classic research by Messick and Thorngate (1967), that revealed that aversive tendencies toward ensuring that the other does not attain greater outcomes than oneself are stronger than "appetitive" tendencies toward attaining greater outcomes for oneself. In most situations, a violation of equality caused by the other's noncooperative behavior may not only hinder or frustrate an individual's interaction goals, but also negatively influence a person's pride, honor, or self-esteem (i.e., two consequences that are likely to instigate anger; see Averill, 1982).

It is interesting that responses to aggressive acts (specifically, offenses) have recently received greater attention in studies on interpersonal forgiveness (e.g., Finkel, Rusbult, Hannon, Kumashiro, & Childs, 2002; McCullough, Worthington, & Rachal, 1997). In support of the notion that (aggressive) offenses often are violations of justice, it has been shown that forgiving is effectively promoted by a compensatory act or apology by the offender (McCullough et al., 1997). If such amends are not made, forgiving is less likely to happen, especially when justice concerns remain prominent. Such processes may lead to an inability to forgive, which in turn may challenge the quality of relationhips and undermine psychological well-being (Karremans, Van Lange, Ouwerkerk, & Kluwer, 2003). Aggression may also be a response to some form of misunderstanding—for example, when a given act is misinterpreted in terms of self-interest, neglect, or exploitation (see Van Lange, Ouwerkerk, & Tazelaar, 2002). Each of us can probably generate an example of a situation in which some unintended error (e.g., accidentally saying the wrong thing) led to aggressive responses, which in turn evoked relatively enduring interpersonal conflict.

Aggression is, of course, by no means confined to dyads or small groups. In large-scale social dilemmas, aggression, or at least subtle forms of aggression, may account for patterns of reactance, resistance, protest, and so on. Such aggression is often evoked by the behavior of specific group members, managers, or local and global authorities. Much research on large-scale social dilemmas has focused on individuals' willingness to contribute or cooperate, which may be regarded as a line of research that would benefit from greater attention for the opposite side of the coin: that is, examining the psychological aspects of individuals' readiness to aggress in subtle or more explicit ways. Also, the topic of forgiveness is, of course, of great relevance to resolving conflict between large groups. To conclude, it is surprising that aggression has received so little attention in social dilemmas, because—unless research suggest otherwise—aggression seems to be an important orientation in social dilemmas, albeit one that seems activated primarily by the behavior of others.

CONCLUDING COMMENTS

This chapter reviewed several conceptually independent orientations—altruism, cooperation, egalitarianism, individualism, competition, and aggression—providing good evidence in support of the existence of each of these orientations, thereby illuminating how and why they may affect behavior and interactions the way they do. We now turn to some issues for further discussion, theorizing, and speculation.

First, we begin by noting that the psychology of interpersonal orientations, while inherently social psychological, cuts across several shifts in the dominant theoretical paradigms of the past as well as integrates several fields of psychology—which is arguably important for any scientific topic to grow, bloom, and progress to yield cumulative knowledge (e.g., Kruglanski, 2006; Mischel, 2004; Van Lange, 2006). It is closely connected with almost any interpersonal process that is relevant to social interaction. The list is endlessly long, and is illustrated by (but by no means limited to) concepts such as altruism, generosity, fairness, equality, cooperation, forgiveness, sacrifice, trust, conflict, aggression, hostility, reactance, competition, suspicion, retaliation, and so on. Most of these topics are essential to understanding relationship processes underlying interactions among kin, friends, close partners, or colleagues, as well as group processes underlying interactions among members of teams, work units, interest groups, and even nations.

Second, the fact that the six orientations need to be distinguished from a theoretical perspective is not to imply that they are independent from an empirical perspective. In fact, there is good evidence in support of the so-called integrative model of interpersonal orientations (see Van Lange, 1999), which reveals that egalitarianism and cooperation tend to go hand in hand. Seeking good outcomes for all tends to be accompanied by seeking equality in outcomes, and vice versa. As such, there is good evidence to suggest a five-categorty typology of orientation, in which prosocial orientation represents cooperation *and* egalitarianism (for further evidence, see Van Lange et al., in press).

Third, there is good reason to believe that interpersonal orientations can be distally activated by interpersonal dispositions, relationship-specific variables, or broad social norms (Rusbult & Van Lange, 2003). For example, based on biological differences and histories of social interaction experiences, people may be more likely to apply one decision rule rather than another. For example, people who had a greater number of siblings (especially sisters) may be more likely to use a prosocial decision rule than an individualistic or a competitive one (see Van Lange, Otten, De Bruin, & Joireman, 1997). Interpersonal orientations should also be strongly shaped by relationship-specific variables, such as relationship differences in terms of commitment, attachment, or closeness. For example, in highly committed relationships, prosocial orientations and perhaps altruistic orientations should be more probable than individualistic orientations. The same may be argued for differences between communal and exchange relationships (Clark & Mills, 1993). Finally, social norms often prescribe specific rules such as the norm of social responsibility (e.g., helping the poor and the sick) or specific behavioral responses (e.g., the norm of reciprocity) that can be understood in terms of interpersonal orientations (e.g., equality).

Fourth, the orientations may have (unintentionally) been described in this chapter as if they are adopted and used in a conscious, well-reasoned, and rational manner. I hope not. In fact, there is good reason to believe that behavior that is guided by these motivational orientations is more often (than not) fairly habitual, a consequence of heuristic (vs. systematic) processing, and accompanied by reactions that tend to be "colored" by some emotion. Indeed, I used the concept of "interpersonal orientation" to convey, at least implicity, some regularity and stability, while at the same time acknowledging flexibility, especially in response to the situation and the behavior of others in that situation. In other words, interpersonal orientations are assumed to exert their effects by influencing cognitive and affective processes in social dilemmas, and giving rise to stable, pattern-contingent transformational tendencies (for an extended discussion, see Van Lange et al., in press).

Indeed, we wish to close by noting that interpersonal orientations are strongly guided by cognitions and affect, a topic that has not yet received much empirical attention. The theorizing regarding interpersonal orientations is most directly rooted in Kelley and Thibaut's (1978) *transformational analysis*, which assumes that individuals may, depending on their orientations, transform a given situation into "an effective situation" that guides behavior and interactions. Part of such transformation processes are the cognitions and emotions that may help individuals "to make sense" of situations—often in a goal-oriented (yet not necessarily conscious) manner. Social dilemmas, in particular, afford multiple and conflicting cognitions (for many, they are dilemmas) and emotions that may guide behavior, and that summarize interaction outcomes (the reader is reminded of the spontaneous comments by participants, reported by Dawes et al. [1977], and quoted earlier in this chapter). For example, people may interpret social dilemmas in terms of classic dimensions of judgment and impression formation, perceiving them in terms of moral evaluation, strength and weakness, intelligence, and the like (Osgood, Suci, & Tannenbaum, 1957; Rosenberg & Sedlak, 1972; Van Lange & Kuhlman, 1994). Also, the anticipation of experiencing guilt may prompt prosocial individuals to behave cooperatively, so as to avoid taking advantage of the other's cooperation, or to avoid being accused of such tendencies (Frank, 1988). It goes without saying that feelings of anger, disappointment, and regret may be experienced when the individual discovers that he or she is the only one who cooperated. Conversely, feelings of interpersonal liking, enjoyment, and gratification may be experienced when individuals have developed stable patterns of mutual cooperation. Indeed, as noted by Ketelaar (2004), cognitions and certainly emotions often "make sense" in that they serve to counteract tempting tendencies toward cheating, deception, and otherwise hurtful forms of "rational" self-interest. Thus situations characterized by conflicts between self-interest and collective interest may well be one of the key places where different interpersonal orientations, emotions, and cognitions are crucially important—after all, they are situations where the intrapersonal and the interpersonal really meet . . . and matter!

ACKNOWLEDGMENTS

This research was supported by Grant No. R-57-178 to Paul Van Lange from the Netherlands Organization of Scientific Research (NWO).

REFERENCES

Allison, S. T., & Messick, D. M. (1990). Social decision heuristics in the use of shared resources. *Journal of Behavioral Decision Making, 3,* 23–42.

Averill, J. R. (1982). *Anger and aggression: An essay on emotion.* New York: Springer.

Axelrod, R. (1984). *The evolution of cooperation.* New York: Basic Books.

Batson, C. D. (1994). Why act for the public good—4 answers. *Personality and Social Psychology Bulletin, 20,* 603–610.

Batson, C. D. (1998). Altruism and prosocial behavior. In D. T. Gilbert, S. T. Fiske, & G. Lindzey (Eds.), *The handbook of social psychology* (pp. 282–316). New York: McGraw-Hill.

Batson, C. D., & Ahmad, N. (2001). Empathy-induced altruism in a prisoner's dilemma: II. What if the target of empathy has defected? *European Journal of Social Psychology, 31,* 25–36.

Batson, C. D., Batson, J. G., Todd, R. M., Brummett, B. H., Shaw, L. L., & Aldeguer, C. M. R. (1995). Empathy and collective good: Caring for one of the others in a social dilemma. *Journal of Personality and Social Psychology, 68,* 619–631.

Blau, P. M. (1964). *Exchange and power in social life.* New York: Wiley.

Brewer, M. B., & Kramer, R. M. (1986). Choice behavior in social dilemmas: Effects of social identity, group size, and decision framing. *Journal of Personality and Social Psychology, 50,* 543–549.

Camerer, C., & Thaler, R. H. (1995). Anomalies: Ultimatums, dictators and manners. *Journal of Economic Perspectives, 9,* 209–219.

Caporael, L. R., Dawes, R. M., Orbell, J. M., & Van de Kragt, A. J. C. (1989). Selfishness examined: Cooperation in the absence of egoistic incentives. *Behavioral and Brain Sciences, 12,* 683–739.

Clark, M. S., & Mills, J. (1993). The difference between communal and exchange relationships: What it is and is not. *Personality and Social Psychology Bulletin, 19,* 684–691.

Dawes, R. M., McTavish, J., & Shaklee, H. (1977). Behavior, communication, and assumptions about other people's behavior in a commons dilemma situation. *Journal of Personality and Social Psychology, 35,* 1–11.

De Cremer, D., & Tyler, T. R. (2005). Managing group behavior: The interplay between procedural justice, sense of self, and cooperation. In M. Zanna (Ed.), *Advances in experimental social psychology* (Vol. 37, pp. 151–218). San Diego, CA: Academic Press.

Deutsch, M. (1975). Equity, equality, and need: What determines which value will be used as the basis of distributive justice? *Journal of Social Issues, 31,* 137–149.

Fehr, E., & Gächter, S. (2002). Altruistic punishment in humans. *Nature, 415,* 137–140.

Finkel, E. J., Rusbult, C. E., Hannon, P. A., Kumashiro, M., & Childs, N. M. (2002). Does commitment promote forgiveness of betrayal? *Journal of Personality and Social Psychology, 82,* 956–974.

Fiske, S. T. (1980). Attention and weight in person perception: The impact of negative and extreme behavior. *Journal of Personality and Social Psychology, 38,* 889–906.

Frank, R. H. (1988). *Passions within reason: The strategic role of the emotions.* New York: Norton.

Gallucci, M., & Perugini, M. (2003). Information seeking and reciprocity: A transformational analysis. *European Journal of Social Psychology, 33,* 473–495.

Grzelak, J. L. (1982). Preferences and cognitive processes in interdependence situations: A theoretical analysis of cooperation. In V. Derlage & J. Grzelak (Eds.), *Cooperation and helping behavior* (pp. 95–122). New York: Academic Press.

Güth, W., Schmittberger, R., & Schwarze, B. (1982). An experimental analysis of ultimatum games. *Journal of Economic Behavior and Organization, 3,* 367–388.

Higgins, E. T. (1998). Promotion and prevention: Regulatory focus as a motivational principle. In M. P. Zanna (Ed.), *Advances in experimental social psychology* (Vol. 30, pp. 1–46). New York: Academic Press.

Homans, G. C. (1961). *Social behavior: Its elementary forms.* New York: Harcourt, Brace & World.

Iedema, J., & Poppe, M. (1994). Effects of social value orientation on expecting and learning others' orientations. *European Journal of Social Psychology, 24,* 565–579.

Kahneman, D., & Tversky, A. (1979). Prospect theory: An analysis of decision under risk. *Econometrica, 47,* 263–292.

Karremans, J. C., Van Lange, P. A. M., Ouwerkerk, J. W., & Kluwer, E. S. (2003). When forgiving enhances psychological well-being: The role of interpersonal commitment. *Journal of Personality and Social Psychology, 84,* 1011–1026.

Kelley, H. H., Holmes, J. W., Kerr, N. L., Reis, H. T., Rusbult, C. E., & Van Lange, P. A. M. (2003). *An atlas of interpersonal situations.* New York: Cambridge University Press.

Kelley, H. H., & Stahelski, A. J. (1970). Social interaction basis of cooperators' and competitors' beliefs about others. *Journal of Personality and Social Psychology, 16,* 66–91.

Kelley, H. H., & Thibaut, J. W. (1978). *Interpersonal relations: A theory of interdependence.* New York: Wiley.

Ketelaar, T. (2004). Ancestral emotions, current decisions: Using evolutionary game theory to explore the role of emotions in decision making. In C. Crawford & C. Salmon (Eds.), *Evolutionary psychology, public policy, and personal decisions* (pp. 145–168). Mahwah, NJ: Erlbaum.

Knight, G. P., & Dubro, A. F. (1984). Cooperative, competitive, and individualistic social values: An individualized regression and clustering approach. *Journal of Personality and Social Psychology, 46,* 98–105.

Kramer, R. M., & Brewer, M. B. (1984). Effects of group identity on resource use in a simulated commons dilemma. *Journal of Personality and Social Psychology, 46,* 1044–1057.

Kruglanski, A. (2006). Theories as bridges. In P. A. M. Van Lange (Ed.), *Bridging social psychology: Benefits of transdisciplinary approaches*. Mahwah, NJ: Erlbaum.

Kuhlman, D. M., & Marshello, A. (1975). Individual differences in game motivation as moderators of preprogrammed strategic effects in prisoner's dilemma. *Journal of Personality and Social Psychology, 32,* 922–931.

Liebrand, W. B. G., Jansen, R. W. T. L., Rijken, V. M., & Suhre, C. J. M. (1986). Might over morality: Social values and the perception of other players in experimental games. *Journal of Experimental Social Psychology, 22,* 203–215.

Liebrand, W. B. G., & Van Run, G. J. (1985). The effects of social motives on behavior in social dilemmas in two cultures. *Journal of Experimental Social Psychology, 21,* 86–102.

Lind, E. A. (2001). Fairness heuristic theory: Justice judgments as pivotal cognitions in organizational relations. In J. Greenberg & R. Cropanzano (Eds.), *Advances in organizational justice* (pp. 56–88). Stanford, CA: Stanford University Press.

Luce, R. D., & Raiffa, H. (1957). *Games and decisions: Introduction and critical survey.* London: Wiley.

Maki, J. E., & McClintock, C. G. (1983). The accuracy of social value prediction: Actor and observer influences. *Journal of Personality and Social Psychology, 45,* 829–838.

Mansbridge, J. J. (1990). *Beyond self-interest.* Chicago: University of Chicago Press.

McClintock, C. G. (1972). Social motivation—a set of propositions. *Behavioral Science, 17,* 438–454.

McClintock, C. G., & Moskowitz, J. M. (1976). Children's preference for individualistic, cooperative, and competitive outcomes. *Journal of Personality and Social Psychology, 34,* 543–555.

McCullough, M. E., Worthington, E. L. Jr., & Rachal, K. C. (1997). Interpersonal forgiving in close relationships. *Journal of Personality and Social Psychology, 73,* 321–336.

Messick, D. M., Bloom, S., Boldizar, J. P., & Samuelson, C. D. (1985). Why we are fairer than others. *Journal of Experimental Social Psychology, 21,* 480–500.

Messick, D. M., & McClintock, C. G. (1968). Motivational bases of choice in experimental games. *Journal of Experimental Social Psychology, 4,* 1–25.

Messick, D. M., & Thorngate, W. B. (1967). Relative gain maximization in experimental games. *Journal of Experimental Social Psychology, 3,* 85–101.

Mikula, G., Petri, B., & Tanzer, N. K. (1990). What people regard as unjust: Types and structures of everyday experiences of injustice. *European Journal of Social Psychology, 20,* 133–149.

Miller, D. T. (1999). The norm of self-interest. *American Psychologist, 54,* 1053–1060.

Miller, D. T., & Ratner, R. K. (1998). The disparity between the actual and assumed power of self-interest. *Journal of Personality and Social Psychology, 74,* 53–62.

Mischel, W. (2004). Toward an integrative science of the person. *Annual Review of Psychology, 55,* 1–22.

Murray, S. L., & Holmes, J. G. (1993). Seeing virtues as faults: Negativity and the transformation of interpersonal narratives in close relationships. *Journal of Personality and Social Psychology, 65,* 707–722.

Olweus, D. (1979). Stability of aggression patterns in males: A review. *Psychological Bulletin, 86,* 852–875.

Osgood, C. E., Suci, G. J., & Tannenbaum, P. H. (1957). *The measurement of meaning.* Urbana: University of Illinois Press.

Poppe, M., & Valkenberg, H. (2003). Effects of gain versus loss and certain versus probable outcomes on social value orientations. *European Journal of Social Psychology, 33,* 331–337.

Ratner, R., & Miller, D. T. (2001). The norm of self-interest and its effects on social action. *Journal of Personality and Social Psychology, 81,* 5–16.

Rosenberg, S., & Sedlak, A. (1972). Structural representations of implicit personality theory. In L. Berkowitz (Ed.), *Advances in experimental social psychology* (Vol. 6, pp. 235–297). San Diego, CA: Academic Press.

Rusbult, C. E., & Van Lange, P. A. M. (2003). Interdependence, interaction, and relationships. *Annual Review of Psychology, 54,* 351–375.

Skowronski, J. J., & Carlston, D. E. (1989). Negativity and extremity biases in impression formation: A review of explanations. *Psychological Bulletin, 105,* 131–142.

Thibaut, J. W., & Kelley, H. H. (1959). *The social psychology of groups.* New York: Wiley.

Thibaut, J. W., & Walker, L. (1975). *Procedural justice: A psychological analysis.* Hillsdale, NJ: Erlbaum.

Tullock, G. (1976). *The vote motive.* London: Institute for Economic Affairs.

Tyler, T. R., & Degoey, P. (1995). Collective restraint in social dilemmas: Procedural justice and social identification effects on support for authorities. *Journal of Personality and Social Psychology, 69,* 482–497.

Tyler, T. R., & Lind, E. A. (1992). A relational model of authority in groups. In M. Zanna (Ed.), *Advances in experimental social psychology* (Vol. 25, pp. 115–191). New York: Academic Press.

Tyler, T. R., Rasinski, K., & Spodick, N. (1985). The influence of voice on satisfaction with leaders: Exploring the meaning of process control. *Journal of Personality and Social Psychology, 48,* 72–81.

Van den Bos, K., Wilke, H. A. M., & Lind, E. A. (1998). When do we need procedural fairness?: The role of trust in authority. *Journal of Personality and Social Psychology, 75,* 1449–1458.

Van Dijk, E., De Cremer, D., & Handgraaf, M. (2004). Social value orientations and the strategic use of fairness in ultimatum bargaining. *Journal of Experimental Social Psychology, 40,* 697–707.

Van Dijk, E., & Wilke, H. (2000). Decision-induced focusing in social dilemmas: Give-some, keep-some, take-some and leave-some dilemmas. *Journal of Personality and Social Psychology, 78,* 92–104.

Van Goozen, S. H. M., Frijda, N. H., & Van de Poll, N. E. (1995). Anger and aggression during role playing: Gender differences between hormonally treated male and female transexuals and controls. *Aggressive Behavior, 21,* 257–273.

Van Lange, P. A. M. (Ed.) (2006). *Bridging social psychology: Benefits of transdisciplinary approaches.* Mahwah, NJ: Erlbaum.

Van Lange, P. A. M. (1999). The pursuit of joint outcomes and equality in outcomes: An integrative model of social value orientation. *Journal of Personality and Social Psychology, 77,* 337–349.

Van Lange, P. A. M., & Kuhlman, D. M. (1994). Social value orientations and impressions of a partner's honesty and intelligence: A test of the might versus morality effect. *Journal of Personality and Social Psychology, 67,* 126–141.

Van Lange, P. A. M., Otten, W., De Bruin, E. N. M., & Joireman, J. A. (1997). Development of prosocial, individualistic, and competitive orientations: Theory and preliminary evidence. *Journal of Personality and Social Psychology, 73,* 733–746.

Van Lange, P. A. M., Ouwerkerk, J. W., & Tazelaar, M. J. A. (2002). How to overcome the detrimental effects of noise in social interaction: The benefits of generosity. *Journal of Personality and Social Psychology, 82,* 768–780.

Van Vugt, M., & Hart, C. M. (2004). Social identity as social glue: The origins of group loyalty. *Journal of Personality and Social Psychology, 86,* 585–598.

Van Vugt, M., & Van Lange, P. A. M. (in press). Psychological adaptations for prosocial behaviour: The altruism puzzle. In M. Schaller, D. Kenrick, & J. Simpson (Eds.), *Evolution and social psychology.* New York: Psychology Press.

Von Neuman, J., & Morgenstern, O. (1947). *Theory of games and economic behavior.* Princeton, NJ: Princeton University Press.

PART II
RELATIONSHIPS → SELF

INTERDEPENDENCE: OVERARCHING PERSPECTIVES

CHAPTER 11

A Functional, Evolutionary Analysis of the Impact of Interpersonal Events on Intrapersonal Self-Processes

MARK R. LEARY

From the beginning of scholarly discussions of the self, theorists have wrestled with how to explain the fact that intrapersonal processes involving self-awareness, self-evaluation, and identity are so intimately entwined with people's interpersonal behavior. Although James (1890) generally talked about the self as if it were an internal, psychological structure, his oft-quoted statement about a person having "as many social selves as there are individuals who recognize him and carry an image of him in their mind" (p. 179) hinted at a complex relationship between intrapersonal and interpersonal processes. However, James made little effort to explain how or why the self is so fundamentally interpersonal in nature. Cooley (1902) expressed the relationship between the inner self and the outer social world in his metaphor of the "looking-glass self," but he too sidestepped the question of why other people's perceptions and judgments of the individual come to be reflected in people's private self-conceptions. Later, Goffman (1959) tried to resolve the issue in a quite different way, denying the existence of the psychological self and suggesting that the so-called self actually resides in the eye of the beholder rather than in the psyche of the behaving individual. Not surprisingly, Goffman's notion that the self exists only in the minds of observers did not catch on among psychologists.

When the self returned as a popular topic in personality and social psychology in the 1980s, many theorists revisited this question by explicitly distinguishing the private (intrapersonal) self from the public (interpersonal) self. Greenwald and Breckler (1985), for example, suggested that the "public self" is sensitive to the evaluations of others and seeks to win approval, whereas the "private self" monitors and regulates the person's behavior with respect to his or her internal standards (see also Buss, 1980; Schlenker, 1985). Although this distinction between the private and the public self reflected a genuine difference between two separate processes, referring to both of them as "selves" (or even as aspects of the self) clouded the issue more than clarified it.

Most theorists concur that there is, in fact, only one self, and it is private. However they define it, most writers agree that the "self" is a psychological structure or process that is involved in attending to, thinking about, evaluating, and regulating the individual. In contrast, the so-called public self is not a self at all but rather a person's thoughts about his or her image in other people's eyes (or, sometimes, other people's image of him or her). Thus, James's (1890) claim that people have multiple selves is a bit misleading. It seems more accurate to say that people possess a single self but that they may perceive, evaluate, and present themselves differently depending upon the person with whom they are interacting.

Although previous discussions have offered important insights into ways in which inner self-processes relate to the outer social world, the relationship between the self and interpersonal behavior remains poorly understood. The goal of this chapter is to address the question of why interpersonal events have such strong effects on self processes by focusing on possible functions of the self. If we can ascertain why people have a self to begin with, we may better understand how and why the self is so strongly affected by interpersonal situations.

THE EVOLUTION OF THE SELF

One promising approach to understanding the relationship between a particular psychological process and some aspect of behavior is to consider the possible adaptive functions of the mechanisms involved. Biologists concur that understanding any animal's behavior requires consideration of the adaptive significance of the mechanism that undergirds and mediates that behavior. Specifically, how does that mechanism help the animal adapt to its environment? This approach does not maintain that all behavior is adaptive. Indeed, we must be very careful not to infer function where there is none. Yet, even when examining behavior that itself could not have evolved in its current form, understanding the platform on which that behavior is built may shed light on the behavior. For example, dogs did not evolve to interact with human beings, yet the pet dog that responds to its owner as if he or she were the alpha male of its pack is improvising on an evolved mechanism. Human beings likely do the same thing, and, if so, we might better understand particular human behaviors by asking what they evolved to do. Social and personality psychologists have typically not adopted this approach to understanding human social behavior, but it may lead us in fruitful directions (Buss, 1995).

Evolutionary psychologists argue that many psychological processes are built upon adaptations that facilitated individuals' ability to deal with their physical and social environments throughout the course of human evolution. In the case of navigating the physical world, all animals, including human beings, possess mechanisms that allow them to perceive and react to various opportunities and challenges in their environments (Pinker, 1997). In addition, social animals possess mechanisms that allow them to interact with other members of their species—for example, mechanisms that mediate behaviors involving mating, bonding, dominance, appeasement, and relations with kin.

As is well known, a few species of great apes show a rudimentary ability to self-reflect (e.g., they can recognize themselves in a mirror; Mitchell, 2003), but no other animal appears to be able to think about itself in the complex, symbolic, and abstract ways that are characteristic of human beings. Something noteworthy happened during human cognitive evolution that allowed human beings, and perhaps their hominid ancestors, to think consciously about themselves—that is, to possess a self. Thus considering the question of what the self evolved to do may help us understand its heavily interpersonal nature.

Three opinions exist regarding when the modern human self first emerged. One position is that the modern capacity for self-awareness was present in *Homo erectus* as long as 1.7 million years ago (Sedikides & Skowronski, 1997, 2002). Anthropologists and paleontologists agree that the appearance of *H. erectus* was associated with important changes in cognition and lifestyle (such as improved tools, the use of fire, and larger communities; see Donald, 1991), but it is less clear that *H. erectus* had a fully functioning self with the same capacities for abstract and symbolic self-thought as people have today. If the hominids who lived 1.7 million years ago possessed a fully modern self, they left no concrete evidence to indicate it (Leary & Buttermore, 2003).

The second position is that the modern self appeared much more recently (Leary & Buttermore, 2003). Only after the Middle–Upper Paleolithic transition, approximately 40,000–60,000 years ago, do we find archeological evidence to suggest that people then were essentially like modern human beings. Around this time we find the first evidence of culture (including indications of group-based identity), bodily adornment (indicating that people could think about how they were viewed by others and engaged in tactical self-presentation), long-range building and construction projects (reflecting an ability to imagine oneself in the distal future), major advances in tool-making technology (suggesting that people had greater foresight into how to design tools for particular uses), and belief in an afterlife (which presumably requires both an ability to imagine oneself in the future and to think about oneself in very abstract ways). After millions of years of living as intelligent apes, the hominids suddenly began to display evidence of abstract self-thought around 50,000 years ago.

The third position proposes that people were not fully self-aware until the last 3,000 years or so (Jaynes, 1976). Most experts dispute this possibility, although the evidence of a shift in consciousness or thought around 500 B.C.E. is intriguing. Something psychologically important did appear to occur in several ancient civilizations at the time of the "axial age" (Jaspers, 1953), but it does not appear to have been the appearance of self-awareness per se. As noted, evidence of self-awareness appears in the archeological record by at least 50,000 years ago (Leary & Buttermore, 2003).

In part, disagreements regarding the evolution of the self may stem from differing conceptualizations of "self" and "self-awareness." Importantly, the ability to think about oneself may not be a unitary cognitive ability. For example, being able to think about oneself in the future (what Neisser [1988] called the "extended self") may involve different cognitive abilities than introspecting on one's own feelings, goals, and thoughts (the "private self"), which in turn may involve different processes than conceptualizing and evaluating oneself in abstract, symbolic ways (the "conceptual" or "symbolic" self). Evidence suggests that these three self abilities may have evolved at different times (Leary & Buttermore, 2003).

Whichever date one prefers for the evolution of the self, a key question that may shed light on the link between self processes and interpersonal behavior involves why the capacity for self-awareness and self-evaluation evolved. Clearly, the ability to think consciously about oneself is beneficial and, in fact, self-awareness may be responsible for much of the wide gulf between the capacities of human beings and those of other animals today (Leary, 2004a). But what function did conscious self-thought initially serve? What was the primary adaptive benefit of thinking about and imagining oneself in one's own mind? Most speculations on this question have centered on one of two benefits of self-awareness.

First, the ability to think about oneself in temporal terms—for example, to remember the past and plan for the future—allowed people to capitalize on time. Animals live in the continual present, making behavioral decisions on a moment-by-moment basis, with no ability to contemplate the past or the future consciously. Even chimpanzees, who have a rudimentary ability to self-reflect, appear to be able to think only a few minutes into the future (Kohler, 1925). The evolution of self-awareness allowed prehistoric hominids to imagine themselves in the distant future, and thus to plan more than a few minutes ahead. Clearly, being able to think about oneself in the future provided considerable benefit because it permitted individuals to imagine consequences of their behavior, prepare for anticipated circumstances, avoid future dangers, and plan projects that required a long span of time to complete. Paleontological evidence suggests that the "extended-self ability" may have been one of the first aspects of self-awareness to appear (Leary & Buttermore, 2003). *Homo habilis*, which lived 2 million years ago, carried tools and tool-making materials over long distances, suggesting that they were able to imagine themselves using or making tools in the future (Potts, 1984). Certain other animals use tools, but they pick them up as needed and do not carry them around in anticipation of future need (Savage-Rumbaugh, 1994).

This ability to think about oneself in a temporal perspective may have also allowed people to control their own actions through volition—that is, to self-regulate. The behavior of self-less animals is determined by their biological predispositions, individual experiences, present environment, and current state, and they can not deliberately choose to behave in ways that are contrary to their natural inclinations. In contrast, human beings, partly because they can imagine themselves in the future, can often control their own behavior. Imagining possible future outcomes of various behaviors can serve as incentives that guide one's actions in the current situation.

The second possible adaptive benefit of self-awareness is a social one. Several theorists have suggested that the ability to introspect on one's thoughts, feelings, intentions, and other states—what some have called the "private self" (Neisser, 1988)—evolved to allow people to infer the mental states of others (see Humphrey, 1982, 1986; Lewis & Mitchell, 1994; Povinelli & Prince, 1998). Humphrey (1986), for example, proposed that self-reflection evolved because it permitted people to imagine what others were thinking and feeling. People can make inferences about other people only by extrapolating from their own experiences. We can infer how others feel in a particular situation because we can imagine how we would feel. We can infer others' intentions only because we can introspect on what our intentions would be if we were in the other person's place. Gallup's (1982, 1997) reproductive hypothesis makes essentially the same point, suggesting that self-awareness allowed people to cooperate and compete more effectively because they could think about others' thoughts, feelings, and intentions.

Several pieces of evidence support a link between self-awareness and the ability to infer others' perspectives. Developmentally, the ability to take other people's perspectives—for example, the ability to realize that another person's visual perspective on a scene differs from one's own, to infer others' emotions, and to imagine (and worry) about other people's judgments—emerge in children at about the same time as self-awareness (Kagan, 1998; Lewis & Brooks-Gunn, 1979). Likewise, the only other animals that show any evidence of being able to take others' perspectives are those that also demonstrate rudimentary self-awareness (de Waal, 1982; Whiten & Byrne, 1988). Further-more, experimental studies show that a momentary reduction or loss of self-awareness—deindividuation—is accompanied by a failure to monitor and react to other people's evaluations (Diener, 1980). Together, such evidence supports the idea that self-awareness is involved in making inferences about other people. Even if one dismisses the notion that self-awareness evolved specifically because it promoted the ability to get into the minds of other peo-ple, no one could doubt that the self is deeply involved in making interper-sonal inferences.

Taking this line of thinking a step further, we can ask what it is that peo-ple are interested in knowing about others—the primary social inferences they are likely to make about other individuals for which self-awareness is a necessary tool. Today we draw all sorts of inferences about other people, inferences about their intelligence, education, political attitudes, abilities, income, emotional states, religion, nationality, sexual orientation, intentions, mental stability, honesty, healthfulness, personality traits, and so on. How-ever, before the appearance of civilization, many of these characteristics did not exist (e.g., educational level, income, political affiliation) and others would have been irrelevant to survival and reproduction. Because evolution would not have selected for inferential abilities that did not enhance inclusive fit-ness, we are left with the question of the nature of the inferences for which the self might have evolved.

Evolutionary biologists and psychologists agree that mechanisms (often called "modules") evolve to handle very specific adaptive problems, although they may later be appropriated to deal with other issues as well (Samuels, 2000). If so, the module for private self-reflection would not have evolved sim-ply to allow people to get into other people's heads in a global, abstract way. Rather, it would have evolved initially to solve one particular type of interper-sonal problem with implications for survival and reproduction.

One could make the case for several candidates, but one promising possi-bility involves the notion that the private self evolved to draw inferences about other people's intentions toward the individual. Specifically, if we knew noth-ing else about another person, we would want to know whether that person intends to cause us harm or can be counted on as a source of help and support. Until that issue is resolved, interpersonal interaction can not easily proceed, and most other inferences about the other person are moot. This question would have been as important to our prehistoric ancestors as it is to us today, if not more so. If self-awareness (or at least certain facets of self-awareness) evolved to facilitate making inferences about others' intentions, then the self is inherently tied into mechanisms that monitor and respond to other people's likely reactions toward the individual.

Even before the appearance of self-awareness, social animals probably possessed some means for assessing, in an automatic and nonconscious fashion, the potential reactions of conspecifics. Although it may be too strong to suggest that animals infer one another's "intentions" per se, they do react to behavioral cues that reflect another animal's stance toward them—for example, whether the other appears to be friendly, agonistic, or dominant. For animals without the capacity for self-reflection, these inferences are neither consciously articulated nor tied to the perceiving animal's thoughts about itself. Yet self-less animals clearly possess mechanisms that attempt to gauge the reactions of other members of their species. Presumably, these mechanisms operate like those that monitor other kinds of threats and opportunities in an animal's environment—by eliciting contextually appropriate emotions and motives (i.e., action tendencies) when certain cues are detected. For example, cues indicating friendly affiliation in a conspecific seem to elicit calmness and approach, whereas those reflecting threat elicit fear and either withdrawal or attack.

Given that other species can monitor other individuals' reactions to them, it is reasonable to assume that early hominids possessed such an automatic mechanism even before the emergence of self-awareness. We must be careful at this point, however, because few other species display patterns of social behavior and relationships that resemble those of human beings, and thus do not possess monitoring systems quite like those of human beings. Chimpanzees resemble us in many ways, but their social structure is far more hierarchical than ours. Thus chimps may not provide a good model for thinking about interpersonal mechanisms in human beings. Bonobos—once called "pygmy chimpanzees"—come closer. Bonobos live in stable social groups consisting of multiple males and females, and their social structure is more egalitarian than that of common chimps, with individuals' status and dominance shifting as contexts change, much as it does among human beings. Furthermore, the sexes are more equal in status among bonobos, males participate in childcare, and males and females develop strong intersex bonds (de Waal & Lanting, 1997; Savage-Rumbaugh, 1994). Curiously, unlike other nonhuman primates (but like human beings), female bonobos are sexually receptive throughout their cycle, and bonobos are the only other mammal that mates face-to-face. Physically, bonobos also resemble early hominids such as Australopithecus more closely than chimpanzees do. My point is not that bonobos are like prehistoric human ancestors (although others have made this case; see Zihlman, Cronin, Cramer, & Sarich, 1978), but rather that they may provide a possible model for how human beings responded to one another before the appearance of full-blown self-awareness.

Like human beings, both common chimpanzees and bonobos are highly motivated to belong to social groups and likewise seem sensitive to being shunned or rejected (Gilbert & Trower, 1990; Gruter & Masters, 1986). Clearly, even animals with only a rudimentary ability for self-reflection are attuned to whether they are being accepted by others, and it seems likely that this characteristic would have been present in the common ancestor that chimpanzees, bonobos, and human beings shared approximately 6 million years ago. Thus, even before they were self-aware, our hominid ancestors likely possessed one or more mechanisms for monitoring others' reactions to them. Elsewhere, I have suggested that one of these mechanisms can be described as a "sociometer," a psychological mechanism that monitors and responds to cues that have implications for the degree to which the individual is likely to be accepted versus rejected by other people.

THE SOCIOMETER

Many theorists have stressed the importance of group living, interpersonal acceptance, and social support to the evolutionary success of the hominids. Human beings and their ancestors were too weak and vulnerable to fend for themselves and survived primarily because they lived in cooperative groups and provided one another with assistance and support (Barash, 1977; Buss, 1991). Social acceptance was literally vital for obtaining ongoing assistance and avoiding the isolation that might leave one vulnerable to predators, accident, or illness. In addition, interpersonal rejection often involves a significant threat in its own right. People are rarely harmed by those who value and accept them, but once one is rejected the likelihood of being harmed is much greater (Leary, Twenge, & Quinlivan, in press). Thus people are concerned about rejection not only because it leaves them without social support but also because it may portend callousness or, worse, malevolence on the part of others.

As a result of selection pressures that favored those who were accepted and integrated into a supportive group, human beings (and presumably their hominid ancestors) evolved a strong need to develop and maintain supportive relationships of various kinds (Baumeister & Leary, 1995), along with systems that monitor their social acceptance by other people (Leary & Baumeister, 2000; Tooby & Cosmides, 1996). At first, the sociometer would have operated nonconsciously and affectively, eliciting negative emotions when potential rejection was detected and motivating behaviors to deal with the threat. As Ford (1987) observed, "In both evolutionary and ontological terms, affective experiences precede the development of evaluative thought as regulatory processes" (p. 638). However, with the appearance of self-awareness—which, as discussed earlier, facilitates drawing inferences about others (Humphrey, 1982)—the sociometer became intimately linked to conscious self-related thought. Armed with the capacity to think consciously about themselves, human beings could contemplate other people's reactions to them.

Like other systems that detect and process threats of evolutionary significance (see McNally, 1987), the sociometer operates nonconsciously in "background mode" to monitor the social environment for cues that are relevant to one's relational value in other people's eyes. People detect indications that others are displeased with them automatically and easily even when they are not thinking consciously about others' reactions (Ohman, 1986). Poised, secure interaction may suddenly falter when a frown, look of boredom or disinterest, expression of displeasure, or indication of disapproval evokes a negative emotional response, induces an acute state of self-awareness, and leads the person to think consciously about his or her interpersonal predicament. Thus, in modern human beings, the sociometer involves both the primitive monitoring system (that operates automatically outside of awareness) and the more recent self system by which people think consciously about how others are responding to them.

Importantly, people think not only about how they are perceived and evaluated at the present time but also about their prospects for acceptance in the future (Leary & Baumeister, 2000). By using both the ability to think about their personal reactions to events (i.e., private-self ability) and the ability to think about themselves in the future (i.e., extended-self ability), people can think about how others are likely to respond to them in the future (Leary & Buttermore, 2003). Such an ability has obvious benefits for regulating one's behavior in ways that will lead others to respond as one desires.

As I have discussed elsewhere, the sociometer system that monitors social acceptance and rejection (or, more precisely, one's relational value) appears to be inextricably connected to self-esteem (for reviews, see Leary, 1999; Leary & Baumeister; 2000; Leary & MacDonald, 2003). Although theorists have traditionally viewed self-esteem as a personal evaluation of oneself that is based on a comparison of one's behavior or characteristics to one's personal standards, the evidence does not strongly support this intrapersonal perspective. Rather, what we call "self-esteem" seems to involve an assessment of one's relational value and acceptability in other people's eyes.

Research has repeatedly shown, for example, that perceived changes in interpersonal evaluations and social acceptance are accompanied by changes in state self-esteem. The kinds of events that most strongly affect self-esteem—failure, criticism, disapproval, moral lapses, and ostracism, for example—nearly always have real or potential implications for the degree to which people believe that others value and accept them (Leary, Cottrell, & Phillips, 2002; Leary, Haupt, Strausser, & Chokel, 1998; Leary, Tambor, Terdal, & Downs, 1995). Furthermore, the primary predictors of self-esteem—such as self-perceived competence, physical attractiveness, likeability, and possession of socially desirable attributes—are precisely those characteristics that connote high relational value to other people (MacDonald, Saltzman, & Leary, 2003). Put simply, state self-esteem seems to function as a gauge of social acceptance and rejection, providing people with feedback regarding their standing in other people's eyes (for reviews, see Leary, 1999,

2002, 2004b; Leary & Baumeister, 2000). Furthermore, individual differences in perceived acceptance are related to trait self-esteem (see Leary & MacDonald, 2003, for a review). A history of feeling that one is valued and accepted by other people leads to a dispositional tendency to see oneself as generally valuable and acceptable, and thus to high trait self-esteem.

When people think consciously about others' evaluations of them, they not only try to infer others' likely reactions but also to determine the source of those reactions. In judging how to respond to others' disinterest, disapproval, or devaluation, people need to know whether the other's reaction is in response to something about them or to other factors. Unfortunately, social feedback is often ambiguous and open to many interpretations. Is my partner ignoring me because she is unhappy with me or because she is distracted by stresses at work? Does the audience seem bored with my speech because I'm a bad speaker or because it's lunch time? Was I passed over for the promotion because I'm incompetent or because the boss was under pressure to promote someone else? People who perceive disinterest, disapproval, or displeasure often consider the possibility that something about their own behavior or characteristics is responsible for others' rejecting reactions, and, given the high degree of attributional ambiguity, they often can identify something about themselves that may have contributed to the other person's reaction.

Thus it is a small step from perceiving that one is being devalued or rejected to concluding that others' reactions are at least partly due to one's own actions or attributes. The result is a negatively tainted self-evaluation, experienced as lowered self-esteem. In contrast, when the self is not implicated in a rejection (e.g., when one is rejected at random or because of mistaken identity), people may be frustrated at losing whatever benefits might be associated with being accepted, but they do not experience a drop in self-esteem (Leary, Rice, & Schreindorfer, 2004; Leary, Tambor, et al., 1995).

As noted, traditional theories of self-esteem have conceptualized self-esteem as a person's private self-evaluation. However, theories that view self-esteem as only a private self-evaluation have a great deal of difficulty explaining why public events have a much greater impact on self-esteem than private events that are known only by the person (Leary & Baumeister, 2000). (Violations of one's personal standards should lower self-esteem whether or not other people know about them.) Furthermore, traditional theories of self-esteem have difficulty explaining why people's self-evaluations and self-related feelings are so strongly affected by social feedback. Several theorists have suggested that people whose self-esteem is influenced by other people's judgments possess inauthentic or contingent self-esteem or are dysfunctionally concerned with others' approval and acceptance (e.g., Deci & Ryan, 1995; May 1983). If so, however, we must conclude that virtually everyone—perhaps with the exception of those with sociopathic personalities—possesses unhealthy self-esteem. The effects of real, anticipated, and imagined rejection on self-esteem are so strong and pervasive that it seems inconceivable that the natural, healthy state is to be unaffected by others' judgments. In fact, even people who vehemently deny that their self-esteem is affected by disapproval and rejection nonetheless show decrements in self-esteem when they receive negative social feedback (Leary et al., 2003).

In contrast, sociometer theory easily explains why people's feelings about themselves are so strongly related to their perceptions of others' evaluations. In some ways, the term "self-esteem" may be a misnomer because self-esteem is not fundamentally about one's esteem for oneself. Rather, what we call "self-esteem" is an internal readout of one's relational value in others' eyes and, by implication, the degree to which one is likely to be accepted and supported by others. Certainly, people may overreact to disapproval and devaluation, but the sociometer seems designed to evoke negative affect and a careful examination of oneself when events occur that have implications for one's social acceptance.

THE SELF-ESTEEM MOTIVE

Psychologists have been interested in self-esteem for two primary reasons. The first is that high self-esteem seemed to hold promise for understanding personal adjustment and success. However, not only are the positive effects associated with self-esteem far less extensive than most people imagined (Baumeister, Campbell, Krueger, & Vohs, 2003), but the effects that do exist appear to be due to social acceptance rather than merely feeling good about oneself (Leary, 1999; Leary, Schreindorfer, & Haupt, 1995).

The second source of psychologists' widespread fascination with self-esteem is the fact that the need for self-esteem was touted as a fundamental and important motive that was responsible for a wide array of behavior. Many psychologists agreed with Markus's (1980) suggestion that the "notion that we will go to great lengths to protect our ego or preserve our self-esteem is . . . probably one of the great psychological truths" (p. 127). Behaviors as diverse as conformity, self-presentation, delinquency, eating disorders, attitude change, social comparison, self-serving attributions, risk-taking behavior, promiscuity, aggression, and prejudice have been attributed to people's efforts to bolster or protect their self-esteem.

The theoretical status of the self-esteem motive continues to be problematic, however. Most generally, it is not at all clear that people "need" self-esteem in any meaningful sense of the word. The concept of need implies not only that the individual is strongly motivated to pursue the outcome in question but also that his or her long-term well-being is compromised in important ways (that go beyond mere emotional distress) when deprived of it. Yet there is growing agreement that, although high self-esteem is associated with slightly more positive emotions than low self-esteem (by definition), evidence that self-esteem strongly relates to other positive behavioral and social outcomes is weak (Baumeister et al., 2003; Mecca, Smelser, & Vasconcellos, 1989). The data suggest that, if people do indeed need self-esteem, they don't need it very much.

Furthermore, the concept of need implies a fundamental motivational system that evolved because it facilitated inclusive fitness during the course of evolution. All species evolved in such a way that they need certain things to function optimally. Clearly, people need air, water, and certain nutrients, and probably also need certain psychological affordances such as belongingness (social isolation produces serious long-term physical and psychological dysfunctions). However, it is far less clear that the human nervous system evolved in a way that made people need to feel good about themselves. There is little question that people *prefer* to feel good rather than bad about themselves, but it is not clear that this preference is the result of an evolved need.

In fact, although holding very positive views of oneself is sometimes beneficial, particularly in terms of lowered emotional distress and persistence on difficult tasks (Baumeister et al., 2003; Leary, Schreindorfer, & Haupt, 1995), natural selection is unlikely to have favored animals whose cognitive systems were biased to make themselves feel better than they deserved to feel. If anything, evolution seems to have selected for animals that were threat-sensitive (and thus felt worse than they actually needed to feel) because underestimating threats is far more likely to be disastrous than overestimating them. As Festinger (1954) observed, "inaccurate appraisals of one's abilities can be punishing or even fatal in many situations" (p. 117). In contrast, most self-serving biases that have been attributed to the self-esteem motive involve overestimating one's capabilities and underestimating the threats that one faces. The general tendency for people to strive for self-esteem is very unlikely to have arisen as an evolutionary adaptation.

My claim that people do not have a need for self-esteem may seem to fly in the face of decades of research that has shown that people consistently show self-serving, egotistical biases in their perceptions of themselves and others. If people don't need self-esteem, why do they do this?

I offer two answers to this question. The first is that, as sociometer theory suggests, self-esteem seems to operate as a gauge of relational value or social acceptance. As people seek relational value, they may appear to be pursuing self-esteem but only because self-esteem is an indicator of their relational value. Thus, when people seem to feed their self-esteem through self-serving attributions, downward social comparisons, and other ego-defensive reactions, they are often engaging in behaviors that they believe will enhance their relational value in other people's eyes. Even in what seem to be nonrelational domains, such as achievement, people's outcomes have implications for other people's perceptions, evaluations, and acceptance of them, so spinning events in a self-serving way may have interpersonal benefits.

Elsewhere, I have suggested that the situation is analogous to filling one's car with gasoline (Leary & Downs, 1995). Although an observer from another planet who knew nothing about cars might conclude that a gas-pumping human was trying to move the fuel gauge from empty to full, we know that people stop at gas stations in order to fill their tanks and not just to make the fuel indicator move upward. Likewise, people do not seek self-esteem for its own sake but rather behave in ways that maintain social acceptance, which, if successful, increases their self-esteem because it is the gauge that reflects the contents of their interpersonal gas tank.

People also seek self-esteem for a secondary, hedonistic, and largely non-functional reason. Sometimes people simply try to feel good about themselves even in the absence of the interpersonal events that would normally produce positive self-feelings. Once human beings acquired the ability to think consciously about themselves, they could use this ability to manipulate information about themselves in their own minds. Often this self-related thinking is in the service of analyzing problems and one's capabilities to deal with them, but it can also be used to construe the state of affairs in ways that make the person feel better without actually confronting the problem. Unlike other animals, people can construe self-relevant information in ways that enhance positive affect and self-esteem in the absence of the environmental conditions that naturally evoke those reactions. So, for example, people may convince themselves that they are more successful, important, or likeable than they really are; make self-serving attributions for their behavior; or engage in downward social comparisons that make them feel better about themselves. In essence, they are using their sophisticated powers of self-cognition to create a mental world that is more to their liking than the real one. However, the goal is not to satisfy some "need" for self-esteem but simply to foster positive affect artificially.

Some critics of sociometer theory have suggested that the existence of these private, self-serving biases argues against the possibility that self-esteem is part of an evolved mechanism designed to detect threats to social acceptance. However, there are many instances in which people capitalize on mechanisms that originally evolved for an adaptive purpose simply to make themselves feel good. In such instances (which include drug use, eating nonnutritious but tasty food, and masturbation), people foster pleasure and satisfaction using mechanisms that developed to promote inclusive fitness but without satisfying the original purpose for which the mechanism evolved. The fact that people bolster their self-esteem cognitively, even in the absence of actual social acceptance, does not argue against the notion that the self-esteem system evolved to promote interpersonal acceptance anymore than the fact that people masturbate suggests that sexual pleasure did not originally evolve to promote reproduction.

CONCLUSIONS

A comprehensive review of the extensive literature on "the self," broadly construed, would likely reveal that most self-related processes—such as those reflected in constructs such as self-awareness, self-concept, self-schema, self-evaluation, self-esteem, self-verification, and so on—have typically been conceptualized in a decidedly nonsocial fashion. To be sure, these self-related phenomena have been theoretically and empirically connected to a wide array of interpersonal behaviors, yet most processes that involve self-awareness, self-representation, self-evaluation, and self-regulation have been construed in a decontextualized, purely psychological way. The implicit assumption seems to be that, as a cognitive structure or process, a person's self exists quite apart from the world in which the person lives, although we may certainly find many ways in which those self processes influence, and are influenced by, what happens in the person's social environment.

The approach taken in this chapter suggests that viewing the self as a psychological process without considering its interpersonal functions and origins may lead to an impoverished perspective on self processes. An evolutionary analysis suggests that the self is related to interpersonal behavior in part because certain aspects of the self evolved to monitor other people's thoughts and intentions vis-à-vis the individual. Prior to the emergence of self-awareness, hominids presumably monitored others' reactions to them in an automatic and nonconscious fashion, but they could not think consciously about how others perceived them or intentionally modify their behavior to evoke certain responses from others. However, after people could think consciously about themselves and their own internal experiences, they could think about other people's reactions to them. Thus people's perceptions of and feelings about themselves became inherently tied to their inferences about others' appraisals of them.

I should stress that the cognitive abilities that allow people to think about themselves through the eyes of other people do not capture everything that the self does. As noted earlier, what we call "the self" probably involves a number of distinct mental abilities, including the ability to think about oneself across time (extended-self ability), introspect on one's private states (private-self ability), and represent oneself in one's mind (and to others) in abstract, symbolic ways (conceptual-self ability) (see Leary & Buttermore, 2003; Neisser, 1988). Most of what I have said in this chapter primarily involves the ability to reflect on one's private states, and thus to extrapolate from one's own inner experience to inferences regarding what others are thinking, feeling, and intending with regard to oneself. These inferences also involve thinking about oneself over time ("She disliked me last week, but perhaps I can make a better impression next week.") and in a symbolic, conceptual fashion ("He thinks that I am rigid in my political views."), but at heart they require me to imagine how I would think, feel, or respond to me if I were someone else, with adjustments made for idiosyncratic reactions and situational influences. Even though not all self-thought is interpersonal, a great deal of it is, and an evolutionary analysis suggests why this is the case.

REFERENCES

Barash, D. P. (1977). *Sociobiology and behavior*. New York: Elsevier.

Baumeister, R. D., Campbell, J. D., Krueger, J. I., & Vohs, K. D. (2003). Does high self-esteem cause better performance, interpersonal success, happiness, or healthier lifestyles? *Psychological Science in the Public Interest, 4*, 1–44.

Baumeister, R. F., & Leary, M. R. (1995). The need to belong: Desire for interpersonal attachments as a fundamental human motivation. *Psychological Bulletin, 117*, 497–529.

Buss, A. H. (1980). *Self-consciousness and social anxiety*. San Francisco: Freeman.

Buss, D. M. (1991). Evolutionary personality psychology. *Annual Review of Psychology, 42*, 459–491.

Buss, D. M. (1995). Evolutionary psychology: A new paradigm for psychological science. *Psychological Inquiry, 6*, 1–49.

Cooley, C. H. (1902). *Human nature and the social order*. New York: Scribner.

Deci, E. L., & Ryan, R. M. (1995). Human agency: The basis for true self-esteem. In M. H. Kernis (Ed.), *Efficacy, agency, and self-esteem* (pp. 31–50). New York: Plenum Press.

de Waal, F. B. M. (1982). *Chimpanzee politics: Power and sex among apes*. New York: Harper & Row.

de Waal, F. B. M., & Lanting, F. (1997). *Bonobos: The forgotten ape*. Berkeley and Los Angeles: University of California Press.

Diener, E. (1980). Deindividuation: The absence of self-awareness and self-regulation in group members. In P. Paulus (Ed.), *The psychology of group influence*. Hillsdale, NJ: Erlbaum.

Donald, M. (1991). *Origins of the modern mind*. Cambridge, MA: Harvard University Press.

Festinger, L. (1954). A theory of social comparison processes. *Human Relations, 7*, 117–140.

Ford, D. H. (1987). *Humans as self-constructing living systems*. Hillsdale, NJ: Erlbaum.

Gallup, G. G. Jr. (1982). Self-awareness and the emergence of mind in primates. *American Journal of Primatology, 2*, 237–248.

Gallup, G. G. Jr. (1997). On the rise and fall of self-conception in primates. In J. G. Snodgrass & R. L. Thompson (Eds.), *The self across psychology* (pp. 73–82). New York: New York Academy of Sciences.

Gilbert, P., & Trower, P. (1990). The evolution and manifestation of social anxiety. In W. R. Crozier (Ed.), *Shyness and embarrassment* (pp. 144–177). New York: Cambridge University Press.

Goffman, E. (1959). *The presentation of self in everyday life*. Garden City, NY: Doubleday.

Greenwald, A. G., & Breckler, S. (1985). To whom is the self presented? In B. R. Schlenker (Ed.), *The self and social life* (pp. 126–145). New York: McGraw-Hill.

Gruter, M., & Masters, R. (1986). Ostracism as a social and biological phenomenon: An introduction. *Ethology and Sociobiology, 7*, 149–158.

Humphrey, N. (1982, August 19). Consciousness: A just-so story. *New Scientist*, pp. 474–477.

Humphrey, N. (1986). *The inner eye*. London: Faber & Faber.

James, W. (1890). *The principles of psychology*. New York: Dover Publications.

Jaspers, K. (1953). *Origin and goal of history*. New Haven, CT: Yale University Press.

Jaynes, J. (1976). *The origin of consciousness in the breakdown of the bicameral mind*. Boston: Houghton Mifflin.

Kagan, J. (1998). Is there a self in infancy? In M. Ferrari & R. J. Sternberg (Eds.), *Self-awareness: Its nature and development* (pp. 137–147). New York: Guilford Press.

Kohler, W. (1925). *The mentality of apes*. New York: Harcourt, Brace, & Co.

Leary, M. R. (1999). The social and psychological importance of self-esteem. In R. M. Kowalski & M. R. Leary (Eds.), *The social psychology of emotional and behavioral problems: Interfaces of social and clinical psychology* (pp. 197–221). Washington, DC: American Psychological Association.

Leary, M. R. (2002). The interpersonal basis of self-esteem: Death, devaluation, or deference? In J. Forgas & K. D. Williams (Eds.), *The social self: Cognitive, interpersonal, and intergroup perspectives* (pp. 143–159). New York: Psychology Press.

Leary, M. R. (2004a). *The curse of the self: Self-awareness, egotism and the quality of human life*. New York: Oxford University Press.

Leary, M. R. (2004b). The sociometer, self-esteem, and the regulation of interpersonal behavior. In R. F. Baumeister & K. D. Vohs (Eds.), *Handbook of self-regulation* (pp. 373–391). New York: Guilford Press.

Leary, M. R., & Baumeister, R. F. (2000). The nature and function of self-esteem: Sociometer theory. In M. P. Zanna (Ed.), *Advances in experimental social psychology* (Vol. 33, pp. 1–62). San Diego, CA: Academic Press.

Leary, M. R., & Buttermore, N. R. (2003). The evolution of the human self: Tracing the natural history of self-awareness. *Journal for the Theory of Social Behaviour, 33*, 365–404.

Leary, M. R., Cottrell, C. A., & Phillips, M. (2001). Deconfounding the effects of dominance and social acceptance on self-esteem. *Journal of Personality and Social Psychology, 81*, 898–909.

Leary, M. R., & Downs, D. L. (1995). Interpersonal functions of the self-esteem motive: The self-esteem system as a sociometer. In M. Kernis (Ed.), *Efficacy, agency, and self-esteem* (pp. 123–144). New York: Plenum Press.

Leary, M. R., Gallagher, B., Fors, E. H., Buttermore, N., Baldwin, E., Lane, K. K., & Mills, A. (2003). The invalidity of personal claims about self-esteem. *Personality and Social Psychology Bulletin, 29*, 623–636.

Leary, M. R., Haupt, A., Strausser, K., & Chokel, J. (1998). Calibrating the sociometer: The relationship between interpersonal appraisals and state self-esteem. *Journal of Personality and Social Psychology, 74*, 1290–1299.

Leary, M. R., & MacDonald, G. (2003). Individual differences in self-esteem: A review and theoretical integration. In M. R. Leary & J. P. Tangney (Eds.), *Handbook of self and identity* (pp. 401–418). New York: Guilford Press.

Leary, M. R., Rice, S. C., & Schreindorfer, L. S. (2004). *Distinguishing the effects of social exclusion and low relational evaluation on reactions to interpersonal rejection.* Unpublished manuscript, Department of Psychology, Wake Forest University, Winston-Salem, NC.

Leary, M. R., Schreindorfer, L. S., & Haupt, A. L. (1995). The role of self-esteem in emotional and behavioral problems: Why is low self-esteem dysfunctional? *Journal of Social and Clinical Psychology, 14*, 297–314.

Leary, M. R., Tambor, E. S., Terdal, S. K., & Downs, D. L. (1995). Self-esteem as an interpersonal monitor: The sociometer hypothesis. *Journal of Personality and Social Psychology, 68*, 518–530.

Leary, M. R., Twenge, J. M., & Quinlivan, E. (in press). Interpersonal rejection as a determinant of anger and aggression. *Personality and Social Psychology Bulletin.*

Lewis, C., & Mitchell, P. (Eds.). (1994). *Children's early understanding of mind: Origins and development.* Hove, UK: Erlbaum.

Lewis, M., & Brooks-Gunn, J. (1979). *Social cognition and the acquisition of self.* New York: Plenum Press.

MacDonald, G., Saltzman, J. L., & Leary, M. R. (2003). Social approval and trait self-esteem. *Journal of Research in Personality, 37*, 23–40.

Markus, H. (1980). The self in thought and memory. In D. M. Wegner & R. R. Vallacher (Eds.), *The self in social psychology* (pp. 102–130). New York: Oxford University Press.

May, R. (1983). *The discovery of being.* New York: Norton.

McNally, R. J. (1987). Preparedness and phobias: A review. *Psychological Bulletin, 101*, 283–303.

Mecca, A. M., Smelser, N. J., & Vasconcellos, J. (Eds.). (1989). *The social importance of self-esteem.* Berkeley and Los Angeles: University of California Press.

Mitchell, R. W. (2003). Subjectivity and self-recognition in animals. In M. R. Leary & J. P. Tangney (Eds.), *Handbook of self and identity* (pp. 567–593). New York: Guilford Press.

Neisser, U. (1988). Five kinds of self-knowledge. *Philosophical Psychology, 1*, 35–59.

Ohman, A. (1986). Face the beast and fear the face: Animal and social fears as prototypes for evolutionary analyses of emotion. *Psychophysiology, 23*, 123–145.

Pinker, S. (1997). *How the mind works.* New York: Norton.

Potts, R. B. (1984). Home bases and early hominids. *Scientific American, 250*, 60–69.

Povinelli, D. J., & Prince, C. G. (1998). When self met other. In M. Ferrari & R. J. Sternberg (Eds.), *Self-awareness: Its nature and development* (pp. 37–107). New York: Guilford Press.

Samuels, R. (2000). Massively modular minds: Evolutionary psychology and cognitive architecture. In P. Carruthers & A. Chamberlain (Eds.), *Evolution and the human mind* (pp. 13–46). Cambridge, UK: Cambridge University Press.

Savage-Rumbaugh, S. (1994). Hominid evolution: Looking to modern apes for clues. In D. Quiatt & J. Itani (Eds.), *Hominid culture in primate perspective* (pp. 7–49). Niwot: University Press of Colorado.

Schlenker, B. R. (1985). Identity and self-identification. In B. R. Schlenker (Ed.), *The self and social life* (pp. 65–99). New York: McGraw-Hill.

Sedikides, C., & Skowronski, J. J. (1997). The symbolic self in evolutionary context. *Personality and Social Psychology Review, 1,* 80–102.

Sedikides, C., & Skowronski, J. J. (2002). Evolution of the symbolic self: Issues and prospects. In M. R. Leary & J. P. Tangney (Eds.), *Handbook of self and identity* (pp. 594–609). New York: Guilford Press.

Tooby, J., & Cosmides, L. (1996). Friendship and the banker's paradox: Other pathways to the evolution of adaptations for altruism. *Proceedings of the British Academy, 88,* 119–143.

Whiten, A., & Byrne, R. W. (1988). The Machiavellian intelligence hypothesis: Editorial. In R. Byrne & A. Whiten (Eds.), *Machiavellian intelligence: Social expertise and the evolution of intellect in monkeys, apes, and humans* (pp. 1–9). Oxford, UK: Clarendon Press.

Zihlman, A. L., Cronin, J. E., Cramer, D. L., & Sarich, V. M. (1978). Pygmy chimpanzee as a possible prototype for the common ancestor of humans and gorillas. *Nature, 275,* 744–746.

CHAPTER 12

Rejection's Impact on Self-Defeating, Prosocial, Antisocial, and Self-Regulatory Behaviors

GINETTE C. BLACKHART
ROY F. BAUMEISTER
JEAN M. TWENGE

One key to understanding human nature is to recognize that what exists and what happens *inside* the individual is largely there in order to serve what happens *between* people (e.g., Baumeister, 2005). The intrapsychic serves the interpersonal. Most likely this is because nature has designed human beings to seek connections with other people as their principal means of getting what they want. Unlike most other species, human beings obtain most of their food and information from each other rather than directly from the physical environment.

The purpose of this chapter is to explore a particularly challenging and troubling link between inner and interpersonal processes. Specifically, we cover a recent program of research designed to study how self-defeating responses follow from interpersonal rejection and exclusion. Rejection thwarts the need to belong and is therefore profoundly problematic to an organism that is overwhelmingly designed to seek acceptance. Self-defeating behavior thwarts the rational pursuit of enlightened self-interest and is therefore profoundly problematic to any organism that seeks to survive and flourish.

Humans' innate motivation to belong is demonstrated by the "pervasive drive to form and maintain at least a minimum quantity of lasting, positive, and significant interpersonal relationships" (Baumeister & Leary, 1995, p. 497). This belongingness motive appears to have an evolutionary basis. Forming and maintaining social bonds would have had both survival and reproductive benefits (see Baumeister & Leary, 1995). Humans are not born with the ability to survive on their own, and as a result they must depend on others for food, water, and protection. Small groups could share food, fight off enemies, help care for offspring, and provide protection for one another, thereby increasing the chances of survival for everyone in the group. Those who formed attachments to others were more likely to reproduce than those who did not form those attachments, and, if long-term attachments were formed, the chances of survival for their offspring increased (see Baumeister & Leary, 1995).

Even today, humans are dependent on others for survival. People need others to care for them when they are very young, when they are sick or injured, and when they are very old. Families and friends share resources to enable survival in the everyday struggles all people experience. In fact, research has shown that those with strong social support networks are less likely to suffer from psychological disorders (e.g., Joiner, 1997). Among those with psychological disorders, a strong social support network is associated with less severe symptoms and better recovery rates (e.g., Hann et al., 2002). Even those with cancer and other life-threatening physical disorders are more likely to survive if they have a strong social support network (e.g., Michael, Berkman, Colditz, Holmes, & Kawachi, 2002).

Because of humans' innate motivation to form and maintain social bonds, threats to their need to belong should result in increased efforts to obtain social acceptance. Thus when one is socially rejected, one should increase prosocial behaviors in order to garner social acceptance and belonging. In addition, one's self-regulation should increase in order to enable one to alter his or her behaviors to conform to the ideals, expectations, values, norms, and other standards that the social group holds. This increase in self-regulatory and prosocial behaviors would increase social acceptance from the group, thereby increasing the likelihood that one would be accepted (either by the group that initially rejected the person or by a new group). Laboratory research, however, has shown quite an opposite pattern of results. After being socially rejected or being told they will end up alone later in life, research participants actually exhibit an increase in selfish and self-defeating behaviors, including a decrease in prosocial behaviors and an increase in antisocial behaviors.

It may be argued that exhibiting less prosocial behavior and acting aggressively toward others is in and of itself self-defeating. If a person's need to belong is threatened by interpersonal rejection, that person should theoretically want to behave in such a way as to be socially accepted by others. Decreased prosocial behaviors, such as helping, and increased aggression toward others would not generally have the desired effect—if anything, they would have the opposite effect of decreasing social acceptance. Instead of finding that rejection causes people to be more prosocial, however, several studies from our labs have shown that socially rejected individuals are in fact less prosocial and more antisocial. These behaviors are self-defeating in general because they reduce a person's chances of securing desired social acceptance. As a result, this chapter not only discusses research indicating that social rejection causes increases in self-defeating behaviors, but also research showing that social rejection causes decreased prosocial behavior, increased aggression, and decreased self-control.

INCREASES IN SELF-DEFEATING BEHAVIOR

Research has shown that once a person has been socially rejected by others, he or she will exhibit increases in self-destructive and self-defeating behavior. For instance, Twenge, Catanese, and Baumeister (2002, 2003) found that socially rejected participants were more likely to make irrational and risky decisions, were more likely to engage in unhealthy behaviors, engaged in more procrastination, and were less likely to delay gratification than non-rejected participants.

The methods for the ensuing studies followed a similar pattern: Participants first completed the Eysenck Personality Questionnaire (EPQ; Eysenck & Eysenck, 1975) and were given accurate feedback about their score on the Extraversion scale by the experimenter. Participants were then told that their level of Extraversion/Introversion was (1) bad for relationships, and they would end up alone later in life (future alone condition); (2) good for relationships, and they would always have friends and people who care about them (future belonging condition); or (3) indicative of being accident-prone, and they would have a lot of accidents later in life (misfortune control condition). The misfortune control condition was included because it described a negative outcome that was not related to relationships or social exclusion.

After giving the participants bogus feedback, Twenge and colleagues (2002) offered them a choice between two lotteries. This procedure had been developed by Leith and Baumeister (1996) to study self-defeating behavior in the form of taking foolish risks. Participants were told that if they won the lottery, they would win money. If they lost the lottery, however, not only would they not win any money, but they would also be subjected to a 3-minute audiotape of fingernails scraping against a chalkboard. Lottery A offered a 70% chance of winning $2 and a 30% chance of winning no money and being subjected to the noise on the audiotape. Lottery B offered a 2% chance of winning $25 and a 98% chance of winning no money and being subjected to the noise on the audiotape. Although the maximum gains expected from winning

Lottery B were substantially larger than the gains expected from winning Lottery A, the chances of winning Lottery B were so low it would be logical to conclude that most people would choose Lottery A to increase their chances of winning money and to substantially decrease their chances of being subjected to an intolerable noise. If one calculates expected gain by multiplying probabilities by outcomes, it is obvious that Lottery A was the more rational choice. In that sense, choosing Lottery B qualifies as a self-defeating behavior (Leith & Baumeister, 1996).

Those participants given feedback that they would end up alone later in life made a poorer and riskier decision on the lottery choice paradigm than participants in the other groups, choosing the lottery that only gave them a 2% chance of winning (Lottery B) over the lottery that gave them a 70% chance of winning (Lottery A). In fact, while only 6% of those in the future belonging condition chose Lottery B, over 60% of those in the future alone condition chose Lottery B. This choice is self-defeating, insofar as rejected participants chose the lottery that gave them little chance of reward and great chance for punishment.

Receiving the future alone feedback also affected participants' choices between healthy and unhealthy behaviors (Twenge et al., 2002). After receiving bogus feedback (that they would end up alone later in life, would always have people who cared about them, or were accident-prone), participants were first given a choice between a candy bar or a lower fat granola bar. Participants next were told that they needed to wait in the lab for a period of time. While they were waiting, they could choose either to fill out a health survey that would help them improve their health or read entertainment magazines (e.g., *People*, *Entertainment Weekly*). Then the experimenter told participants that she needed to take their pulse as a measurement of their overall health: Participants could choose either to have their resting pulse or their running pulse taken. Participants were told that the running pulse would require them to run in place for 2 minutes, but that it was a better measure of their overall health than a resting pulse measurement. Participants given future alone feedback were significantly more likely than those in the future belonging or accident-prone groups to choose the three unhealthy behaviors over the healthy ones. That is, they were more likely to choose the candy bar over the granola bar, to read entertainment magazines rather than complete the health questionnaire, and to have their resting pulse taken rather than their running pulse. Choosing to engage in unhealthy behaviors over healthy ones is self-defeating in that the unhealthy behaviors portend negative long-term consequences.

Procrastination is another important form of self-defeating behavior insofar as it causes health problems, stress, and inferior performance (Tice & Baumeister, 1997). Procrastination is also increased by rejection experiences (Twenge et al., 2002). Participants were told that they would be taking a nonverbal intelligence test that would consist of arithmetic problems assessing the participant's skills on quantitative reasoning, analytical abilities, and fluid thinking. Participants were subsequently told that they would have the opportunity to practice these types of problems before the test. The experimenter explained that previous research indicated that practicing the arithmetic problems for 10–15 minutes would significantly improve their performance on the nonverbal intelligence test. Participants were informed that they would have 15 minutes to practice, and that at least some of that time should be spent practicing the arithmetic problems. They were also told, however, that if they did not want to practice the equations the whole time, they could engage in a number of other tasks, such as playing a handheld video game (Nintendo Game Boy with Tetris) or reading entertaining magazines (e.g., *Cosmopolitan*, *Maxim*). Participants given feedback that they would be alone later in life procrastinated more than participants who received belonging or accident-prone feedback. Participants in the future alone condition chose to engage in pleasurable activities, such as playing the video game or reading the magazines, rather than completing math problems that would improve their performance on the upcoming intelligence test.

The negative impact of interpersonal rejection on delay of gratification was also shown by Twenge and colleagues (2003). Delay of gratification is a crucial trait in many spheres of human success, from farming to obtaining higher education. Thus failure to delay gratification is a potentially costly and self-defeating pattern. In the Twenge and colleagues study, an experimental manipulation different from that used in the previous studies was employed. Participants arrived in groups of four to six, all of the same gender. After a 15-minute introductory session, participants were told that they would be paired with another participant to work on a task, and all were asked to indicate the two people from the group they most wanted to work with on this next task. Participants were next told that either (1) no one chose to work with them (rejected condition) or (2) everyone chose to work with them (accepted condition). After being given this bogus feedback, participants read a scenario in which they were asked to imagine that a friend had received two job offers. One job offered a higher beginning salary, but little opportunity for advancement or a better income, therefore favoring a short-term gain at the expense of a long-term gain. The other job offered a considerably lower beginning salary, but the possibility of substantial advancement and a higher income later, therefore favoring a long-term gain over a short-term gain (which requires a higher delay of gratification). When given the choice to advise the friend to take one of these two jobs, rejected condition participants were more likely than accepted condition participants to advise the friend to take the job with a higher salary but little opportunity for advancement, thereby favoring short-term rewards over long-term benefits.

In summary, these studies indicate that when participants are led to believe that they have been rejected by others or will end up alone later in life, they engage in self-defeating and self-destructive behaviors. Rejected participants made an irrational, risky decision in a lottery paradigm, choosing the lottery that had a greater payout but a very low chance of winning over a lottery with a lower payout but a greater chance of winning (and of avoiding an unbearable noise). Rejected participants also chose unhealthy behaviors over healthy ones, such as choosing a candy bar over a granola bar, opting to read entertainment magazines over taking a health survey that could help them increase healthy behaviors, and deciding to have their resting pulse taken over their running pulse. Rejected participants also procrastinated prior to an upcoming test, insofar as they read entertaining magazines or played video games rather than practicing for the exam. In addition, rejected participants said they would advise a friend to take a job with a high starting salary but little possibility for future advancement over a job with a lower starting salary but with opportunities for substantial advancements in the future, a clear sign of inability to delay gratification.

DECREASE IN PROSOCIAL BEHAVIORS

As discussed earlier, decreased prosocial behavior following rejection is self-defeating if an individual has the goal of gaining acceptance and inclusion. Prosocial behaviors include a wide range of actions, such as sharing, helping, giving, and comforting. Although it would be expected that socially rejected individuals would increase their prosocial behaviors to gain acceptance from others, research has shown that social rejection leads to significant decreases in prosocial behavior. For instance, Twenge, Ciarocco, Cuervo, Bartels, and Baumeister (2005) found that socially excluded participants donated less money to an important cause, were unwilling to volunteer for future studies, were less helpful, and cooperated less with others, as compared to participants who were accepted by others.

In this study, after completing the EPQ, participants received the same bogus feedback used by Twenge and colleagues (2002, 2003)—that is, they were given future alone feedback, future belonging feedback, and accident-prone control feedback. Participants then received $2.00 in quarters as payment for participation in the experiment. After receiving payment, participants were given the opportunity to donate money to a "Student Emergency Fund." Participants in the future alone condition donated significantly less money to the fund than participants in the other two groups.

In another study conducted by Twenge and colleagues (2005), after participants were given the same bogus feedback, the experimenter knocked a cup of pencils onto the floor, giving participants the opportunity to help the experimenter pick up the pencils (based on a bystander intervention study by Latané & Dabbs, 1975). Participants in the future alone condition were less likely to help the experimenter pick up pencils after the cup of pencils fell to the floor than those in the other groups. In fact, only 15% of future alone participants helped the experimenter pick up pencils, as compared to 64% of those in the other groups.

Participants who had been led to expect a lonely life were also less likely to cooperate on a prisoner's dilemma game (Twenge et al., 2005). The prisoner's dilemma game (Rapoport & Chammah, 1965) is a widely used research method that involves a non-zero-sum game in which each player must choose between two responses. One response option is to cooperate with the opponent in the pursuit of maximum mutual gain, but this option exposes the player to the risk of being exploited by the other person. The second response option protects the individual against exploitation and creates the possibility of maximum individual gain; however, if both players choose this option, both of them lose. Only by mutual cooperation can both players achieve favorable outcomes. As a result, cooperating is considered a prosocial behavior that in this case benefits the self as well as others. Participants were told they were playing the game with another participant, but in actuality they were playing against a computer.

In this study, the computer was programmed to defect on the first turn and every fourth turn thereafter. On any of the other turns, the computer was programmed to mimic the participant's response on the subsequent turn. For example, if the participant defected on his or her first turn, the computer would then defect on its next turn. If the participant cooperated on his or her first turn, then the computer cooperated on the next turn.

The results showed that participants in the future alone condition were more likely to defect and less likely to cooperate during the game than participants in the other conditions, thus showing less prosocial behavior toward their supposed opponent. This was true even when the opponent (the computer) cooperated on the first turn and participants played for money rather than for points. These same results were still apparent when participants received feedback (future alone, future belonging, or accident-prone) on a piece of paper rather than orally from the experimenter and the experimenter was blind to the condition. Thus, even when the opponent cooperated, when the participant was motivated by money, or when the experimenter was blind to the condition the participant was assigned to, socially rejected participants were still less likely to cooperate than those in the other groups.

Social rejection also had an impact on participants' helpfulness (Twenge et al., 2005). Participants arrived in groups of four to six and, after a brief interaction period, were given feedback consistent with rejection or acceptance by others in the group. After being given feedback, participants were then presented the option of leaving or participating in one, two, or three more experiments to help out the experimenter. Participants receiving rejection feedback volunteered to participate in significantly fewer experiments than those receiving acceptance feedback.

These studies illustrate that after people have been rejected by others, they engage in less prosocial behavior. Excluded participants donated less money to an important cause, were less likely to help the experimenter after a mishap, were less cooperative, and volunteered to participate in fewer studies to help the experimenter than accepted or control participants.

INCREASE IN ANTISOCIAL AND AGGRESSIVE BEHAVIORS

Antisocial and aggressive behavior may also be considered self-defeating insofar as an individual wishes to befriend and gain acceptance from other people. A number of studies have shown that after being socially rejected, people exhibit an increase in antisocial behaviors toward other people. For instance, Bourgeois and Leary (2001) found that participants who were chosen last by a team captain displayed significantly more disparagement toward the team captain than those who were chosen first. In addition, Murray, Rose, Bellavia, Holmes, and Kusche (2002) found that when faced with the threat of rejection from their romantic partners, low self-esteem participants derogated their partners and reduced closeness to their partners.

Participants also have been found to act aggressively toward others following rejection (Twenge, Baumeister, Tice, & Stucke, 2001). In this experiment, participants arrived in pairs and then filled out the EPQ. Next, they wrote an essay expressing their opinion on the abortion issue (they were required to choose one side of the issue). Participants next evaluated an essay supposedly written by the other participant (it was actually written by the experimenter) expressing views opposite to the participant's own views. After evaluating the essay, participants received feedback on the EPQ and were placed into either the future alone condition, the future belonging condition, the accident-prone control condition, or a no feedback condition. After receiving either positive ("a very good essay!") or negative ("one of the worst essays I've read!") feedback from the other "participant" regarding their own essay, participants evaluated the other participant on 10 statements. Those in the future alone condition who received negative feedback on their essay were significantly more negative in their evaluations of the other participant than those in any of the other conditions. This indicates that anticipating a lonely future caused people to be harsh and aggressive toward someone who had recently criticized them.

Rejected participants were also aggressive toward others when playing a computer game (Twenge et al., 2001). After arriving in groups of four to six people and a period of interaction with the group, participants were told that either no one wanted to work with them or that everyone wanted to work with them on the next task. They were next informed that they would complete a task with another person who was *not* in the group with which they had previously interacted. Participants received negative feedback on an essay they had written, ostensibly from the person they would be working with on the next task. Participants were then told they would play a computer game with this participant (participants were actually playing against the computer, which was programmed to mimic the participant's responses). In this game, participants were given the goal of pressing a button as fast as they could. Whoever lost the turn would hear a blast of white noise through headphones. The participant administered white noise blasts to the other "participant" whenever the other player lost. Participants were also able to control the duration and intensity of the noise blast when administering it to the other player.

Participants in the rejected group were considerably more aggressive toward their supposed opponent in that the duration of the noise blasts were significantly longer and the intensity was significantly greater than those administered by participants in the accepted condition. This finding occurred even when the participant believed the person they were playing against had not given them negative feedback and was therefore a neutral, innocent third-party. Thus aggression toward another person occurred even without direct provocation. These results were further supported by Twenge and Campbell (2003), who reported that social exclusion produced exceptionally high levels of aggression among people who scored high in narcissism. Similar results were also reported by Kirkpatrick, Waugh, Valencia, and Webster (2002), who found that participants lower in self-reported social inclusion were more aggressive (assigning higher portions of hot sauce to tasters who were known not to like spicy food) toward their supposed opponents, as compared to participants who reported more social connectedness.

Support for the idea that social rejection leads to antisocial behavior and aggression toward others has also been reported in studies of children who have been rejected by their peers. Several studies have found that children rejected by their peers are aggressive and antisocial (see McDougall, Hymel, Vaillencourt, & Mercer, 2001, for a review). For instance, Leary, Kowalski, Smith, and Phillips (2003) examined the cases of children involved in school shootings. They found that in all but two of the cases that occurred between 1995 and 2001 that they examined, the children who had committed the violence against their peers had experienced acute or chronic social rejection in the form of ostracism, bullying, and/or romantic rejection. In a longitudinal study, Ialongo, Vaden-Kiernan, and Kellum (1998) found that early peer rejection was a significant predictor of aggressive behavior in later childhood and adolescence. Additionally, Hubbard (2001) found that when children who reported being rejected or accepted by their peers played competitive games with a confederate, rejected children displayed more facial and verbal anger after unfavorable outcomes than accepted children. Thus the pattern of social rejection leading to increased aggression and antisocial behavior can be seen in both laboratory studies and observational and longitudinal studies in both children and adults.

Thus far, this chapter has discussed literature suggesting that interpersonal rejection leads to selfish and self-destructive behavior. Rejection from others leads people to act in a self-defeating manner, such as procrastinating, engaging in unhealthy behaviors, making risky decisions, and not delaying gratification. These self-defeating behaviors also include acting aggressively toward others and not engaging in prosocial behaviors inasmuch as the self desires to be included and accepted by others. As a lack of self-regulation has been implicated in many of these behaviors, it is suggested that social rejection leads to deficits in self-regulation, thus causing self-defeating behavior following rejection by others.

DECREASE IN SELF-REGULATION

The ability to control and regulate impulses, desires, wishes, emotions, and other behaviors is a core feature of the self. In fact, many vital functions of the self involve regulation, such as making decisions, inhibiting and initiating behavior, taking responsibility, and making and carrying out plans (Baumeister, 1998). Recent research, however, has shown that social rejection cause deficits in self-regulation.

As discussed, rejected participants were less likely to delay gratification than accepted participants, which in itself is a form of self-regulation failure. Rejected participants have also shown deficits in self-regulation in other laboratory studies. For instance, after giving participants bogus feedback about their future following completion of the EPQ (see Twenge et al., 2002), participants in the future alone condition drank less of a bad-tasting yet healthy beverage than participants in the future belonging, accident-prone control, and no feedback control conditions (Baumeister, DeWall, Ciarocco, & Twenge, 2005). Participants in the future alone condition also gave up significantly faster when trying to solve unsolvable puzzles and committed significantly more errors on a dichotic listening task as compared to participants in the other three conditions (Baumeister et al., 2005).

Rejection also influenced participants' inhibition in terms of not eating unhealthy food. Participants arrived at the laboratory in groups of four to six people. After an introductory session, they were given feedback consistent with their placement into either the rejected or the accepted conditions. Participants were subsequently told that they were going to perform a taste-testing task. Participants were given a bowl of 35 bite-size chocolate chip cookies and instructed to eat as many cookies as necessary in order to accurately evaluate the smell, taste, and texture of the cookies. Participants in the rejected condition ate significantly more cookies during the taste-testing task as compared to accepted participants. These results are noteworthy given that Tice, Bratslavsky, and Baumeister (2001) found that participants in a similar sample viewed eating cookies as an unhealthy and undesirable behavior that should be regulated by the self. In addition, Vohs and Heatherton (2000) found that self-regulatory resource depletion led to increased consumption of ice cream, indicating that overeating is a reliable indicator of self-control failure. When participants were rejected, their self-regulation deteriorated, and they ate more cookies.

In an observational study, rejection by peers also had a negative impact on learning-disabled children's attentiveness and hyperactivity, a behavioral pattern that learning-disabled children who had not been socially rejected did not display (Kistner & Gatlin, 1989). Recent research has suggested, however, that the effects of social exclusion on self-regulation may depend on the prospect of future acceptance by others (DeWall, Baumeister, & Vohs, 2005). Participants in two studies were either given future alone or future belonging bogus feedback after completing the EPQ (similar to that used by Twenge et al., 2002, 2003). Participants in a third study were either told that a research assistant did not want to work with them on a task (rejection condition) or that the research assistant had to leave unexpectedly (control condition). Participants next completed self-regulation tasks (i.e., playing the game Operation, in which performance is judged by both speed and accuracy, the Stroop color-word task, or a dichotic listening task). Before engaging in these tasks, half of the participants were told that better performance on these tasks were diagnostic indicators of interpersonally helpful traits, such as empathy and social sensitivity, or were predictive of healthy and successful relationships, including the quality and quantity of friendships. Consistent with past research, among participants not given this information prior to completing the self-regulation tasks, rejected participants performed worse on the task than nonrejected participants. For those participants told that performance on the self-regulation task was indicative of good social skills or healthy relationships, however, rejected participants performed better on the task than nonrejected participants. These results suggest that social rejection only causes a reduction in self-regulation if participants do not believe self-regulation will lead to increased acceptance by others. When motivated by the chance of social acceptance, rejected people can overcome the temptation to fail at self-regulation.

Research has thus shown that when people are socially rejected, they exhibit decrements in self-regulation as demonstrated by less persistence on unsolvable puzzles, committing more errors on a dichotic listening task, exhibiting less ability to delay gratification, displaying deficits in attention, drinking less of a bad-tasting but healthy beverage, and consuming more cookies during a taste test than nonrejected participants. It appears that the only time social rejection does not cause deficits in self-regulation is when participants believe that exhibiting self-control will increase social acceptance. Because social rejection consistently led to decreased self-control, with the one exception, could self-regulation act as a mediating factor between social rejection and self-defeating behaviors?

POSSIBLE MEDIATORS

Several variables have been suggested as mediators between social rejection and self-defeating behaviors. One variable that has been suggested is mood or affect. Belongingness theory (Baumeister & Leary, 1995) states that when one is socially rejected or excluded, one should experience a significant amount of distress and/or negative affect. Laboratory studies examining reactions to rejection in nondepressed samples, however, have failed to find increased distress or negative affect following rejection (e.g., Bourgeois & Leary, 2001; Twenge et al., 2002, 2003). In addition, several studies examining negative affect as a possible mediating factor have shown that mood does not mediate the relationship between social rejection and self-defeating behavior (Baumeister, Twenge, & Nuss, 2002; Twenge et al., 2001, 2002, 2003, 2005). Several other variables, such as self-esteem, belongingness, trust in others, sense of control, and self-awareness have also been tested as possible mediators. Twenge and colleagues (2005) reported, however, that none of these variables were significant mediators of the relationship between social rejection and self-defeating behaviors.

Another possible factor that may mediate the relationship between social rejection and self-defeating behaviors is self-regulation. Given that recent studies have indicated that social rejection leads to deficits in self-regulation (DeWall et al., 2005), it is plausible that deficits in self-regulation increase self-defeating behaviors. For instance, Feldman, Rosenthal, Brown, and Canning (1995) found that children who were rejected by their peers in the sixth grade reported having a greater number of sexual partners 4 years later, which was mediated by self-restraint. In addition, Ayduk and colleagues (2000) found that greater ability in delay of gratification actually buffered participants from interpersonal difficulties (e.g., aggression) following perceived or actual rejection.

Self-regulation may act as a possible mediator because self-regulation failure is implicated in antisocial behavior, aggression, a lack of prosocial behavior, and self-defeating behaviors, such as procrastination, inability to delay gratification, choosing unhealthy over healthy behaviors, and the like. Future laboratory studies, however, will need to examine in greater depth whether self-regulation acts as a mediating factor between rejection and self-defeating behaviors. In addition, research will need to investigate whether self-regulation mediates only unidirectional or bidirectional relationships.

That is, does self-regulation act as a mediator when social rejection leads to greater aggression, as well as when aggressive behavior leads to social rejection by peers? As no research has been conducted to directly test self-regulation as a mediating factor in the relationship between social rejection and self-defeating behaviors, it is suggested that future studies focus on this area. In addition, other possible mediating factors should be examined as well, such as physiological and/or biological variables.

DIRECTION OF CAUSALITY

Research has shown that social rejection leads to an increase in a number of selfish and self-defeating behaviors, as well as deficits in self-regulation and self-control. Do these processes influence each other mutually or is causality unidirectional? That is, is it the case that social rejection causes these behaviors, or can engaging in self-defeating behaviors and exhibiting deficits in self-regulation actually cause rejection by others as well? Research has suggested that perhaps there is a bidirectional relationship between social rejection and aggression/antisocial behavior (including decreases in prosocial behavior), as well as between rejection and self-regulation.

Although there is well-documented support for the idea that social rejection leads to increases in aggression and antisocial behavior, several studies also suggest that those who display antisocial behaviors and who are aggressive toward others are likely to be rejected by their peers. Both physical and verbal aggression have been closely linked to peer rejection in children in the United States (Crick & Grotpeter, 1995; Wood, Cowan, & Baker, 2002) and in Italy (Tomada & Schneider, 1997). In a prospective study, Little and Garber (1995) found that aggression directly predicted peer rejection 3 months later in fifth and sixth graders. Based on these findings, it would appear that while social rejection can predict an increase in aggressive and antisocial behavior, as well as a decrease in prosocial behavior, aggressive and antisocial behavior also predicts later rejection by peers.

Additional studies suggest that the relationship between social rejection and self-control is bidirectional as well. For instance, Ferrer and Krantz (1987) found that self-control negatively correlated with social rejection in third and fifth graders, in that those who were rejected by their peers also displayed less self-control. Wood and colleagues (2002) also reported that, in preschool-age children, those who were rejected by their peers were also noncompliant and hyperactive. Because these studies are strictly correlational, however, direction cannot be determined on the basis of these results alone. A longitudinal study (Feldman et al., 1995) found, however, that sixth graders who were socially rejected by their peers reported a greater number of sexual partners in adolescence. Feldman and colleagues (1995) also reported that those sixth graders who were low in self-restraint were more likely to be rejected by their peers than those with greater self-restraint. It would appear, based on this research, that not only can social exclusion predict a decrease in self-regulation, but deficits in self-regulation also predict social rejection.

Asking whether these relationships influence each other mutually or if the causality is unidirectional is important for understanding how these relationships operate. Although rejection leads to aggression, aggression toward others can also lead to rejection by others. While being rejected by others may lead us to decrease prosocial behaviors toward others, such as helping, not helping others may appear rude to others and therefore cause someone to be rejected. While failures in self-regulation and self-control may lead to rejection by others, being rejected by others can also cause failures in self-regulation. Even self-defeating behaviors, such as procrastination, can lead to rejection by others, but being rejected can increase procrastination. Thus it is not merely that interpersonal rejection causes selfish and self-destructive behaviors, but in fact that these self-destructive and selfish behaviors also lead to rejection by others. This research thus indicates that the behaviors people display *after* being rejected, such as aggression, less prosocial behavior, self-defeating behaviors, and deficits in self-regulatory behaviors, may actually bring about further rejection by others.

CONCLUSION

Several lines of research have shown that social rejection has deleterious effects on well-being by increasing the occurrence of self-destructive and selfish behaviors. When rejected by others, people consequently make poor and risky choices, engage in unhealthy behaviors, procrastinate, and are unable to delay gratification. In addition, rejected participants are reluctant to donate money to an important cause, are unwilling to volunteer for future studies, are unhelpful after a mishap, are uncooperative, and display aggressive behavior toward others.

This increase in self-defeating behavior following social rejection may be mediated by self-regulation. A number of studies have shown that following interpersonal rejection, participants displayed significant deficits on several different self-regulation tasks (there was one exception: when participants believed that self-regulation could lead to an increase in acceptance by others, rejected participants exhibited self-control). In addition, it is important to consider self-regulation as a possible mediator because self-regulation failure has been implicated in antisocial behavior, aggression, a lack of prosocial behavior, and self-defeating behaviors such as procrastination, inability to delay gratification, and choosing unhealthy over healthy behaviors. Further research will be needed in order to determine whether self-regulation does in fact act as a mediator in the relationship between social rejection and self-destructive behaviors.

Research has also indicated that perhaps social rejection and self-defeating behaviors (including aggressive and prosocial behaviors) influence each other in a bidirectional fashion. Following social rejection, rejected individuals are aggressive toward others, but those exhibiting aggressive and antisocial behaviors are also more likely to be rejected by their peers. Rejected individuals are less prosocial, but exhibiting less prosocial behaviors, such as helping, may be considered rude and can therefore elicit rejection by others. Engaging in certain self-defeating behaviors may lead to rejection by others, and, conversely, interpersonal rejection increases the likelihood that one will commit self-defeating acts. Those who are rejected additionally exhibit deficits on self-regulatory tasks, while deficits in self-regulation may also lead individuals to be rejected by their peers. Whereas rejection may lead to increased selfish and self-destructive behaviors and deficits in self-regulation, these behaviors in turn may lead to further rejection by others.

The significance of these findings, that social exclusion leads to self-defeating behaviors, is that if people are to increase their chances of being accepted by others, they need to increase prosocial and decrease antisocial behaviors toward others as well as exhibit greater self-regulation and self-control. It appears, however, that when socially rejected individuals believe that exhibiting greater self-regulation will gain them more acceptance by others, they are motivated to self-regulate. A majority of the studies reviewed, however, indicated that when people are socially rejected, they instead engage in behaviors that not only hurt themselves, but that also hurt their chances of being accepted by others. Perhaps future research will be able to uncover additional factors that may prevent individuals from engaging in self-defeating behaviors once they have been socially rejected, therefore enabling people to gain acceptance from others even following rejection.

REFERENCES

Ayduk, O., Mendoza-Denton, R., Mischel, W., Downey, G., Peake, P. K., & Rodriguez, M. (2000). Regulating the interpersonal self: Strategic self-regulation for coping with rejection sensitivity. *Journal of Personality and Social Psychology, 79*, 776–792.

Baumeister, R. F. (1998). The self. In D. T. Gilbert, S. T. Fiske, & G. Lindzey (Eds.), *Handbook of social psychology* (4th ed., pp. 680–740). New York: McGraw-Hill.

Baumeister, R. F. (2005). *The cultural animal: Human nature, meaning, and social life*. New York: Oxford University Press.

Baumeister, R. F., DeWall, C. N., Ciarocco, N. J., & Twenge, J. M. (2005). Social exclusion impairs self-regulation. *Journal of Personality and Social Psychology, 88*, 589–604.

Baumeister, R. F., & Leary, M. R. (1995). The need to belong: Desire for interpersonal attachments as a fundamental human motivation. *Psychological Bulletin, 117,* 497–529.

Baumeister, R. F., Twenge, J. M., & Nuss, C. K. (2002). Effects of social exclusion on cognitive processes: Anticipated aloneness reduces intelligent thought. *Journal of Personality and Social Psychology, 83,* 817–827.

Bourgeois, K. S., & Leary, M. R. (2001). Coping with rejection: Derogating those who choose us last. *Motivation and Emotion, 25,* 101–111.

Crick, N. R., & Grotpeter, J. K. (1995). Relational aggression, gender, and social-psychological adjustment. *Child Development, 66,* 710–722.

DeWall, C. N., Baumeister, R. F., & Vohs, K. D. (2005). *Recovering from rejection: Undoing the self-regulation deficits stemming from social exclusion.* Manuscript submitted for publication.

Feldman, S. S., Rosenthal, D. R., Brown, N. L., & Canning, R. D. (1995). Predicting sexual experience in adolescent boys from peer rejection and acceptance during childhood. *Journal of Research on Adolescence, 5,* 387–411.

Ferrer, M., & Krantz, M. (1987). Self-control, locus of control and social status in children. *Psychological Reports, 60,* 355–358.

Hann, D., Baker, F., Denniston, M., Gesme, D., Reding, D., Flynn, T., et al. (2002). The influence of social support on depressive symptoms in cancer patients: Age and gender differences. *Journal of Psychosomatic Research, 52,* 279–283.

Hubbard, J. A. (2001). Emotion expression processes in children's peer interaction: The role of peer rejection, aggression, and gender. *Child Development, 72,* 1426–1438.

Ialongo, N. S., Vaden-Kiernan, N., & Kellam, S. (1998). Early peer rejection and aggression: Longitudinal relations with adolescent behavior. *Journal of Developmental and Physical Abilities, 10,* 199–213.

Joiner, T. E. Jr. (1997). Shyness and low social support as interactive diatheses, with loneliness as mediator: Testing an interpersonal–personality view of vulnerability to depressive symptoms. *Journal of Abnormal Psychology, 106,* 386–394.

Kirkpatrick, L. A., Waugh, C. E., Valencia, A., & Webster, G. D. (2002). The functional domain specificity of self-esteem and the differential prediction of aggression. *Journal of Personality and Social Psychology, 82,* 756–767.

Kistner, J. A., & Gatlin, D. (1989). Correlates of peer rejection among children with learning disabilities. *Learning Disability Quarterly, 12,* 133–140.

Latané, B., & Dabbs, J. M. Jr. (1975). Sex, group size, and helping in three cities. *Sociometry, 38,* 180–194.

Leary, M. R., Kowalski, R. M., Smith, L., & Phillips, S. (2003). Teasing, rejection, and violence: Case studies of the school shootings. *Aggressive Behavior, 29,* 202–214.

Leith, K. P., & Baumeister, R. F. (1996). Why do bad moods increase self-defeating behavior?: Emotion, risk taking, and self-regulation. *Journal of Personality and Social Psychology, 71,* 1250–1267.

Little, S. A., & Garber, J. (1995). Aggression, depression, and stressful life events predicting peer rejection in children. *Development and Psychopathology, 7,* 845–856.

McDougall, P., Hymel, S., Vaillancourt, T., & Mercer, L. (2001). The consequences of childhood peer rejection. In M. R. Leary (Ed.), *Interpersonal rejection* (pp. 213–247). London: Oxford University Press.

Michael, Y. L., Berkman, L. F., Colditz, G. A., Holmes, M. D., & Kawachi, I. (2002). Social networks and health-related quality of life in breast cancer survivors: A prospective study. *Journal of Psychosomatic Research, 52*, 285–293.

Murray, S. L., Rose, P., Bellavia, G. M., Holmes, J. G., & Kusche, A. G. (2002). When rejection stings: How self-esteem constrains relationship-enhancement processes. *Journal of Personality and Social Psychology, 83*, 556–573.

Rapoport, A., & Chammah, A. M. (1965). *Prisoner's dilemma*. Ann Arbor: University of Michigan Press.

Tice, D. M., & Baumeister, R. F. (1997). Longitudinal study of procrastination, performance, stress, and health: The costs and benefits of dawdling. *Psychological Science, 8*, 454–458.

Tice, D. M., Bratslavsky, E., & Baumeister, R. F. (2001). Emotional distress regulation takes precedence over impulse control: If you feel bad, do it! *Journal of Personality and Social Psychology, 80*, 53–67.

Tomada, G., & Schneider, B. H. (1997). Relational aggression, gender, and peer acceptance: Invariance across culture, stability over time, and concordance among informants. *Developmental Psychology, 33*, 601–609.

Twenge, J. M., Baumeister, R. F., Tice, D. M., & Stucke, T. S. (2001). If you can't join them, beat them: Effects of social exclusion on aggressive behavior. *Journal of Personality and Social Psychology, 81*, 1058–1069.

Twenge, J. M., & Campbell, W. K. (2003). "Isn't it fun to get the respect that we're going to deserve?": Narcissism, social rejection, and aggression. *Personality and Social Psychology Bulletin, 29*, 261–272.

Twenge, J. M., Catanese, K. R., & Baumeister, R. F. (2002). Social exclusion causes self-defeating behavior. *Journal of Personality and Social Psychology, 83*, 606–615.

Twenge, J. M., Catanese, K. R., & Baumeister, R. F. (2003). Social exclusion and the deconstructed state: Time perception, meaninglessness, lethargy, lack of emotion, and self-awareness. *Journal of Personality and Social Psychology, 85*, 409–423.

Twenge, J. M., Ciarocco, N. J., Cuervo, D., Bartels, J. M., & Baumeister, R. F. (2005). *Social exclusion decreases prosocial behavior*. Manuscript submitted for publication.

Vohs, K. D., & Heatherton, T. F. (2000). Self-regulatory failure: A resource-depletion approach. *Psychological Science, 11*, 249–254.

Wood, J. J., Cowan, P. A., & Baker, B. L. (2002). Behavior problems and peer rejection in preschool boys and girls. *Journal of Genetic Psychology, 163*, 72–88.

Does the Existence
of Social Relationships Matter
for Subjective Well-Being?

RICHARD E. LUCAS
PORTIA S. DYRENFORTH

Subjective well-being (SWB) researchers examine quality of life from the respondent's perspective. A quick examination of the major reviews in this area would likely lead to the following impressions: First, heritable personality factors have relatively strong effects on well-being (Diener & Lucas, 1999; Lykken & Tellegen, 1996). Second, most demographic factors including one's income, level of education, gender, age, and health status have only very weak associations with SWB (Diener, Suh, Lucas, & Smith, 1999). And third, among those factors that people can control, social relationships seem to matter most. In his broad review of the SWB literature, Argyle (2001) stated that "social relationships have a powerful effect on happiness and other aspects of well-being, and are perhaps its greatest single cause" (p. 71). Myers called the link between friendship and well-being a "deep truth" (1992, p. 154) and stated that although "age, gender, and income . . . give little clue to someone's happiness, . . . better clues come from knowing . . . whether [people] enjoy a supportive network of close relationships" (2000, p. 65). If these reviews are correct, people seeking to maximize happiness should forego the pursuit of money, beauty, and material possessions, and instead devote their lives to developing and maintaining close personal relationships.

However, close examination of these reviews reveals that authors rarely address the link between the *existence* of social relationships and greater well-being. Instead, they focus on whether people are satisfied with their relationships or whether they value relationships over and above other life goals. For example, in his review of the literature on close relationships and SWB, Myers (1999) discussed individuals "who feel satisfied with their love life," "who enjoy close relationships," who value "having close friends and a close marriage," and who say they have friends who "support their goals by frequently expressing interest and offering help and encouragement" (p. 378). However, he only cited one study that examined individuals who actually report having more (or fewer) friends. In this chapter, we focus specifically on the question of whether the existence of social relationships is associated with higher levels of SWB. We review the literature on the associations between relationships and happiness and discuss the mechanisms that may be able to account for these links.

DEFINITIONAL ISSUES

Before beginning, it is important to address various definitional issues. Foremost among these concerns the definition of SWB. The field of SWB deals with a broad collection of constructs that are linked by their focus on individuals' evaluations of their lives. The field is guided by three general principles. First, SWB researchers focus on evaluations of life from the respondent's own perspective. Second, SWB research is the study of both positive and negative aspects of life. And finally, SWB researchers are generally interested in individuals' lives as a whole.

The specific variables that SWB researchers study are arranged in a loose hierarchical structure (Diener, Scollon, & Lucas, 2004). At the highest level is the construct of SWB itself, which reflects a very broad, abstract, subjective evaluation of an individual's life. However, this broad construct is multidimensional and somewhat difficult to define in any concise way. Therefore SWB researchers often break the construct down into more easily definable and easily measurable constructs. For instance, SWB researchers are often interested in individual's cognitive judgment of their life satisfaction. To assess life satisfaction, researchers usually ask participants directly whether they believe that their life is a good one. This variable is assumed to reflect the conditions in an individual's life including the quality of his or her health, relationships, income, and job (see Campbell, Converse, & Rodgers, 1976; though also see Schwarz & Strack, 1999).

Satisfaction measures tap conscious attitudes about an individual's life. However, if his or her life is going well, it is also likely that that person will experience high levels of positive emotions and low levels of negative emotions. For that reason, SWB researchers often tap affective variables in addition to cognitive variables. Specifically, SWB researchers may track levels of emotion over time to determine how a person feels on average. Because positive and negative emotions are separable, if not independent (Diener & Emmons, 1984; Watson & Tellegen, 1985), it is best to measure positive emotions such as happiness, joy, and excitement separately from negative emotions such as sadness, fear, and anxiety. In certain cases, it is also useful to measure specific emotions separately, as they may have different effects on outcome variables and may result from different processes.

Although these well-being components are moderately to strongly correlated with one another, they are theoretically and empirically distinguishable (Lucas, Diener, & Suh, 1996). Therefore, to get a complete sense of an individual's SWB, the various components (life satisfaction, positive affect, and negative affect) must be measured separately. As we shall see, various predictors of well-being (including social relationships) may affect these components in different ways. In this chapter we specify which components are most relevant to the processes and mechanisms under discussion when the existing research literature permits.

Definitional issues also arise when discussing the concept of relationships. As Berscheid and Reis (1998) pointed out, there is much ambiguity in the term "relationship," and different researchers use the term in different ways. Although most people would agree that the bond that an individual shares with a romantic partner counts as a relationship, interactions that an individual has with other individuals are often not so clear. For instance, if someone has a brief discussion with a stranger on the street, is a new relationship formed? Do routinized, script-based interactions that occur on a regular basis (e.g., interactions with a checkout clerk at the grocery store) represent a meaningful, albeit nonintimate, relationship?

Berscheid and Reis (1998) noted that various criteria have been proposed to determine what is and what is not a relationship. Some researchers have suggested that any simple interaction between two or more people counts as a relationship. Others argue that only repeated patterns of contact count. Still others maintain that the relationship partners must develop a mental schema of the relationship before a relationship can be said to exist. For the purposes of this chapter, we follow Reis's (2001) definition in which *relationship* is defined as "an enduring association between two persons" (p. 61). Reis goes on to note that

> the existence of a relationship implies that these persons have established an ongoing connection with each other; that their bond has special properties, including a sense of history and some awareness of the nature of the relationship; that they influence each other's thoughts, feelings, and behavior; and that they expect to interact again in the future. (p. 61)

Reis also distinguishes the term *relationship* from the term *interaction*, which refers to a single social event. It is important to note, however, that social interactions (with both relationship partners and mere acquaintances) may be an important mechanism by which social relationships operate. For this reason, we review literature on social interactions as well as social relationships. This allows us to consider more fully the processes by which relationships affect well-being.

WHY SHOULD RELATIONSHIPS MATTER?

The theoretical links between social relationships and well-being are relatively straightforward. Most theories start with the premise that relationship partners provide resources that individuals may not be able to acquire on their own. Each individual has limited skills, intelligence, information, strength, and energy. Pooling resources can often lead to non-zero-sum outcomes that benefit all. Some theorists posit that these tangible benefits directly affect the happiness of relationship partners. Other theorists argue that the survival benefits that social relationships provided for our ancestors have led to an enduring human need for relationships. Still other theorists maintain that one's relationship history affects future interactions, which, in turn affect well-being. Each of these theories has different implications for empirical research on the benefits of social relationships.

For instance, Wills (1985) documented six different types of support that individuals can receive from social relationships. The two most basic of these—instrumental support and informational support—provide tangible benefits in times of need. *Instrumental support* refers to the assistance that one receives from others; this form of support from others ranges from lending money, to helping with household chores, to providing material resources such as food, housing, or tools. *Informational support*, on the other hand, refers to the information and guidance that one receives from others in difficult times. In addition to these tangible forms of support, relationships also provide *psychological* benefits for the relationship partners. For instance, relationships partners may provide motivational support, "encouraging persons to persist in their efforts at problem solution, reassuring them that their efforts will ultimately be successful and that better things will come, helping them to endure frustration, and communicating their belief that 'we can ride it through'" (Wills, 1985, p. 74). Relationships may also provide esteem support and status support. *Esteem support* provides people with the feeling that they are accepted and valued in spite of their problems and weaknesses; *status support* provides a signal to others that a person is valuable and capable of fulfilling his or her role obligations. Finally, *social companionship* itself is pleasant and the emotional benefits of this pleasant activity may constitute a form of support. If these forms of support are responsible for the link between social relationships and well-being, measures of these constructs should mediate the association. Thus the task for relationship researchers would simply be to assess these forms of support and determine which were responsible for the link with happiness.

It may also be true that in addition to evaluating the resources that we receive from others, we also evaluate the resources that we must give up. We may feel happy and satisfied when we believe that the relationship is fair and equitable (Wills, 1985); or we may be happiest in communal relationships where reciprocal exchanges are not expected (Clark & Mills, 1979). Thus there may be relationship-level variables concerning resource transactions that affect the individual relationship partners' happiness. A variety of patterns of interdependence can be examined (Rusbult & Van Lange, 1996), and these patterns may affect happiness and satisfaction in distinct ways. Again, according to these theories, concrete measures of resources and resource transactions should provide considerable insight into the effects of relationships on well-being.

However, a second class of theories adds a complicating factor to relationship research. Evolutionary theories posit that the existence of strong relationships has historically been correlated with positive outcomes. Those individuals who valued relationships would be more likely to accrue the benefits that these relationships provide. In turn, they would be more likely to survive and reproduce. Thus a strong desire for relationships would be adaptive and this trait would be passed on to future generations (Buss, 1990, 2000). Importantly, our ancestors did not need to recognize the correlation between relationships and resources for these evolutionary advantages to accrue. Simply desiring and pursuing relationships would lead to the selective advantage. Thus it is the desire for the relationships rather than the desire for the resources that gets passed on. Individuals may desire—and be happy in—relationships even when these relationships provide very few tangible benefits.

In their comprehensive review, Baumeister and Leary (1995) suggested that these evolutionary pressures have led to a universal need to belong. They posited that this need cannot be satisfied by mere social contact. Instead, relationships that are "marked by stability, affective concern, and continuation into the foreseeable future" are needed (p. 500). If the existence of close relationships is a fundamental need, then individuals should experience distress and anxiety when the need is not met and happiness and joy when it is met. Furthermore, Baumeister and Leary suggested that it is not just immediate affective reactions that are affected. If a need is fundamental, the success with which it is fulfilled should have far-reaching implications for health and well-being. Consistent with evolutionary theories, Baumeister and Leary posited that if the need for belongingness is fundamental, it should be nonderivative.

In other words, the desire for relationships should not result from a more basic desire for the resources that relationships provide. Baumeister and Leary join with various other need and motive theorists in positing a central role for the need for close, supportive relationships (e.g., Deci & Ryan, 2000; Maslow, 1970; Ryan & Deci, 2002).

A final possibility regarding the links between social relationships and well-being concerns an individual's past history with relationships. Specifically, attachment theorists posit that past relationship experiences affect our working models of ourselves and others, and these working models affect current relationships and current emotional experiences (Bowlby, 1969; Reis & Patrick, 1996). Like evolutionary theorists, attachment theorists believe that humans have an innate need to form close emotional bonds, and that this need is manifested even in very early stages in life. Because human infants cannot protect and care for themselves, they need to maintain close proximity to caregivers. Those who do are more likely to survive. In addition, infants need to explore their environment to learn. Attachment theorists posit that exploration and proximity maintenance are regulated through emotional processes. When danger is perceived, infants feel fear and anxiety and retreat to the relative comfort of the caregiver. When the environment seems safe, the infant feels secure and is willing to explore. Bowlby also thought that early attachment experiences led to the formation of working models of relationships, which in turn guide future relationship experiences. Thus one's early relationship history could affect one's view of oneself, one's view of potential relationship partners, and one's expectation about new relationships, and together these expectations could affect current relationship patterns and current levels of SWB.

EMPIRICAL LINKS BETWEEN SOCIAL RELATIONSHIPS AND SUBJECTIVE WELL-BEING

Social relationships are often held up as the single most important correlate of SWB (Argyle, 2001). Many reviewers note the predictive power of relationships when compared to other pieces of information about an individual's life (e.g., Myers, 2000). Yet effect sizes for various predictors are rarely compared directly. We wanted to determine whether the effect sizes for social relationships are truly bigger than the effect sizes for other commonly investigated factors. As a point of comparison, we chose to focus on one correlation that has received quite a bit of attention: the correlation between income and SWB.

To estimate the size of the income effect, we turned to four different sources. First, Diener and Biswas-Diener (2002) recently conducted a review of within-nation correlations between income and SWB. They listed results from 11 different studies. Correlations ranged from −.02 to .45, with an unweighted average across all studies of .20. Pinquart and Sörensen (2000) presented a more thorough review, conducting a meta-analysis of the association between socioeconomic status and well-being among the elderly. They found an average correlation of .21 between income and happiness and an average correlation of .18 between income and life satisfaction. An earlier meta-analysis by Haring, Stock, and Okun (1984) found an average correlation of .17 between SWB and income. Finally, we turned to the General Social Survey (Davis, Smith, & Marsden, 2003) to assess the correlation between SWB and real income in 1986 dollars among over 30,000 Americans assessed between 1972 and 1998. The correlation in this sample was .18. Thus various sources consistently show that the average correlation between income and happiness is somewhere between .17 and .21. These correlations will serve as a reference point when we discuss the effects of social relationships.

We divide our discussion into three sections. First, we focus on general measures of sociability and social activity. Next, we investigate more specific measures that assess the number of friends that an individual has and his or her frequency of contact with other people. Finally, we investigate the associations between marital status and well-being.

Sociability and Social Activity

One of the oldest lines of research within the field of SWB investigates the links between sociability and happiness. In the 1930s, for example, Watson (1930) and Jasper (1930) found that the personality trait of extraversion (which assesses an individual's degree of sociability, among other characteristics) correlates positively with emotional well-being. In 1967, Wilson conducted a comprehensive review of the correlates of "avowed happiness" and found that social relationships and feelings of sociability are consistent predictors of happiness. In 1969, Bradburn found that pleasant affect (but not unpleasant affect) is related to sociability. These initial findings led to at least two streams of research that have informed our understanding of the role of social relationships in SWB.

On the one hand, researchers have followed up on Watson's (1930) and Jasper's (1930) findings that extraverts are happier than introverts. Costa and McCrae (1980), for instance, replicated this effect, showing that extraversion was related to positive but not to negative affect, neuroticism was related to negative but not to positive affect, and that both extraversion and neuroticism affected life satisfaction through the affective variables. Since Costa and McCrae published their paper, numerous studies have replicated these findings (see Lucas & Fujita, 2000, and Watson & Clark, 1997, for reviews). In a meta-analysis, Lucas and Fujita (2000) found that the weighted average correlation between extraversion and positive affect was .37. The correlation was slightly lower, but still moderate, when different sources (self- vs. informant reports) were used to assess extraversion and pleasant affect ($r = .25$) and when daily or moment reports of pleasant affect were used ($r = .28$). In addition, Lucas and Fujita conducted a series of studies showing that when multiple measures of extraversion and positive affect were assessed and modeled using structural equation modeling techniques, the association between the two traits was very strong, often approaching .80. Together these results show that the association is not the result of shared method variance. The correlation between extraversion and positive affect is thus one of the strongest and most robust correlations in SWB research, much stronger than the effects of demographic factors like income.

Research into the links between extraversion and positive affect shows that personality traits that index sociability are moderately to strongly correlated with SWB variables. Early theorists suggested that extraverts were happier than introverts because extraverts spent so much time in enjoyable social interaction (e.g., Eysenck & Eysenck, 1985). However, a simple correlation between extraversion and well-being does not show that it is social relationships per se that affect well-being. Thus a second line of research has addressed this question directly, focusing on the links between social contact and well-being. These studies also provide evidence that social interaction matters. For instance, Argyle and Lu (1990) constructed a list of 37 common activities and asked participants how much they enjoyed each activity and how often they participated in each activity. After separating the list into groups of related activities, Argyle and Lu found that ratings of happiness correlated moderately (r's ranged from .20 to .43) with both enjoyment of and participation in social activities.

Argyle and Lu's (1990) study provides support for the idea that participation in social activity is important for happiness, but their methods were limited by a reliance on retrospective measures of social activity. But additional studies show that even when more rigorous methods are used, this association holds up well. For instance, researchers can use experience sampling methods (Bolger, Davis, & Rafaeli, 2003; Reis & Gable, 2000) to track social activity as it occurs. This strategy eliminates both memory problems and problems with the reconstruction of events. A number of researchers have used these techniques to document the association between social activity and well-being. For instance, Watson, Clark, and colleagues (Clark & Watson, 1988; Watson, 1988; Watson, Clark, McIntyre, & Hamaker, 1992) used daily diary methods to assess various types of social activities. They repeatedly showed that the amount of time an individual spends in social activities is moderately correlated (r's in the range of .30) with the amount of positive affect that he or she experiences. Consistent with research on extraversion, social activity is usually less strongly correlated or even uncorrelated with negative affect.

Studies that assess trait levels of extraversion or aggregated levels of social contact deal with questions at the level of the person—for example, Are people who participate in more social activity happier than those who participate in less social activity? This question is related to, but distinct from, questions about the extent to which individuals are happier when they are with others than when they are alone. This question can be answered by tracking changes in emotions across social and nonsocial situations using experience sampling and other diary methods. Consistent with research at the person level, these within-person studies show, again, that social interactions are associated with greater positive affect. For instance, Watson and colleagues (1992, Study 2) assessed a variety of mood and social activity variables over a 6- to 7-week period in a daily diary study (see also Clark & Watson, 1988; Gable, Reis, & Elliot, 2000; Larson & Csikszentmihalyi, 1983; Pavot, Diener, & Fujita, 1990; Watson, 1988). They found that daily levels of affect correlated .26 with daily social activity. However, the size of the correlation varied for different types of social activity. For instance, social activities related to "social entertainment" (e.g., going to a movie, playing cards, going shopping) and "active participation" (e.g., romantic activity, going to a party, getting a drink with friends) were significantly associated with within-person positive affect, but social activities related to "social responsibility" (e.g., having a serious discussion, running errands, or studying) were not. Interestingly, these associations were not always the same at the between-person level. Aggregated levels of social responsibility were more strongly correlated with positive affect than were aggregated levels of the other two social activity variables. This shows that between- and within-person analyses often provide different information about the nature of the association between social activity and well-being.

Studies examining the links between SWB and sociability provide support for the idea that social relationships matter for global levels of SWB. Extraverts are happier than introverts, and this greater happiness appears to be due in part to extraverts' greater social activity. People are happier when they are with others than when they are alone, and people who spend a lot of time with others are happier than those who spend more time alone. These correlations tend to be larger than correlations between SWB and income, and thus these studies provide support for the idea that social activity is a particularly important correlate. However, these studies also have a number of limitations. First, experience sampling studies generally focus on the amount of social contact an individual experiences during a short period of time (from a week to a few months). Short-term social activity is then used to predict affect that an individual experiences over the same period. Although such short-term affective variables are relevant to SWB research, they do not capture the "life-as-a-whole" aspect of SWB. It is possible that short-term levels of social activity provide an immediate boost to happiness, while long-term levels of social relationships play less of a role.

Second, research on general social activity cannot determine whether contact with close individuals is particularly beneficial. In their need-to-belong theory, Baumeister and Leary (1995) explicitly stated that everyday social interaction will not satisfy the basic need to belong. Instead, close, supportive relationships are necessary. Similarly, in his review of the literature on relationships and well-being, Myers (1999) noted that it is close, supportive relationships that seem to be most beneficial. Thus additional research is needed to determine whether close relationships are particularly important for SWB.

Friends and Family

Regarding the links between social relationships and well-being, a variety of variables can be examined. For instance, it is possible that the number of friends that an individual has is critical. Alternatively, it may be the amount of contact with friends that plays the most important role. A third possibility is that neither the number of friends nor the amount of contact with friends drives the relationship. Instead, it may be that certain types of relationships are particularly important. For instance, Pennebaker (1990) has shown that opening up to individuals about one's problems has beneficial health consequences. It may be that having a friend in whom one can confide provides the strongest benefits. For this reason, we discuss these different aspects of relationships separately.

As an initial investigation, we again turned to the General Social Survey. Between 1983 and 1987, over 6,000 respondents were asked to indicate the number of close friends that they had. If social relationships matter, those individuals who report having more close friends should also report higher levels of well-being. Consistent with existing reviews of the field, the number of friends that an individual reports does correlate significantly with his or her report of general happiness. However, the effect is not strong. The correlation between these two variables is only .13. This effect is actually smaller than the effect of income within the same sample ($r = .18$).

These results are quite typical of the literature on social relationships. In 1984, Okun, Stock, Haring, and Witter published a meta-analysis of research on social activity and well-being. Their analysis shows that the scope of an individual's social contact (which, according to their definition, includes the size of his or her social network) correlates just .16 with happiness and life satisfaction. In a more recent meta-analysis of research conducted with older adults, Pinquart and Sörensen (2000) found that quantity of social activity (including the number of relationships and the frequency of contact) only correlated .12 with life satisfaction and .17 with happiness. These numbers were only slightly higher (r's $= .14$ and .23) when relationships with friends were analyzed separately from relationships with adult children, family members, or other kin.

Evidence also suggests that frequency of contact does no better than number of friends as a predictor of SWB. For instance, in the General Social Survey, respondents were asked to indicate the frequency with which they spend a social evening with relatives, neighbors, friends, parents, and siblings. In addition, participants were asked how frequently they visited their closest friend and how often they called their closest friend on the phone. Correlations between these variables and happiness were all very small, with none exceeding .06. Similarly, when Okun and colleagues (1984) separated frequency of contact from scope of contact, they found that the correlations were lower when frequency measures were used. Frequency of social activity only correlated .13 with measures of SWB.

It is also possible that it is not having friends per se that is associated with well-being, but having someone to count on when times are difficult. Again, the General Social Survey provides evidence that this is not the case. Respondents were asked to indicate the number of people on whom they can call when they have problems. Again, the correlation with well-being was low, only .05.

Results from the General Social Survey and the meta-analyses of social activity are at odds with the evidence reviewed in the previous section. Experience sampling studies show that people who spend more time with others tend to experience greater levels of happiness, whereas survey research shows that the size of an individual's social network and the frequency of contact play a very small role. However, there are at least four differences between the studies reviewed in the two sections. First, experience sampling studies tend to use student samples, and these effects may vary for different age groups. Second, measures of well-being tend to differ across the two types of studies. Large surveys tend to use short (often single-item) measures of global happiness or life satisfaction, whereas experience sampling studies often include multiple-item measures of positive and negative affect. Social activity tends to correlate more strongly with positive affect than with negative affect, and large-scale survey research may find higher correlations if different measures were used. A third difference concerns the type of social activity that is assessed. Many experience sampling studies assess the percentage of time that an individual spends in social activity, whereas survey research often asks about the frequency with which specific social interactions occur. It is possible that social companionship matters more than close social relationships, and that experience sampling studies are more likely to tap this general social activity. Finally, as noted above, experience sampling studies often focus on social activity and well-being over relatively short periods of time. Social activity may provide a short-lived boost in affect, but this boost may not add up to long-term changes in global well-being. In any case, these different studies provide contradictory evidence. The field would be well served by an up-to-date meta-analysis that explicitly addresses potential moderators of these effects.

Marital Status and Well-Being

The final topic we address concerns the link between SWB and marital status. Studies from a variety of fields in the social sciences, using an array of measures, and across a range of nations, have consistently found an association between marital history and well-being (Johnson & Wu, 2002; Mastekaasa, 1994). Married people report the highest well-being scores; they are followed by the continuously single, and then by the widowed and divorced (e.g., Barrett, 2000; Hope, Rodgers, & Power, 1999). For instance, Mastekaasa (1994) used data from 19 nations to examine differences among married, divorced, widowed, and never married respondents. The married group was consistently highest in well-being while the divorced and widowed group was consistently lowest. Although some variations in the specific patterns of association between well-being measures and marital status surfaced, this large cross-sectional design provided clear evidence that well-being is related to marital status across a variety of nations. Two different meta-analyses have confirmed the existence of this reliable association (Haring-Hidore, Stock, Okun, & Witter, 1985; Wood, Rhodes, & Whelan, 1989).

However, as with social relationships in general, the effect of marital status is not strong. In the General Social Survey, for instance, marital status accounts for about 5% of the variance in reports of happiness. This corresponds to a correlation of approximately .23, just slightly higher than the correlation between well-being and income. Results from the meta-analyses show even smaller correlations. For instance, Haring-Hidore and colleagues (1985) reported an average correlation of just .14 between happiness and marital status. This effect was reduced even further when analyses were restricted to comparisons between married and never married respondents ($r = .09$). Thus we can conclude that marriage matters, but the effect is not large (also see DePaulo & Morris, 2005).

As they have with social relationships in general, researchers have attempted to determine the underlying causes of the association between marital status and SWB. Three classes of explanations have been proposed: crisis explanations, role explanations, and selection effects. *Crisis explanations* posit that role transitions create temporary changes in well-being that subside over time. For marriage, this temporary change would be positive; for divorce and widowhood, it would be negative. If the crisis explanation is correct, the association between happiness and well-being should disappear once time since the marital event is controlled.

If the effects of marriage are long lasting, then additional processes are needed to account for these effects. For instance, *role explanations* posit that the effects of marriage result from permanent changes in an individual's social role. The role of a divorced or widowed person may be more difficult than the role of someone with the support and resources provided by marriage (Johnson & Wu, 2002). The social role argument suggests that divorce and widowhood lead to permanent increases in stress that result in lasting negative effects beyond the period of initial separation. Permanent life strains may include economic hardship, additional childcare responsibilities, and the loss of social support provided by a spouse. If the social role explanation is correct, people should show permanent changes in happiness following marriage, divorce, or widowhood.

The final explanation that has been suggested concerns *selection effects*. It is possible that individuals who possess certain characteristics are also predisposed to particular marital outcomes. For instance, happy people may be easier to live with and may be more likely to attract and hold on to a partner. If selection effects exist, differences between groups should emerge long before any marital event has occurred. For instance, longitudinal studies should show that happily married individuals were happier than divorced individuals long before the individuals in either group got married.

Support for all three explanations is mixed. For instance, Booth and Amato (1991) used data from a three-wave panel study to look at the effects of divorce on psychological stress. The 8-year study showed that stress levels rise prior to the actual divorce and begin to decrease afterward. In support of the crisis explanation, divorced individuals eventually returned to levels of well-being that were similar to those of people who remained married. However, two additional studies suggest that divorce can be associated with permanent changes in well-being. Mastekaasa (1995) used an 8-year Norwegian panel study to examine SWB following divorce. Consistent with the findings of Booth and Amato's study, reported distress began to increase prior to divorce or separation. However, in Mastekaasa's study, distress levels were about the same whether measured in the first 4 years after divorce or 4–8 years later. Similarly, Johnson and Wu (2002) found no evidence that distress abated in the period following divorce. Interestingly, Johnson and Wu used the same panel study (with an additional wave of data and a different analytic technique) that Booth and Amato had used, yet the two studies arrived at different conclusions about crisis effects.

Support for crisis explanations also vary depending on the specific marital event that is examined. Recently, we used data from a 15-year longitudinal study to simultaneously examine crisis, role, and selection explanations of the marital status/SWB association. By following large groups of individuals for long periods of time, the entire time course of relation formation and dissolution could be tracked. Results from our first study (Lucas, Clark, Georgellis, & Diener, 2003) showed that the pattern of reactions following widowhood supports a crisis explanation. Specifically, respondents dropped about 1.5 points on an 11-point scale (which is very large considering that most people fall within a point or two of the average), they took about 8 years to reach their maximum postevent levels of happiness, and these levels were not quite as high as before they lost their spouse. Adaptation did occur, but it took a long time and was somewhat incomplete.

Similarly, results showed that marriage itself was not associated with long-lasting changes in happiness. Instead, life satisfaction ratings went up slightly in the years before marriage, reached a peak during the year of marriage, and then declined relatively quickly in the subsequent years. In fact, married respondents returned to their premarriage level of happiness in just 2 years, on average. These results suggest that the association between marital status and happiness is due more to the effects of divorce and widowhood than to the effect of marriage itself.

Finally, studies also find support for selection effects. For instance, individuals who eventually marry have lower initial psychiatric symptoms than those who remain single (Hope et al., 1999). Lucas and colleagues (2003; Lucas, in press) found that married people were happier than average long before they married, and that people who would eventually divorce were less happy than people who would stay married long before the individuals in either group got married. Stutzer and Frey (2003) tested selection effects explicitly (using the same German data set that Lucas used). They found that happy singles were in fact more likely than unhappy singles to get married in the near future.

Although preexisting differences between people who will eventually marry and those who will not (and between people who will stay married and those who will divorce) provide support for selection effects, these are not the only studies to do so. In addition, a recent behavioral genetic analysis indicated that propensity to marry is heritable (Johnson, McGue, Krueger, & Bouchard, 2004). Therefore, it is possible that those who are genetically predisposed to emotional well-being may also be individuals who are most likely to marry. Further evidence of possible self-selection into stable marriages for individuals high in well-being are found in the personality literature where traits such as extraversion are found to correlate with rates of divorce (Jockin, McGue, & Lykken, 1996).

These results suggest that crisis, social role, and selection effects may play different roles for different marital events. The higher levels of happiness among married people seem to be due in part to selection effects and to the short-lived boost that recently married individuals receive. In addition, divorced people seem to be less happy than married people even before individuals in either group marry. Finally, both divorce and widowhood have long-lasting effects on happiness and it appears that divorced people never quite return to baseline levels of happiness.

SUMMARY

The evidence reviewed in this chapter shows that social relationships do predict SWB. People who are sociable and extraverted experience more positive affect than those who are not. People who spend more time with others are happier than those who spend a lot of time alone. People who have many friends are happier than those who have only a few. And people who are married are happier than those who are divorced or widowed. However, the size of these effects does not support the conclusion that the existence of social relationships is a particularly strong correlate. Correlations with extraversion tend to be moderate to large, but extraverts' greater social activity can only partially explain their greater happiness. Correlations with marital status, number of friends, frequency of visits with friends, and other measures of actual social activity tend to be small, generally falling between .10 and .20. In fact, these correlations tend to be weaker than the effect of income, an effect that has been described as miniscule.

Why, then, have social relationships been held up as "the single greatest cause" of SWB (Argyle, 2001, p. 71) when most effect sizes are very small? We believe that there are three reasons, all of which are speculative at this time. First, most of the research reviewed in this chapter relied on large-scale nationally representative surveys or meta-analyses of existing research. The former generally include single-item measures of happiness or life satisfaction; the latter tend to aggregate across a variety of well-being measures including happiness, satisfaction, positive affect, and negative affect. Although on average effect sizes tend to be small, there is some evidence that they are larger when analyses focus specifically on measures of positive affect. Thus future research must examine these variables separately to clarify the size of this effect.

A second possible reason is that the beneficial effects of social relationships on SWB are generally discussed in the context of outcomes from a wide variety of domains. Reviewers often point out that social relationships are not only linked with happiness and life satisfaction, they also predict risk for mental illness, poor physical health, and even death (e.g., Berkman & Syme, 1979; House, Landis, & Umberson, 1988; House, Robbins, & Metzner, 1982). Thus the robustness of these effects and the variety of domains in which social relationships seem to matter is impressive, even if the size of the effects within these domains is not. Social relationships may have wide-reaching but subtle effects that together make them important for people's physical and mental health.

A final factor concerns the fact that relationship quality may be more important for well-being than the mere existence of relationships or the frequency with which individuals engage in social contact. In addition to measuring the existence of social relationships, researchers often assess satisfaction with relationships or the extent to which an individual values strong relationships over other outcomes in his or her life, and it is these variables that may have the strongest effects (Myers, 1999). Presumably, these measures tap additional information about the quality of people's relationships—information that is not reflected in simple measures of quantity. Our review focused on the existence of social relationships, so we cannot draw any conclusions about the importance of these additional characteristics. We believe that the quality of people's relationships should matter for well-being, and therefore these variables are important and interesting.

However, measures of these constructs must also be interpreted cautiously. For instance, no one would interpret a measure of income satisfaction as providing additional information about the "quality" of an individual's income. These satisfaction measures may provide valid information about a person's relative income (compared to salient others) or the value that a person places on income, but they do not provide any information about the objective characteristics of the income itself. Yet researchers often do interpret relationship satisfaction ratings as indicators of some characteristic of the relationship. Unfortunately, these relationship satisfaction ratings are likely to tap a general tendency to be satisfied with various other domains in life. This additional variance will inflate correlations with global measures of well-being. Strong conclusions can only be drawn from studies that use sophisticated methods to assess relationship quality. Thus simple measures of self-reported relationship satisfaction must be interpreted cautiously.

Because of these limitations in existing research, future studies should focus on clarifying the size of the correlations when various types of social relationship measures are used. Updated meta-analyses that are guided by strong theories will help to clarify which social relationships are most important for well-being. In addition, multiple-method studies of relationship quality can clarify whether additional characteristics beyond the existence of relationships are responsible for their beneficial effects. Finally, sophisticated research designs including behavior genetic analyses (e.g., Jockin et al., 1996; Johnson et al., 2004) and longitudinal studies (Johnson & Wu, 2002; Lucas et al., 2003; Stutzer & Frey, 2003) can help to rule out alternative explanations of these effects.

On a final note, we should clarify that we are not saying that the existence of social relationships is unimportant—just that the effect sizes are small by traditional standards. As we have argued elsewhere (Lucas & Dyrenforth, 2005), these small effects can be extremely important. For instance, the effect sizes for relationships tend to be at least as high as the effect of the nicotine patch on smoking cessation ($r = .18$), slightly higher than the effect of antihistamines on a runny nose ($r = .11$), and much higher than the effect of aspirin on the reduced risk of death by heart attack ($r = .02$; see Meyer et al., 2001, for a summary of effect sizes from many different fields). Thus, even if the true effect size is around .20, relationships can have a powerful effect on well-being.

REFERENCES

Argyle, M. (2001). *The psychology of happiness* (2nd ed.). New York: Routledge.

Argyle, M., & Lu, L. (1990). The happiness of extraverts. *Personality and Individual Differences, 11*(10), 1011–1017.

Berscheid, E., & Reis, H. T. (1998). Attraction and close relationships. In D. T. Gilbert, S. T. Fiske, & G. Lindzey (Eds.), *The handbook of social psychology* (4th ed., pp. 193–281). New York: McGraw-Hill.

Barrett, A. E. (2000). Marital trajectories and mental health. *Journal of Health and Social Behavior, 41*, 451–464.

Baumeister, R. F., & Leary, M. R. (1995). The need to belong: Desire for interpersonal attachments as a fundamental human motivation. *Psychological Bulletin, 117*(3), 497–529.

Berkman, L. F., & Syme, S. L. (1979). Social networks, host resistance, and mortality: A nine-year follow-up study of Alameda County residents. *American Journal of Epidemiology, 109*(2), 186–204.

Bolger, N., Davis, A., & Rafaeli, E. (2003). Diary methods: Capturing life as it is lived. *Annual Review of Psychology, 54*, 579–616.

Booth, A., & Amato, P. (1991). Divorce and psychological stress. *Journal of Health and Social Behavior, 32*, 396–407.

Bowlby, J. (1969). *Attachment and loss* (Vol. 1). New York: Basic Books.

Bradburn, N. M. (1969). *The structure of psychological well-being*. Oxford, UK: Aldine.

Buss, D. M. (1990). The evolution of anxiety and social exclusion. *Journal of Social and Clinical Psychology, 9*(2), 196–201.

Buss, D. M. (2000). The evolution of happiness. *American Psychologist, 55*(1), 15–23.

Campbell, A., Converse, P. E., & Rodgers, W. L. (1976). *The quality of American life: Perceptions, evaluations, and satisfactions*. New York: Russell Sage Foundation.

Clark, M. S., & Mills, J. (1979). Interpersonal attraction in exchange and communal relationships. *Journal of Personality and Social Psychology, 37*(1), 12–24.

Clark, M. S., & Watson, L. A. (1988). Mood and the mundane: Relations between daily life events and self-reported mood. *Journal of Personality and Social Psychology, 54*(2), 296–308.

Costa, P. T., & McCrae, R. R. (1980). Influence of extraversion and neuroticism on subjective well-being: Happy and unhappy people. *Journal of Personality and Social Psychology, 38*(4), 668–678.

Davis, J. A., Smith, T. W., & Marsden, P. V. (2003). *General Social Surveys, 1972–2002* [Computer file]. Ann Arbor, MI: Inter-University Consortium for Political and Social Research. Available at webapp.icpsr.umich.edu/GSS/.

Deci, E. L., & Ryan, R. M. (2000). The "what" and "why" of goal pursuits: Human needs and the self-determination of behavior. *Psychologial Inquiry, 11*, 227–268.

DePaulo, B. M., & Morris, W. L. (2005). Singles in society and in science. *Psychological Inquiry, 16*, 57–83.

Diener, E., & Biswas-Diener, R. (2002). Will money increase subjective well-being? *Social Indicators Research, 57*(2), 119–169.

Diener, E., & Emmons, R. (1984). The independence of positive and negative affect. *Journal of Personality and Social Psychology, 47*(5), 1105–1117.

Diener, E., & Lucas, R. E. (1999). Personality and subjective well-being. In D. Kahneman, E. Diener, & N. Schwarz (Eds.), *Well-being: The foundations of hedonic psychology* (pp. 213–229). New York: Russell Sage Foundation.

Diener, E., Scollon, C. N., & Lucas, R. E. (2004). The evolving concept of subjective well-being: The multifaceted nature of happiness. *Advances in Cell Aging and Gerontology, 15*, 187–219.

Diener, E., Suh, E. M., Lucas, R. E., & Smith, H. L. (1999). Subjective well-being: Three decades of progress. *Psychological Bulletin, 125*(2), 276–302.

Eysenck, H. J., & Eysenck, M. W. (1985). *Personality and individual differences*. New York: Plenum Press.

Gable, S. L., Reis, H. T., & Elliot, A. J. (2000). Behavioral activation and inhibition in everyday life. *Journal of Personality and Social Psychology, 78*(6), 1135–1149.

Haring, M., Stock, W. A., & Okun, M. A. (1984). A research synthesis of gender and social class as correlates of subjective well-being. *Human Relations, 37*, 645–657.

Haring-Hidore, M., Stock, W. A., Okun, M. A., & Witter, R. A. (1985). Marital status and subjective well-being: A research synthesis. *Journal of Marriage and the Family, 47*(4), 947–953.

Hope, S., Rodgers, B., & Power, C. (1999). Marital status transitions and psychological distress: Longitudinal evidence from a national population sample. *Psychological Medicine, 29*(2), 381–389.

House, J. S., Landis, K. R., & Umberson, D. (1988). Social relationships and health. *Science, 241*, 540–545.

House, J. S., Robbins, C., & Metzner, H. L. (1982). The association of social relationships and activities with mortality: Prospective evidence from the Tecumseh Community Health Study. *American Journal of Epidemiology, 116*(1), 123–140.

Jasper, H. H. (1930). The measurement of depression–elation and its relation to a measure of extraversion–introversion. *Journal of Abnormal and Social Psychology, 25*, 307–318.

Jockin, V., McGue, M., & Lykken, D. T. (1996). Personality and divorce: A genetic analysis. *Journal of Personality and Social Psychology, 71*(2), 288–299.

Johnson, D. R., & Wu, J. (2002). An empirical test of crisis, social selection, and role explanations of the relationship between marital disruption and psychological distress: A pooled time-series analysis of four-wave panel data. *Journal of Marriage and Family, 64*(1), 211–224.

Johnson, W., McGue, M., Krueger, R. F., & Bouchard, T. J. (2004). Marriage and personality: A genetic analysis. *Journal of Personality and Social Psychology, 85*(2), 285–294.

Larson, R., & Csikszentmihalyi, M. (1983). The experience sampling method. *New Directions for Methodology of Social and Behavioral Science, 15*, 41–56.

Lucas, R. E. (in press). Time does not heal all wounds: A longitudinal study of reaction and adaptation to divorce. *Psychological Science*.

Lucas, R. E., Clark, A. E., Georgellis, Y., & Diener, E. (2003). Reexamining adaptation and the set point model of happiness: Reactions to changes in marital status. *Journal of Personality and Social Psychology, 84*(3), 527–539.

Lucas, R. E., Diener, E., & Suh, E. (1996). Discriminant validity of well-being measures. *Journal of Personality and Social Psychology, 71*(3), 616–628.

Lucas, R. E., & Dyrenforth, P. S. (2005). The myth of marital bliss? *Psychological Inquiry, 16,* 111–115.

Lucas, R. E., & Fujita, F. (2000). Factors influencing the relation between extraversion and pleasant affect. *Journal of Personality and Social Psychology, 79*(6), 1039–1056.

Lykken, D., & Tellegen, A. (1996). Happiness is a stochastic phenomenon. *Psychological Science, 7*(3), 186–189.

Maslow, A. H. (1970). *Motivation and personality* (2nd ed.). New York: Harper & Row.

Mastekaasa, A. (1994). Marital status, distress, and well-being: An international comparison. *Journal of Comparative Family Studies, 25*(2), 183–205.

Mastekaasa, A. (1995). Marital dissolution and subjective distress: Panel evidence. *European Sociological Review, 11*(2), 173–185.

Meyer, G. J., Finn, S. E., Eyde, L. D., Kay, G. G., Moreland, K. L., Dies, R. R., et al. (2001). Psychological testing and psychological assessment: A review of evidence and issues. *American Psychologist, 56*(2), 128–165.

Myers, D. G. (1992). *The pursuit of happiness: Who is happy and why.* New York: Morrow.

Myers, D. G. (1999). Close relationships and quality of life. In D. Kahneman, E. Diener, & N. Schwarz (Eds.), *Well-being: The foundations of hedonic psychology* (pp. 374–391). New York: Russell Sage Foundation.

Myers, D. G. (2000). The funds, friends, and faith of happy people. *American Psychologist, 55*(1), 56–67.

Okun, M. A., Stock, W. A., Haring, M. J., & Witter, R. A. (1984). Health and subjective well-being: A meta-analysis. *International Journal of Aging and Human Development, 19,* 111–132.

Pavot, W., Diener, E., & Fujita, F. (1990). Extraversion and happiness. *Personality and Individual Differences, 11*(12), 1299–1306.

Pennebaker, J. W. (1990). *Opening up: The healing power of confiding in others.* New York: Morrow.

Pinquart, M., & Sörensen, S. (2000). Influences of socioeconomic status, social network, and competence on subjective well-being in later life: A meta-analysis. *Psychology and Aging, 15*(2), 187–224.

Reis, H. T. (2001). Relationship experiences and emotional well-being. In C. D. Ryff & B. H. Singer (Eds.), *Emotion, social relationships and health* (pp. 57–95). New York: Oxford University Press.

Reis, H. T., & Gable, S. L. (2000). Event-sampling and other methods for studying everyday experience. In C. M. Judd & H. T. Reis (Eds.), *Handbook of research methods in social and personality psychology* (pp. 190–222). New York: Cambridge University Press.

Reis, H. T., & Patrick, C. (1996). Attachment and intimacy: Component processes. In E. T. Higgins & A. W. Kruglanski (Eds.), *Social psychology: Handbook of basic principles* (pp. 523–563). New York: Guilford Press.

Rusbult, C. E., & Van Lange, P. A. (1996). Interdependence processes. In E. T. Higgins & A. W. Kruglanski (Eds.), *Social psychology: Handbook of basic principles* (pp. 564–596). New York: Guilford Press.

Ryan, R. M., & Deci, E. L. (2002). Overview of self-determination theory: An organismic-dialectical perspective. In R. M. Ryan & E. L. Deci (Eds.), *Handbook of self-determination research* (pp. 3–33). Rochester, NY: University of Rochester Press.

Schwarz, N., & Strack, F. (1999). Reports of subjective well-being: Judgmental processes and their methodological implications. In D. Kahneman, E. Diener, & N. Schwarz (Eds.), *Well-being: The foundations of hedonic psychology* (pp. 61–84). New York: Russell Sage Foundation.

Stutzer, A., & Frey, B. S. (2003). *Does marriage make people happy, or do happy people get married?* Social Science Research Network. Retrieved August 27, 2004, from ssrn.com/abstract=375960.

Watson, D. (1988). Intraindividual and interindividual analyses of positive and negative affect: Their relation to health complaints, perceived stress, and daily activities. *Journal of Personality and Social Psychology, 54*(6), 1020–1030.

Watson, D., & Clark, L. A. (1997). Extraversion and its positive emotional core. In R. Hogan, J. A. Johnson, & S. Briggs (Eds.), *Handbook of personality psychology* (pp. 767–793). San Diego, CA: Academic Press.

Watson, D., Clark, L. A., McIntyre, C. W., & Hamaker, S. (1992). Affect, personality, and social activity. *Journal of Personality and Social Psychology, 63*(6), 1011–1025.

Watson, D., & Tellegen, A. (1985). Toward a consensual structure of mood. *Psychological Bulletin, 98*(2), 219–235.

Watson, G. B. (1930). Happiness among adult students of education. *Journal of Educational Psychology, 21*, 79–109.

Wills, T. A. (1985). Supportive functions of interpersonal relationships. In S. Cohen & S. L. Syme (Eds.), *Social support and health* (pp. 61–82). Orlando, FL: Academic Press.

Wilson, W. R. (1967). Correlates of avowed happiness. *Psychological Bulletin, 67*(4), 294–306.

Wood, W., Rhodes, N., & Whelan, M. (1989). Sex differences in positive well-being: A consideration of emotional style and marital status. *Psychological Bulletin, 106*(2), 249–264.

CHAPTER 14

Cognitive Interdependence

Considering Self-in-Relationship

CHRISTOPHER R. AGNEW
PAUL E. ETCHEVERRY

Close interpersonal relationships serve as a critical interface between intrapersonal and interpersonal processes. These processes underlying relationships have generally been considered in isolation, though with appreciable success. Within-person approaches to understanding relational phenomena abound, including compelling work on attachment orientations (see Feeney, Chapter 7, this volume), personality dimensions relevant to relationships (see Campbell, Brunell, & Finkel, Chapter 4, this volume), implicit theories of relationships (see Knee & Canevello, Chapter 8, this volume), and self-regulation (Vohs & Ciarocco, 2004; also see Rawn & Vohs, Chapter 2, this volume). Moreover, between-person, relationship-focused approaches considering that which emerges or resides between partners in ongoing involvements, such as relationship satisfaction (Arriaga, 2001), self-expansion (see Strong & Aron, Chapter 17, this volume), or interdependence (Rusbult & Van Lange, 2003; also see Kumashiro, Rusbult, Wolf, & Estrada, Chapter 16, this volume), have also flourished in recent years. Although both intrapersonal and interpersonal approaches provide important knowledge about close relationships, each approach is clearly limited by that which it does not fully consider.

We believe that the concept of *cognitive interdependence*, or the mental state characterized by a pluralistic, collective representation of self-in-relationship, represents a congenial blending of the intrapersonal and the interpersonal. The current chapter reviews the concept of cognitive interdependence, with a particular focus on some implications of the concept for the self. We begin by considering past work on the self, including a discussion of cognitive, affective, and behavioral structures linking relationship partners to the self, before turning our attention to cognitive interdependence. We close with suggested avenues for future work on self-in-relationship.

THE SELF IN RELATION

The study of the self in social psychology is ubiquitous. The very notion of the "self" has evolved as the traditional concept of a unidimensional independent self, socially isolated, has been debunked both theoretically and empirically (Tice & Baumeister, 2001). A growing body of research indicates that the self is both social and contextual. For example, in perhaps the most successful characterization of the self as social, social identity theory (Tajfel & Turner, 1986) has championed the importance of group-level identity, or the ability of group membership to influence views of the self. A large number of empirical studies have supported the importance of the collective self in influencing people's behavior, cognition, and emotional reactions (for a review, see Brewer & Brown, 1998). In addition, research has shown that not all group memberships are equally meaningful to the self. Rather, the chronic importance of group membership and situational changes in relevancy of group membership help determine which aspect of the self will be salient at any given time.

More recently, theorists have begun to consider the possibility of a relational self (Acitelli, Rogers, & Knee, 1999; Andersen & Chen, 2002; Cross & Morris, 2003; Garrido & Acitelli, 1999; Sedikides & Brewer, 2001). The relational self involves a consideration of the interpersonal relationships (primarily dyadic) in which a person is involved and how these relationships are incorporated into the self. A relational self develops when the self becomes defined, at least in part, in terms of interpersonal relationships. By being tied to the self, these relationships and relationship partners gain privileged status to influence behavior, cognition, and affect, as well as perceptions of the self. Of course, a person initiates many relationships over the course of a lifetime, most of which are not incorporated into his or her relational self. An important issue, then, is which relationships will become part of the self. Basing our own ideas on interdependence theory (Kelley & Thibaut, 1978; Rusbult, Arriaga, & Agnew, 2001; Thibaut & Kelley, 1959), we posit that relationships in which two people are highly interdependent such that the actions of one person strongly influence the outcomes of the other will be most likely to become incorporated into a sense of self.

Interdependence theory is a broad yet flexible theory of human social behavior (Rusbult et al., 2001). It provides a set of concepts for characterizing any given dyadic or group situation, and it describes the ways in which differ- ent situations shape motivation and behavior in dyads, including romantically involved couples (Kelley, 1979; Kelley & Thibaut, 1978). *Interdependence* exists between two people when the actions of one person can partially or wholly determine the outcomes of another. The opportunity for influencing each other's outcomes lays the groundwork for developing mutually reward- ing or mutually harmful patterns of interactions and interpersonal contact. However, simple interdependence will unlikely be enough for a relational self to develop. For example, if two cars arrive at a four-way intersection at the same time, the two drivers can be said to be interdependent because a wrong move by either can result in disaster for both (i.e., an accident). However, given the transitory nature of this interdependence, it is unlikely that either driver could be said to have developed much of a relationship with the other. Instead, the level of interdependence needed to begin to develop a relational sense of self is likely to be quite high and would have to last an extended period of time. It is likely that only a few prototypical relationships typically become incorporated into one's sense of self. These might include relation- ships between parents and children, siblings, close friends, and romantic part- ners.

Of course, some less-than-positive interactions can be characterized by a high level of interdependence. For example, a relationship with an annoying roommate, a competitive coworker, or a member of a competing sports team could all have characteristics of high interdependence. But these types of rela- tionships would probably not lead to a relational sense of self that includes that person. Along with a high degree of interdependence, relationships would need to be characterized by a strong *correspondence of outcomes*, in which cooperation and shared benefits are seen as possible between the two members of the dyad in order to be likely to involve an incorporation of the relationship into the self. As a dyad works together to achieve positive out- comes and mutual goals, a sense of a relational self should emerge. However, when the pursuit of outcomes becomes more competitive and members of the dyad are pursuing individualistic goals, a sense of a relational self will not develop or, if already present, may begin to weaken in established relation- ships.

Once a relational sense of self is established, it is important to consider what consequences will result. Consistent with interdependence theory, high levels of interdependence will result in two main consequences relevant to the self. First, the interdependence of the relationship will begin to express itself in the development of *cognitive, affective, and behavioral structures* that are unique to a relationship partner and to the relationship. A hallmark of an interdependent relationship and dependence on a partner will be the impor- tance ascribed to the relationship and the unique relationship motives and structures developed to assist in interaction within the relationship. Second, interdependence of a relationship and correspondence of outcomes in the relationship will lead to consciously *considering the self as part of the relationship*, interconnected with the relationship partner, in a manner that minimizes the distinctions between the individual self and the self in the relationship. Past research on the relational self or self-in-relationships has primarily focused on either one or the other of these aspects (Mashek, Aron, & Boncimino, 2003).

STRUCTURES LINKING RELATIONSHIP PARTNERS TO THE SELF

Several theoretical perspectives have focused on the ability of a relationship or an interdependent partner to influence cognitive, affective, and behavioral structures and uniquely link these to the sense of self. One of the most prominent of these is self-discrepancy theory (Higgins & May, 2001), which incorporates the actual or perceived wishes of important other people (e.g., parent, romantic partner) into self-regulation of personal behavior and affect responses. From this perspective, awareness of the actual or perceived expectations that others have (called the "instrumental actual self") includes those characteristics of the self that enable one to be viewed more or less positively by others. This awareness is assumed to become incorporated into cognitive and behavioral strategies for self-regulation and results in the enactment (or avoidance) of certain behaviors.

Self-discrepancy theory also argues that a person is aware of the wishes and prescriptive expectations that others have regarding him or her. Knowledge of what important others ideally wish one would do or expect that one ought to do can be incorporated into self-regulatory processes designed to achieve these goals. These expectations, especially when they originate from others perceived as important, influence a person's self-regulation, and thus influence cognition, affect, and behavior (Higgins, 1989).

Goals are also relevant to self-regulation. It has been theorized that goals become associated in cognition with the person or persons to whom these goals are relevant (see Shah, Chapter 19, and Fitzsimons, Chapter 3, this volume). A goal may become tied to another person because that person is the target of the goal, the means to achieve that goal, or a person who strongly wishes that goal to be achieved. Research from this perspective has demonstrated that a person who is associated with a goal can help to prime or activate that goal. Once activated, goals influence cognition and behavior in order to allow movement toward the achievement of those goals, both consciously and automatically (Shah, 2003).

Adult attachment theory (Hazan & Shaver, 1987) also discusses the ability of a relationship and a relationship partner to influence cognition and behavior relevant to the self and the relationship. Most often, adult attachment has been discussed in terms of individual differences (Simpson & Rholes, 1998). However, it is important to note that attachment theory assumes a general attachment system with specific needs that a person seeks to satisfy (e.g., safe haven, intimacy). As the interdependence of a relationship increases, members of that relationship will learn how to interact in order to satisfy their attachment needs. Learned patterns of behavior related to general attachment (i.e., attachment styles) will likely change somewhat in response to a specific partner's behavior and the state of the larger relationship. In this way, cognition and behavior relevant to attachment goals will change in response to the interdependent nature of the relationship (Fraley, 2002; Overall, Fletcher, & Friesen, 2003).

All these theories describe how aspects of cognition, affect, and behavior are tied to expectations and knowledge of close personal relationships and the relationship partners. In a social-cognitive account of the relational self, Andersen and Chen (2002) propose a theoretical perspective in which knowledge of the self becomes linked to knowledge of a significant other, thereby forming a relationship self. Since each relationship will be different, the overall set of knowledge of the self, as well as cognitive, affective, and behavioral structures, will be unique to each relationship although overlap will occur across similar relationships. From this perspective, similar to self-discrepancy theory and the notion of automatic activation of goals (Shah, 2003), consideration of the significant other and the relationship with that person will activate the relevant knowledge of the self as well as relevant cognitive, affective, and behavioral structures. This perspective, as with interdependence theory, assumes that the relationship-specific knowledge and patterns of activation will be most common with highly important interpersonal relationships.

The previously discussed perspectives provide important evidence of how highly interdependent people develop sets of knowledge about each other as well as cognitive, affective, and behavioral structures unique to their relationships and partners. However, these perspectives do not assume that the relationship partner has been incorporated into the individual's sense of self. Rather, they describe processes that occur within close intimate relationships but that could also occur across a wide range of relationships. It is our belief that the ability of another person to influence self-perception and to activate cognitive and behavioral structures is a necessary but not a sufficient condition to imply the existence of a relational self. We believe that along with the development of unique relationship knowledge for a particular interpersonal relationship, a relational self also implies that the person in the relationship begins to think of his or her self in terms of the relationship, minimizing the differences between the self, the partner, and the relationship. We now turn to research that has more strongly focused on this sense of a relational self.

BLURRING THE DISTINCTION BETWEEN
THE INTERDEPENDENT RELATIONSHIP AND THE SELF

A relational self implies something more than the development of relationship-specific, self-relevant cognitive, affective, and behavioral structures. Interdependence in a relationship can lead to a sense of a relational self in which members of a relationship think of themselves in terms of the relationship and as connected to the relationship partner, minimizing discrepancies between the individual self, the self in relationships, and the self and the partner. This leads to knowledge of the self being recast in terms of the relationship. The perception of the self-in-relationship should also reinforce the unique cognitive, affective, and behavioral processes associated with that relationship.

This perspective on the relational self as including an explicit redefinition of the self in terms of an interdependent relationship has received theoretical and empirical consideration. Some recent research has proposed that individual differences may exist in the degree to which people define themselves in terms of their interpersonal relationships. For some people, interpersonal relationships may be an important part of their sense of self, but for others the self may be defined much more independently (Cross & Morris, 2003). This view of an interpersonal self has been found to be associated with memory for information about others and organization of information about others in terms of relationships (Cross, Morris, & Gore, 2002).

In a more relationship-specific perspective, proponents of self-expansion theory have argued that people seek to incorporate aspects of their partner into their sense of self. As relationship closeness increases, the partner's characteristics begin to blend with those of the self, leading to actual confusion between the two. This sense of an expanded self can lead to more positive treatment of a partner, as demonstrated in reward allocation games, in which best friends were given more rewards than strangers or casual acquaintances (Mashek et al., 2003). Self-expansion can benefit the relationship as a person initiates self-protective mechanisms to support the relationship and the partner (Goodfriend, 2004).

COMBINING RELATIONSHIP-SPECIFIC STRUCTURES
WITH A RELATIONAL SENSE OF SELF

We argue that the strongest form of an interdependent relational self will include (1) unique relationship-specific cognitive, affective, and behavioral structures; and (2) a consideration of the self in relational terms. We believe that these two factors influence each other in a cyclical fashion, with the relationship-specific development of cognitive, affective, and behavioral structures encouraging the development of a relational sense of self that, in turn, encourages the further shaping of cognition, affect, and behavior via relationship interdependence. Our use of this definition of a relational self is more exclusive than others offered previously (e.g., Andersen & Chen, 2002).

We also believe that the strong interdependence of relationship partners—specifically, the correspondence of outcomes and dependence on the relationship for positive outcomes—is the single greatest predictor of the development of a strong sense of a relational self. We label this relational self that includes relationship-specific cognitive, affective, and behavioral structures, along with an explicit consideration of the self as part of the relationship, *cognitive interdependence*. This label belies our belief that a relational self indicates a cognitive awareness of relational interdependence that blurs the lines between the self, the partner, and the relationship. To understand the development of cognitive interdependence, it is necessary to understand the effects of relational interdependence and the building blocks and outcomes of dependence, including relationship commitment.

INTERDEPENDENCE AND RELATIONSHIP COMMITMENT

Within interdependence theory, the concept of dependence plays a pivotal role. Dependence level describes the degree to which each of two interacting individuals needs a specific relationship for the fulfillment of subjectively valued outcomes. According to the theory, dependence is greater to the degree that the outcomes available in alternative relationships are poorer. To illustrate, consider the relationship of Cathy and Kevin. According to interdependence theory, Kevin's dependence on Cathy will be greater to the extent that he relies uniquely on Cathy for the fulfillment of his needs. These needs may include the need for security, for emotional intimacy, and/or for sexual fulfillment. In contrast, Kevin's dependence on Cathy is reduced to the extent that he believes his needs could be gratified elsewhere (e.g., in an alternative relationship).

The investment model (Le & Agnew, 2003; Rusbult, 1983; Rusbult, Martz, & Agnew, 1998) extends interdependence theory propositions by suggesting that the structural state of dependence produces the psychological experience of commitment (Agnew, Van Lange, Rusbult, & Langston, 1998). The psychological experience of *commitment* is held to include conative, cognitive, and affective components (Arriaga & Agnew, 2001). The *conative component* of commitment is manifested in an individual's intention to persist in a given relationship. For example, Kevin is committed to his relationship with Cathy to the extent that he actively intends to remain in the relationship. The *cognitive component* of commitment is manifested in an individual's long-term orientation toward the relationship: Kevin is committed to Cathy to the extent that he envisions himself as involved in the relationship for the foreseeable future and considers the implications of his current actions for their future outcomes. The *affective component* of commitment is manifested in the degree to which an individual forms a psychological attachment to the partner and the relationship: Kevin is committed to Cathy to the extent that he experiences life in dyadic terms, such that his emotional well-being is linked to Cathy and their relationship.

The three components of commitment are theoretically and empirically distinguishable but tend to co-occur (Arriaga & Agnew, 2001). Overall, commitment may be best thought of as the subjective state that dependent individuals experience on a daily basis. In this sense, commitment may be construed as the subjective sense of allegiance that is established with regard to the source of one's structural dependence. Because Kevin is dependent on his relationship with Cathy, he develops intentions to persist in the relationship, he foresees long-term involvement with Cathy, and he feels affectively linked to Cathy and their relationship. From this perspective, a committed individual clearly sees the world differently than does a noncommitted individual.

How is it that committed individuals come to act and think in a relationship-enhancing manner? The distinction between the given situation and the effective situation, as delineated by interdependence theory, provides a framework for understanding how committed individuals come to think and behave in this way. According to Kelley and Thibaut (1978), the *given situation* refers to each partner's immediate, personal well-being in a specific situation, describing each person's self-centered preferences. Although self-centered behaviors occur in everyday life, behavior is often shaped by broader concerns, including long-term goals or desires to promote both one's own and a partner's well-being. Movement away from given preferences results from *transformation of motivation*, a process that leads individuals to relinquish their immediate self-interest and act on the basis of broader considerations.

For committed relationship partners, transformation of motivation often involves movement away from the desire to maximize one's own immediate self-interest (referred to in interdependence terminology as "MaxOwn"), and coming to see the situation instead on the basis of what is good for the partner ("MaxOther") or good for both partners ("MaxJoint"). The *effective situation* refers to the modified preferences resulting from the transformation process. The theory holds that dyad members' behaviors are based on the transformed, effective situation.

COGNITIVE INTERDEPENDENCE

Interdependence theory assumes that the transformation process is shaped by internal processes accompanying an interpersonal event (cf. Kelley, 1979). Few studies have explicated the role of internal events in the process of adaptation to interdependence structure. Thus our knowledge of the mental concomitants of relationship commitment is limited. We introduced the concept of cognitive interdependence to help fill theoretical gaps. In our view, as individuals become increasingly committed to a relationship, and as they develop relationship-specific cognition, affect, and behavioral responses, they come to think of their partners as part of themselves, and come to regard themselves as part of a collective unit that includes the partner. Consider Kevin and Cathy once again. Over time Kevin may become increasingly committed to continuing his involvement with Cathy, foreseeing an extended future with her in which his well-being rests on Cathy and their relationship. Accordingly, increased commitment is likely to instigate more frequent relationship-relevant cognitive activity, along with a shift in the nature of personal identity and self-representation. Kevin is likely to develop a relatively couple-oriented identity and a relatively pluralistic representation of his self-in-relationship. Kevin will no longer think of himself simply as Kevin. Instead he will regard himself more and more as part of a collective KevinandCathy unit. This pluralistic, collective mental representation of the self-in-relationship is referred to as a state of cognitive interdependence.

Cognitive interdependence may be thought of as a habit of thinking that supports pro-relationship motivation and behavior. The existing literature both indirectly and directly supports the assertion that cognitive interdependence characterizes committed relationships. For example, actor–observer differences in attribution are attenuated for close partners in comparison to strangers, with such attenuation presumably occurring because the distinction between self and partner becomes blurred (Sande, Goethals, & Radloff, 1988). Similarly, individuals tend to "reflect" others' successes when the other is close, but not when the other is a stranger (Tesser, 1988). The existence of reflected experiences of success and parallel patterns of self–partner attribution is compatible with the notion that commitment results in cognitive restructuring, including incorporation of a close partner into one's sense of self.

Past Research on Cognitive Interdependence

To more directly test whether strong commitment to a relationship is associated with a relatively pluralistic, other-inclusive cognitive representation of the self-in-relationship, we conducted two empirical studies, a cross-sectional survey study and a two-wave longitudinal study (Agnew et al., 1998). Of course, to examine commitment-inspired changes in the self, we first had to identify valid methods of measuring the cognitive interdependence construct. We employed three operational definitions of the construct: (1) the spontaneous use of plural pronouns in relationship-relevant cognitions (i.e., exhibiting greater use of first-person-plural personal and possessive pronouns such as "we," "us," "our," or "ours"); (2) the Inclusion of Other in the Self Scale (the IOS Scale; Aron & Aron, 1997; Aron, Aron, & Smollan, 1992); and (3) the self-reported centrality of one's relationship to one's life. These measures have the advantage of being psychometrically diverse: the pronoun measure provides a covert means of tapping relationship-relevant thought structures; the IOS Scale is a graphical measure that assesses how an individual mentally perceives the amount of self–partner overlap in a relationship; and the centrality of relationship measure is a paper-and-pencil self-report of the degree to which a relationship is considered an essential, highly central element of one's life. Collectively, these measures psychometrically triangulate on mental representations of the self-in-relationship.

For romantic relationships, we found that cognitive interdependence increased hand in hand with increases in commitment level. The more romantically committed individuals became, the greater was their tendency to think about the relationship in a pluralistic, other-inclusive manner, as reflected in the spontaneous use of plural pronouns to describe one's self and one's relationship. In addition, the more romantically committed individuals became, the more they came to regard themselves as "blended" with the partner, as revealed in perceived overlap in mental representations of self and partner. Furthermore, romantically committed individuals tended to regard their relationships as relatively central to who they are and what their lives are about.

We also found in our longitudinal study of romantic relationships that the effects of commitment and cognitive interdependence were reciprocal: earlier commitment was significantly associated with increases over time in levels of cognitive interdependence *and* earlier cognitive interdependence was significantly associated with increases over time in commitment level. We anticipated such reciprocal causal associations, in that key processes in ongoing relationships unfold over extended periods of time. Such cyclical patterns could have considerable adaptive value in the context of a generally healthy ongoing involvement. Although the field of social psychology has tended to emphasize models of unidirectional cause and effect, we believe that models of mutual cyclical influence may be a more suitable means of understanding causal processes in ongoing relationships.

Given that commitment to a relationship entails a fundamental restructuring of the individual's cognitive representation of the self-in-relationship, it stands to reason that an unexpected or unwanted breech in commitment would have profound implications for an individual's sense of self. This is precisely the situation faced by an individual who has been left (or "dumped") by his or her partner: In this situation, his or her partner has unilaterally decided to terminate the relationship, despite the fact that he or she still desires the relationship to continue (Agnew, 2000). The abandoned partner is still mentally committed—that is, he or she has cognitively incorporated his or her now-former partner into his or her sense of self. The experience of loss for the abandoned partner is likely to be quite devastating, as he or she discovers that a fundamental part of the self that was once present is now absent.

We sought to further document the existence of cognitive interdependence in committed romantic relationships and also to trace the different cognitive patterns that we believe characterize the thinking of those who choose to remain in a relationship ("stayers"), those who choose to leave a relationship ("leavers"), and those left by their partner (the "abandoned"). To that end, we used data collected from college students involved in relatively newly formed dating relationships (Agnew, 2000). The advantage of utilizing a sample of new romances to study cognitive interdependence was somewhat pragmatic: there was a great likelihood that many of these relationships would end in a reasonably short period of time. Thus we could readily obtain the thoughts of all three categories of relationship members: leavers, stayers, and the abandoned. Moreover, even in relatively new relationships, the experience of relationship loss can be quite intense.

The longitudinal pattern of cognitive interdependence for stayers, leavers, and the abandoned was traced to determine whether levels of this construct changed over time in similar ways for each breakup group or whether the changes varied by group. Consistent with our theoretical stance, commitment level was found to be associated with degree of cognitive interdependence within each time period as well as across time periods (Agnew, 2000). These results provide further evidence of the link between degree of relationship commitment and degree of cognitive incorporation of one's relationship partner into the self.

In addition, over time, leavers were found to become increasingly less committed than were stayers. That these two types of relationship members would differ in commitment is not particularly surprising given the respective fates of their relationships. The results for abandoned individuals were more noteworthy: they did not differ significantly from stayers at any point in time. In other words, abandoned individuals were just as committed to their partners over time as those individuals whose relationships remained intact. Results from analyses of variance show that individuals in the three groups did not differ in their initial degree of cognitive interdependence. However, over time, stayers exhibited increasingly more cognitive interdependence than did leavers. More interestingly, abandoned individuals did not differ from stayers at any point in time. That is, the abandoned evidenced the same degree of cognitive interdependence over time as stayers. From a cognitive perspective, their relationships appear to have never ended.

These results suggest that, for all intents and purposes, abandoned individuals have the same mindset with respect to their relationships as do stayers: these two groups exhibited similar levels of commitment over time. The obvious, but important, difference between these two groups is that abandoned individuals are faced with the unwanted loss of their relationship.

These results help illustrate why people can be so strongly affected by the loss of a specific relationship or relationship partner: abandoned individuals think in terms of an intact relationship, seeing themselves still "as one" with the partner. Their thoughts continue to include the partner, despite the ill fate of their relationship. The residual traces of cognitive interdependence may fuel an ongoing devastating emotional experience.

Consequences of Cognitive Interdependence

In addition to cognitive interdependence, commitment to a relationship has been shown to be associated with a wide range of relationship-promoting cognitions and behaviors, such as (1) disparagement of tempting alternative partners (Simpson, Gangestad, & Lerma, 1990); (2) willingness to sacrifice desired behavioral options for the good of a relationship (Van Lange, Agnew, Harinck, & Steemers, 1997; Van Lange et al., 1997); (3) tendencies to accommodate rather than to retaliate when a partner behaves poorly (Rusbult, Verette, Whitney, Slovik, & Lipkus, 1991); (4) forgiveness (Finkel, Rusbult, Kumashiro, & Hannon, 2002); (5) perceived superiority of one's relationship versus others' relationships (Van Lange, Rusbult, Semin-Goossens, Goerts, & Stalpers, 1999); and (6) trust in one's partner (Wieselquist, Rusbult, Foster, & Agnew, 1999). In sum, the extant social psychological literature supports the contention that committed individuals are willing to exert significant cognitive and behavioral effort toward the goal of maintaining and enhancing their relationships.

In recent work we have sought to expand the known consequences of commitment and the state of cognitive interdependence, hypothesizing that commitment to a relationship and greater cognitive interdependence should also be associated with decreased perceptions of harm stemming from a relationship partner (Agnew & Smoak, 2003, 2004). Believing that one's partner will not harm the self is consistent with many of the known consequences of commitment, including increased trust in one's partner (Wieselquist et al., 1999) and willingness to sacrifice for one's partner (Van Lange et al., 1997). More directly, recent research on reinterpretation of violence in intimate relationships characterized by high commitment supports the notion that commitment fuels a tendency to reduce negative perceptions associated with one's partner (Arriaga, 2002).

Implications for the Self: A Precarious Balancing Act

In the applied realm, decreased perceptions of harm as a consequence of relationship commitment are of particular interest in trying to understand the tendency for committed individuals to report lower rates of protective behavior within their relationships, particularly with respect to sexual behaviors and contraception use. In our work in this area, we combine aspects of theory relevant to commitment processes with balance processes (Heider, 1958). We view this approach as a useful synthesis of interpersonal and intrapersonal perspectives.

The relationship between couple members accounts for one essential element of importance with respect to the possible underpinnings of (non)protective cognitions and behavior. In addition to examining the *interpersonal* context influencing relational behavior, it is also important to understand how *intrapersonal* perceptions of risk status interact with relationship commitment to determine an individual's protective behaviors. Balance theory provides a useful heuristic framework for understanding how increasing levels of commitment can influence an individual's perceptions of relative risk. Balance theory has proven to be one of the more enduring social psychological theories, due likely to the fact that it explicates a fundamental way that people tend to think. The theory has been applied to the further understanding of a number of conceptual domains, including attitudes toward social issues (e.g., Newcomb, 1961), toward friendships (e.g., Aronson & Cope, 1968), and toward political candidates (e.g., Ottati, Fishbein, & Middlestadt, 1988).

Balance theory's main concern is with three types of mental representations (or "elements") and the relations between them: (1) the person in whose experience balance processes are operating (symbolized as P by Heider [1958]); (2) some other perceived person (symbolized as O), and (3) a perceived event, idea, or thing (symbolized as X). Heider used this symbolic notation of elements to analyze structures in which the elements are related to one another. He proposed that two states can exist in these structures: balance and imbalance. When imbalance occurs, a structure is considered unstable and tends to shift over time toward a state of balance. To the extent that people maintain imbalanced states in their cognitions, they tend to experience tension, a tension that motivates a push toward balance.

In applying balance logic to an interpersonal situation involving critical judgments about a relational partner, consider the juxtaposition of elements shown in Figure 14.1 from the perspective of Partner A, who is trying to figure out whether or not he is at risk of acquiring a sexually transmitted disease (STD) from Partner B. Partner A (or P) feels positively about Partner B (or O); let's assume that Partner A feels strongly committed to Partner B (see Link 1, which is positive; this is a "sentiment relation," using Heider's terminology). Partner A's relative positivity toward Partner B may grow over time as relationship commitment continues to develop. In addition, Partner A believes that STDs (symbolized as X) are negative, both in and of themselves and with respect to his or her own disease status (see Link 2, which is negative; this is a "unit relation," using Heider's terminology). The unknown element in this situation, the element that must be "solved" by Partner A, is with respect to Partner B's relationship to STDs (Link 3). In an ideal world, Partner A would have

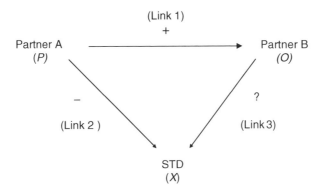

FIGURE 14.1. Combining intra- and interpersonal perspectives regarding perceptions of risk.

objective information to evaluate B's relation to STDs. In the real world, however, Partner B's disease status is unknown to A (and may be unknown to B as well). Accordingly, Partner A can only operate from perception, situated within these elements. From a balance theory perspective, A is likely to assume that B is not an STD threat because of a need for balance—that is, the need to believe that one's beloved partner couldn't possibly be affiliated positively with a negative element. Thus Partner A's strong feelings of commitment toward Partner B would lead him to "solve" Link 3 as negative. Note that this would yield a balanced triad (i.e., multiplication of the signs for each element linkage yields a positive rather than a negative product):

$$(\text{Link } 1 = +) \times (\text{Link } 2 = -) \times (\text{Link } 3 = -) = +$$

Following from interdependence and balance theories, we conducted three studies to test hypotheses regarding the association between relationship commitment level and harm perceptions (Agnew & Smoak, 2003, 2004). We hypothesized that individuals involved in sexual relationships with partners for whom they feel high commitment would be less likely to perceive their partner as a source of harm or risk than would those in less committed relationships because strong feelings of commitment cannot be reconciled with perceiving one's partner as a potential risk. Consistent with our hypotheses, we found significant associations between commitment level and harm perceptions, both generally and in specific harm domains. Moreover, experiments featuring scenario-based versions of the situation depicted in Figure 14.1 also yielded significant results in line with our hypothesized reasoning: greater commitment between partners yielded lower risk assessments with respect to a partner. Thus it appears that the same mindset that helps to keep us linked to a relational partner also may put us in jeopardy by affecting our harm and risk judgments with respect to our close partners.

FUTURE DIRECTIONS

Cognitive interdependence is very useful as an explanatory concept. Thus additional research is needed to examine how cognitive interdependence is influenced by and influences relationship cognition, affect, and behavior. Not surprisingly, given the relative newness of the concept of a relational self, many productive and little-explored avenues exist for future study. Below we drive a bit down a few of these avenues.

Development of Cognitive Interdependence

Additional research is needed to examine what contributes to the development of cognitive interdependence among close relationship partners. As argued previously, a high level of interdependence and correspondence of outcomes are necessary components. However, it is also likely that intra-individual factors play a role in the development of cognitive interdependence. For instance, attachment style may play a role in the ability to develop cognitive interdependence. People high in avoidance will likely find it difficult to develop the sense of relationship focus required for the development of cognitive interdependence. In addition, narcissistic individuals would be unlikely to have the capacity to develop the other and relationship focus found in cognitive interdependence (see Campbell et al., Chapter 4, this volume). Several other individual difference factors, such as the general tendency to define the self in relationship terms (Cross & Morris, 2003), may impact a person's ability to form a relational sense of self. In keeping with the spirit of this book, it is likely that both intrapersonal and interpersonal factors contribute to the development of cognitive interdependence and both are key venues for additional research.

Cognitive Interdependence and Information Processing

Several consequences of cognitive interdependence have already been described. However, one area that is particularly in need of future research is the effect of cognitive interdependence on how members of a romantic relationship process information relevant to their relationship. Consequences of commitment and cognitive interdependence reviewed previously focus primarily on how a member of a romantic relationship views his or her partner (e.g., with greater trust) and on changes in how the person views the relationship (e.g., perceived superiority of the relationship). These processes are important and worthy of future study. However, underlying these consequences appears to be a change in how information relevant to one's partner and the relationship itself is processed by people in the relationship.

Based on interdependence theory, a transformation of motivation can occur in which relationship motives change how situations and outcomes are evaluated. In a similar manner, cognitive interdependence may lead to a change in how information about the relationship is processed. Relationship-specific information may achieve a special status in the same way that information about the self has been argued to have special status in information processing (Baumeister, 1998). Although these ideas are speculative, the implications of this sort of information-processing effect of cognitive interdependence are worth further explicating and investigating.

Negative Implications of Cognitive Interdependence

As touched upon above, it is important to note that there may be negatives associated with a strong relational identity. As the strength of the relational self grows, it may lead to decisions that are good for the relationship (and the relational self) but bad for the individual (and the individual self). The development of a relational self may lead to competition between the quality of the relationship and the well-being of the individual relationship members. Our recent work is but one example: a strong relational identity may decrease the ability to view one's partner as a source of harm and risk. This work highlights the potential negative concomitants of cognitive interdependence.

In a larger sense, a strong relational self may lead to ignoring negative information about one's partner in general. While likely having positive implications for the relationship, negative consequences for the individual could ensue if potentially harmful information is ignored. A person characterized by a high level of cognitive interdependence may be slow to recognize potentially harmful actions by his or her partner, actions that threaten the individual or the relationship. Future research that focuses on potential negative implications of cognitive interdependence is warranted and sorely needed.

Of course, all intimate romantic relationships will end eventually, even those with high levels of cognitive interdependence, if not by choice then by death. A strong sense of a relational self and interdependence with a relationship partner will make the ending particularly hard on the surviving member. If a person has strongly tied his or her sense of who he or she is to the relationship, its ending amounts to a true loss to the person's sense of self. More work is needed to examine how the termination of a relationship that partly defines the self affects surviving members as well as on ways to alleviate the associated distress.

Opportunities Ahead

Finally, additional research is needed to test the generalizability of the concept of cognitive interdependence across relationship types and to further test the underlying assumptions of the construct. In particular, experimental research would add to the understanding of cognitive interdependence by exploring more fully the causal manner in which relationship cognition and behavior are influenced by cognitive interdependence. Careful experimental research could also explore the factors that contribute to the development of cognitive interdependence. Intrapersonal and interpersonal processes within relationships are inherently complex, requiring exacting research to tease apart cause and effect over the course of time. Such opportunities (albeit not without challenges) lie ahead.

REFERENCES

Acitelli, L. K., Rogers, S., & Knee, C. R. (1999). The role of identity in the link between relationship thinking and relationship satisfaction. *Journal of Social and Personal Relationships, 16*, 591–618.

Agnew, C. R. (2000). Cognitive interdependence and the experience of relationship loss. In J. H. Harvey & E. D. Miller (Eds.), *Loss and trauma: General and close relationship perspectives* (pp. 385–398). Philadelphia: Brunner-Routledge.

Agnew, C. R., & Smoak, N. D. (2003, October). *Commitment and harm perceptions.* Paper presented at the annual meeting of the Society for Experimental Social Psychology, Boston.

Agnew, C. R., & Smoak, N. D. (2004, February). *Relationship commitment and perceptions of harm.* Paper presented at the annual meeting of the Society of Personality and Social Psychology, Austin, TX.

Agnew, C. R., Van Lange, P. A. M., Rusbult, C. E., & Langston, C. A. (1998). Cognitive interdependence: Commitment and the mental representation of close relationships. *Journal of Personality and Social Psychology, 74*, 939–954.

Andersen, S. M., & Chen, S. (2002). The relational self: An interpersonal social-cognitive theory. *Psychological Review, 109*, 619–645.

Aron, A., & Aron, E. N. (1997). Self-expansion motivation and including other in the self. In S. Duck (Ed.), *Handbook of personal relationships: Theory, method, and interventions* (2nd ed., pp. 251–270). Chichester, UK: Wiley.

Aron, A., Aron, E. N., & Smollan, D. (1992). Inclusion of Other in the Self Scale and the structure of interpersonal closeness. *Journal of Personality and Social Psychology, 63*, 596–612.

Aronson, E., & Cope, V. (1968). My enemy's enemy is my friend. *Journal of Personality and Social Psychology, 8*, 8–12.

Arriaga, X. B. (2001). The ups and downs of dating: Fluctuations in satisfaction in newly formed romantic relationships. *Journal of Personality and Social Psychology, 80*, 754–765.

Arriaga, X. B. (2002). Joking violence among highly committed individuals. *Journal of Interpersonal Violence, 17,* 591–610.

Arriaga, X. B., & Agnew, C. R. (2001). Being committed: Affective, cognitive, and conative components of relationship commitment. *Personality and Social Psychology Bulletin, 27,* 1190–1203.

Baumeister, R. F. (1998). The self. In D. T. Gilbert, S. T. Fiske, & G. Lindzey (Eds.), *The handbook of social psychology* (Vol. 1, pp. 680–740). New York: Oxford University Press.

Brewer, M. B., & Brown, R. J. (1998). Intergroup relations. In D. T. Gilbert, S. T. Fiske, & G. Lindzey (Eds.), *The handbook of social psychology* (Vol. 2, pp. 554–594). New York: Oxford University Press.

Cross, S. E., & Morris, M. L. (2003). Getting to know you: The relational self-construal, relational cognition, and well-being. *Personality and Social Psychology Bulletin, 29,* 512–523.

Cross, S. E., Morris, M. L., & Gore, J. S. (2002). Thinking about oneself and others: The relational-interdependent self-construal and social cognition. *Journal of Personality and Social Psychology, 82,* 399–418.

Finkel, E. J., Rusbult, C. E., Kumashiro, M., & Hannon, P. A. (2002). Dealing with betrayal in close relationships: Does commitment promote forgiveness? *Journal of Personality and Social Psychology, 82,* 956–974.

Fraley, R. C. (2002). Attachment stability from infancy to adulthood: Meta-analysis and dynamic modeling of developmental mechanisms. *Personality and Social Psychology Review, 6,* 123–151.

Garrido, E. F., & Acitelli, L. K. (1999). Relational identity and the division of household labor. *Journal of Social and Personal Relationships, 16,* 619–637.

Goodfriend, M. R. (2004). *Partner-esteem: Romantic partners in the eyes of biased beholders.* Unpublished doctoral dissertation, Purdue University, West Lafayette, IN.

Hazan, C., & Shaver, P. (1987). Romantic love conceptualized as an attachment process. *Journal of Personality and Social Psychology, 52,* 511–524.

Heider, F. (1958). *The psychology of interpersonal relations.* New York: Wiley.

Higgins, E. T. (1989). Self-discrepancy theory: What patterns of self-beliefs cause people to suffer? In L. Berkowitz (Ed.), *Advances in experimental social psychology* (Vol. 22, pp. 93–136). San Diego, CA: Academic Press.

Higgins, E. T., & May, D. (2001). Individual self-regulatory functions: It's not "we" regulation, but it's still social. In C. Sedikides & M. B. Brewer (Eds.), *Individual self, relational self, collective self* (pp. 47–67). Philadelphia: Psychology Press.

Kelley, H. H. (1979). *Personal relationships: Their structure and processes.* Hillsdale, NJ: Erlbaum.

Kelley, H. H., & Thibaut, J. W. (1978). *Interpersonal relations: A theory of interdependence.* New York: Wiley.

Le, B., & Agnew, C. R. (2003). Commitment and its theorized determinants: A meta-analysis of the investment model. *Personal Relationships, 10,* 37–57.

Mashek, D. J., Aron, A., & Boncimino, M. (2003). Confusions of self with close others. *Personality and Social Psychology Bulletin, 29,* 382–392.

Newcomb, T. M. (1961). *The acquaintance process.* New York: Holt, Rinehart & Winston.

Ottati, V., Fishbein, M., & Middlestadt, S. E. (1988). Determinants of voters' beliefs about the candidates' stands on issues: The role of evaluative bias heuristics and the candidates' expressed message. *Journal of Personality and Social Psychology, 55,* 517–529.

Overall, N. C., Fletcher, G. J., & Friesen, M. D. (2003). Mapping the intimate relationship mind: Comparisons between three models of attachment representations. *Personality and Social Psychology Bulletin, 29,* 1479–1493.

Rusbult, C. E. (1983). A longitudinal test of the investment model: The development (and deterioration) of satisfaction and commitment in heterosexual involvements. *Journal of Personality and Social Psychology, 45,* 101–117.

Rusbult, C. E., Arriaga, X. B., & Agnew, C. R. (2001). Interdependence in close relationships. In G. J. O. Fletcher & M. S. Clark (Eds.), *Blackwell handbook of social psychology: Vol. 2. Interpersonal processes* (pp. 359–387). Oxford, UK: Blackwell.

Rusbult, C. E., Martz, J. M., & Agnew, C. R. (1998). The Investment Model Scale: Measuring commitment level, satisfaction level, quality of alternatives, and investment size. *Personal Relationships, 5,* 357–391.

Rusbult, C. E., & Van Lange, P. A. M. (2003). Interdependence, interaction and relationships. *Annual Review of Psychology, 54,* 351–375.

Rusbult, C. E., Verette, J., Whitney, G. A., Slovik, L. F., & Lipkus, I. (1991). Accommodation processes in close relationships: Theory and preliminary empirical evidence. *Journal of Personality and Social Psychology, 60,* 53–78.

Sande, G. N., Goethals, G. R., & Radloff, C. E. (1988). Perceiving one's own traits and others': The multifaceted self. *Journal of Personality and Social Psychology, 54,* 13–20.

Sedikides, C., & Brewer, M. B. (Eds.). (2001). *Individual self, relational self, collective self.* Philadelphia: Psychology Press.

Shah, J. (2003). The motivational looking glass: How significant others implicitly affect goal appraisals. *Journal of Personality and Social Psychology, 85,* 424–439.

Simpson, J. A., Gangestad, S. W., & Lerma, M. (1990). Perception of physical attractiveness: Mechanisms involved in the maintenance of romantic relationships. *Journal of Personality and Social Psychology, 59,* 1192–1201.

Simpson, J. A., & Rholes, W. S. (Eds). (1998). *Attachment theory and close relationships.* New York: Guilford Press.

Tajfel, H., & Turner, J. C. (1986). The social identity theory of intergroup behavior. In S. Worchel & W. G. Austin (Eds.), *Psychology of intergroup relations* (pp. 7–24). Chicago: Nelson.

Tesser, A. (1988). Toward a self-evaluation maintenance model of social behavior. In L. Berkowitz (Ed.), *Advances in experimental social psychology* (Vol. 21, pp. 181–227). San Diego, CA: Academic Press.

Thibaut, J. W., & Kelley, H. H. (1959). *The social psychology of groups.* New York: Wiley.

Tice, D. M., & Baumeister, R. F. (2001). The primacy of the interpersonal self. In C. Sedikides & M. B. Brewer (Eds.), *Individual self, relational self, collective self* (pp. 71–88). Philadelphia: Psychology Press.

Van Lange, P. A. M., Agnew, C. R., Harinck, F., & Steemers, G. E. M. (1997). From game theory to real life: How social value orientation affects willingness to sacrifice in ongoing close relationships. *Journal of Personality and Social Psychology, 73,* 1330–1344.

Van Lange, P. A. M., Rusbult, C. E., Drigotas, S. M., Arriaga, X. B., Witcher, B. S., & Cox, C. L. (1997). Willingness to sacrifice in close relationships. *Journal of Personality and Social Psychology, 72,* 1373–1395.

Van Lange, P. A. M., Rusbult, C. E., Semin-Goossens, A., Goerts, C. A., & Stalpers, M. (1999). Being better than others but otherwise perfectly normal: Perceptions of uniqueness and similarity in close relationships. *Personal Relationships, 6,* 269–289.

Vohs, K. D., & Ciarocco, N. J. (2004). Interpersonal functioning requires self-regulation. In R. F. Baumeister & K. D. Vohs (Eds.), *Handbook of self-regulation: Research, theory, and applications* (pp. 392–407). New York: Guilford Press.

Wieselquist, J., Rusbult, C. E., Foster, C. A., & Agnew, C. R. (1999). Commitment, pro-relationship behavior, and trust in close relationships. *Journal of Personality and Social Psychology, 77,* 942–966.

SPECIFIC SOCIAL
INTERACTION PROCESSES

CHAPTER 15

High-Maintenance Interaction and Self-Regulation

ELI J. FINKEL
W. KEITH CAMPBELL
AMY B. BRUNELL

Scenario #1. Imagine that you and your spouse have decided to repaint your kitchen. Both of you have experience with domestic painting, so you decide to do the job yourselves rather than hire a professional painter. You know from experience that you (working alone) would be able to apply the first coat of paint in approximately 3 hours, which would leave 2 hours to finish preparing tomorrow's lecture before bedtime. Given that your spouse also has painting experience, you are confident that your estimate of 3 hours is conservative. It soon becomes clear, however, that you and your spouse have learned incompatible painting strategies over the years; despite your best efforts, you keep getting in each other's way. You are forced to exert effort to discern what your partner is doing so the two of you can coordinate your work. This effort offsets the advantage of having two competent painters working together. In the end, the painting does indeed take 3 hours, but when you turn your attention to lecture preparation, you find that your mind is unfocused and your motivation is diminished. You have trouble forcing yourself to spend those 2 hours working hard, and the quality of your work is poor.

Scenario #2. Imagine that two unacquainted white college seniors— Chad and Jake—take the Graduate Record Exam (GRE) at separate exam

297

locations. Chad and Jake both arrive 10 minutes early and find themselves waiting in a room with only one other person in it: a black student who is also waiting to take the GRE. Each pair of students strikes up a conversation about GRE study strategies. After discussing how the GRE is generally a politically correct test, they wind up talking casually about affirmative action more generally before being summoned to take the exam. Chad and Jake are quite similar to one another, except that whereas Chad has minimal prejudice against black people, Jake is strongly prejudiced. When they receive their exam scores, Chad finds that he performs as well as he typically did on his practice tests, but Jake finds that he underperforms relative to his practice tests scores.

In the present chapter, we explore the idea that the preceding scenarios are representative of a recently identified category of interpersonal interactions that impair subsequent self-regulation; we refer to such interactions as *high-maintenance interactions*. The goal of this chapter is to review evidence that effortful social coordination on interpersonal tasks (e.g., painting with others) can impair personal self-regulation on subsequent, unrelated tasks (e.g., maintaining focus and concentration). We first provide a conceptual analysis of social coordination by addressing definitional issues, identifying social coordination as an interdependence phenomenon, and emphasizing the distinction between social coordination and social conflict. We then highlight some relevant developments in the self-regulation literature before reviewing the rapidly expanding evidence supporting the idea that high-maintenance interactions impair self-regulation on subsequent unrelated tasks. Next we advance a model of self-regulation and relationship functioning. We conclude with a discussion of the implications of this work and directions for future research.

SOCIAL COORDINATION

We adopt the following definitions for the terms *social coordination* and *high maintenance* (Finkel, Campbell, Brunell, Dalton, & Chartrand, 2005): "Interpersonal interactions are characterized by effective *social coordination* to the degree that the interacting individuals are able to align their behaviors with one another in an efficient and effortless manner. The term *high-maintenance interaction* refers to the degree to which social coordination on an interpersonal task requires energy exertions beyond those required to perform the task itself." The interracial interaction scenario presented previously is an example of a high-maintenance interaction for Jake (the student with strong prejudice) because facilitating smooth social coordination with his black waiting room companion requires that he exert energy (to inhibit his prejudice in the interest of facilitating smooth interaction) beyond that required by the social interaction itself. The identical situation is not a high-maintenance interaction for Chad (the student with minimal prejudice) because he does not have to exert extra energy to facilitate smooth social interaction. Below we review evidence that differences in the degree to which social coordination experiences are high maintenance affect the degree to which the interactants experience personal self-regulatory failure on subsequent unrelated tasks. In the interracial interaction scenario, for example, Jake's GRE performance would likely suffer after the social interaction whereas Chad's would not.

An Interdependence Theory Analysis of Social Coordination

Interdependence theory researchers define *interdependence* as "the process by which interacting persons influence one another's experiences" (Rusbult & Van Lange, 1996, p. 564; see also Kelley et al., 2003; Kelley & Thibaut, 1978; Thibaut & Kelley, 1959). Although this definition is broad enough to include diverse interdependence phenomena, some topics have been well researched whereas others have been largely neglected. Examples of well-researched topics include how people navigate conflicts of interest (e.g., Finkel, Rusbult, Kumashiro, & Hannon, 2002; Rusbult, Verette, Whitney, Slovik, & Lipkus, 1991; Van Lange, 1999) and how trust develops (e.g., Holmes & Rempel, 1989). We suggest that the self-regulatory consequences of high-maintenance interaction is a central interdependence topic that has been neglected empirically until the last few years. This neglect is surprising given the degree to which effective social coordination promotes enhanced quality of life. Tasks requiring coordination are pervasive, and many tasks are more efficiently accomplished by people working in concert than by individuals working alone. We next examine how efficient versus inefficient social coordination influences the interactants' subsequent self-regulatory success.

Coordination versus Conflict

Although research examining the personal consequences of interpersonal *conflict* has been common over the past several decades, research investigating the personal consequences of poor interpersonal *coordination* has been sparse until the last few years. Rusbult and Van Lange (2003) highlight the distinction between these two topics by presenting two different scenarios for John and Mary as they decide where to spend their summer vacation. In the first, John wants to go to a beach resort and Mary wants to go to Rome. In the second, John and Mary both want to go to Rome. Whereas the first scenario requires that John and Mary make delicate decisions that account for their different preferences, the second does not—after all, they have the same preferences in the first place. Rusbult and Van Lange observe that interaction in the second scenario "is a coordination problem—the two must agree on a date for their vacation, and one person must arrange for travel and lodging. Thus, in comparison to situations with conflicting interests, *situations with corresponding interests are relatively simple. . . .* They entail coordinating in such a manner as to enjoy the good outcomes that are readily available to the pair" (p. 352, emphasis added).

Efficient versus Effortful Coordination

We suggest that such coordination is frequently simple not because coordinating with others is easy (e.g., consider how difficult it would be to program a robot to engage in smooth social coordination), but rather because humans possess remarkable behavioral repertoires for effecting smooth social coordination. Furthermore, once these repertoires are developed, we can generally apply them effortlessly and nonconsciously to diverse social situations. As a result, well-coordinated social interactions are the norm; poor social coordination is the salient exception (Hatfield, Cacioppo, & Rapson, 1994).

Although efficient social coordination is the norm, interactions requiring effortful attention to the nuances of such coordination still exist in everyday life. For example, it is often complicated—and exhausting—for a group of friends to decide which movie to see, even if everybody would be content to see any movie under consideration. We suggest that when people have compatible goals but the interpersonal execution of these goals is inefficient enough to require heightened vigilance to social coordination issues, the interactants' self-regulatory success on subsequent unrelated tasks may well become impaired. Before reviewing the literature examining the effects of high-maintenance interactions on self-regulation, we turn our attention to some recent and relevant developments in the rapidly expanding self-regulation literature.

SELF-REGULATION

We use the term *self-regulation* to refer to what Baumeister (1998, p. 712) has called the self's "executive function," which is the aspect of the self that "makes decisions, initiates actions, and in other ways exerts control over both self and environment." Self-regulation is the psychological process activated when studying on a Friday night rather than going out to a bar with friends or when forcing oneself to concentrate on a difficult task when one's mind begins to wander; it entails efforts by the self to alter its own inner states or responses (Vohs & Baumeister, 2004) in a goal-directed manner. Self-regulation is a superordinate category consisting of many lower level processes, including (1) general self-regulatory effectiveness (e.g., using time well, being responsible), (2) willpower, (3) effective task performance, (4) motivation to perform challenging but potentially rewarding tasks rather than easy tasks with a low likelihood of being satisfying in the long run, and (5) inhibiting inappropriate behavioral tendencies. The present chapter reviews research relevant to all five of these components of self-regulation.

Self-regulation has been an increasingly hot area of research over the last 20 years (see Baumeister & Vohs, 2004, for a comprehensive edited volume on the topic), but most of this research emphasizes processes within a given individual. The research reviewed here builds on this literature by exploring whether the interpersonal process of high-maintenance interaction impairs personal self-regulatory success on subsequent unrelated tasks. This research serves as one illustration of a more general point: A comprehensive theory of self-regulation requires greater insight into the processes by which interpersonal processes influence individuals' self-regulatory success (see also Fitzsimons, Chapter 3; Koole, Kuhl, Jostmann, & Finkenauer, Chapter 18; Kumashiro, Rusbult, Wolf, & Estrada, Chapter 16; Rawn & Vohs, Chapter 2; Seeley & Gardner, Chapter 20; and Shah, Chapter 19, this volume).

Self-Regulatory Strength Depletion and the Two-Task Paradigm

We suggest that a primary mechanism by which high-maintenance interaction impairs self-regulation is by depleting psychological resources. Accumulating evidence suggests that engaging in successful self-regulation requires the individual to tap into a central psychological resource called *self-regulatory strength*, which refers to "the internal resources available to inhibit, override, or alter responses" (Schmeichel & Baumeister, 2004, p. 86). In the context of high-maintenance interactions, tempting responses might include being rude, losing focus, or discontinuing the interaction; striving to achieve efficient coordination in such interactions requires that one exert self-regulatory strength to override these tempting responses. Evidence suggests that self-regulatory strength is a limited and depletable resource that fluctuates in response to previous self-regulatory exertions (for reviews, see Muraven & Baumeister, 2000; Schmeichel & Baumeister, 2004). To the degree that individuals exert self-regulation in a given situation, they will have fewer self-regulatory resources available on a separate task they perform moments later; their "strength" is sapped and they are left in a state of *self-regulatory strength depletion*. An important implication is that "a person can become exhausted from many simultaneous demands and so will sometimes fail at self-control even regarding things at which he or she would otherwise succeed" (Baumeister & Heatherton, 1996, p. 3).

Research on self-regulatory strength depletion typically employs a *two-task paradigm* in which participants perform an initial task that either requires self-regulatory exertion or does not. After completing this first task, all participants complete the identical follow-up task that also requires self-regulatory exertion. Research reveals that relative to participants who first performed a task requiring no self-regulatory exertion, those who first performed a task requiring self-regulatory exertion exhibit impaired performance on the second task (e.g., Baumeister, Bratslavsky, Muraven, & Tice, 1998; Finkel & Campbell, 2001; Muraven, Collins, & Neinhaus, 2002; Muraven, Tice, & Baumeister, 1998; Vohs & Heatherton, 2000; Vohs & Schmeichel, 2003), although experiencing the initial task requiring self-regulatory exertion only impairs performance on follow-up tasks that also require self-regulatory exertion (Schmeichel, Vohs, & Baumeister, 2003). In addition, these depletion effects are not caused by differences across experimental conditions in mood (e.g., Schmeichel et al., 2003; Vohs & Schmeichel, 2003), self-efficacy (Wallace & Baumeister, 2002), or even subjectively experienced depletion (e.g., Muraven & Slessareva, 2003); this raises the possibility that self-regulatory exertion results in depleted self-regulatory strength for follow-up tasks without mediation through high-level conscious processes. The research reviewed here adapts the two-task paradigm to explore the effects of high-maintenance interaction on impaired personal self-regulation on subsequent unrelated tasks.

EMPIRICAL EVIDENCE

Two lines of research have emerged over the past few years to provide support for the idea that high-maintenance interaction results in impaired personal self-regulation on subsequent unrelated tasks. The first emerges from a desire to understand dynamics in romantic relationships and emphasizes the importance of interpersonal coordination. The second emerges from a desire to understand the consequences of being concerned about enacting prejudiced responses during interracial interaction. Together, the two lines of research paint a clear picture: Experiencing high-maintenance interactions results in impaired self-regulation.

Inefficient Social Coordination and Impaired Self-Regulation

In a series of seven studies, Finkel, Campbell, and their colleagues present evidence that coordination difficulties can impair subsequent self-regulation. The first three studies employ correlational procedures to investigate high-maintenance interaction processes in ongoing romantic relationships (Finkel, Campbell, & Sands, 2004), whereas the next four employ experimental procedures to investigate these processes in interactions between strangers (Finkel et al., 2005).

In the first study, participants (all of whom were involved in dating relationships) first completed a new, 12-item measure assessing the degree to which interpersonal coordination with their partner over the preceding 1-month period required effort (Finkel et al., 2004, Study 1). Sample items are "Over the past month, I have had to exert a lot of effort to coordinate things with my partner" and "Over the past month, it has required a lot of effort to understand my partner." Participants then completed a new, 6-item measure of general self-regulatory effectiveness over the same time frame. Sample items from this scale are "I tended to prioritize my time well" and "I was less responsible than I usually am" (reverse-scored). Results revealed a strong negative correlation between high-maintenance interaction and effective self-regulation: Having to exert effort to coordinate with a romantic partner is associated with ineffective self-regulation.

The primary goals of the second study were (1) to replicate the earlier findings with a design that does not depend upon retrospective reports and controls for the effects of five potential confounds and (2) to discern whether high-maintenance interaction is associated with increasingly impaired self-regulation over time (Finkel et al., 2004, Study 2). Willpower served as a new measure of self-regulation, as it strongly predicts effective performance on important self-regulatory tasks (e.g., Mischel, 1974; Mischel, Shoda, & Rodriquez, 1989). In this study, participants (all of whom were involved in dating relationships) completed one-item measures of high-maintenance interaction ("Maintaining efficient and pleasant interaction with my partner requires a lot of energy") and willpower ("I am able to resist temptation and work effectively toward long-term goals") 14 times over a 6-month period (every other week). Results extended findings from the first study by demonstrating that high-maintenance interaction was not only associated with impaired self-regulation, but it also predicted increasingly impaired self-regulation over time. These associations were robust beyond the effects of mood, happiness, vitality, self-deception, and impression management. (Additional results revealed that this effect also works in reverse, with self-regulation predicting increasing perceptions of high-maintenance interaction over time; such evidence of bidirectional causation suggests that the processes of impaired self-regulation and high-maintenance interaction may well exacerbate one another in a vicious cycle.)

The third study set out to replicate the findings from the first two with an entirely different method (Finkel et al., 2004, Study 3). The new procedure (1) employed a specific and behavioral (rather than a general and self-report) measure of self-regulation (GRE performance) and (2) balanced competing demands for internal validity and external validity. To strengthen external validity, high-maintenance interaction was assessed regarding an interaction with the participant's ongoing romantic partner (as in the first two studies) rather than with a stranger. In addition, it was assessed as partners engaged in an unscripted interaction that allowed them to communicate without constraints on what they were allowed to say. To strengthen internal validity, this interaction (with regard to which high-maintenance interaction was assessed) took place in a well-controlled laboratory setting and revolved around a specific dyadic task (described below).

Participants (who were both members of heterosexual romantic couples) engaged in a 4-minute laboratory interaction task, in which one partner instructed the other to place a set of abstract shapes in a specific order determined by the experimenter. The partners were allowed to communicate with one another as much as they liked, but they could not see each other because they were on separate sides of a visual divider. When this 4-minute interaction was over, partners reported the degree to which they experienced it as a high-maintenance interaction. Sample items from the four-item high-maintenance interaction scale are "We had a difficult time communicating" and "It was easy for us to coordinate our efforts" (reverse-scored). Results revealed that the high-maintenance interaction measure was negatively associated with GRE performance, an effect that remained robust beyond the effects of mood and self-efficacy. Although this trend of associations held for both males and females, it was statistically significant only for females.

Although these three studies provide compelling evidence that experiencing high-maintenance interaction with a romantic partner is associated with impaired self-regulation, they are limited insofar as (1) their non-experimental methods do not allow for firm causal conclusions, (2) they depend on self-report measures of high-maintenance interaction, and (3) they examine high-maintenance interaction exclusively in romantic relationships. To address these limitations, the fourth study set out (1) to garner evidence that high-maintenance interaction *causes* impaired self-regulation and (2) to provide additional support for this association without relying on self-report measures to assess either high-maintenance interaction or self-regulation (Finkel et al., 2005, Study 1). Female participants interacted with a same-sex confederate whose behavior rendered the interaction either high maintenance (inefficient, difficult) or low maintenance (efficient, easy) for them. The rationale behind using this method was that high-maintenance interaction is not limited to interactions between previously acquainted individuals; rather, any interaction characterized by inefficient coordination and requiring energy exertion should result in impaired self-regulation. Participants used a joystick to navigate a computer-based maze for 3 minutes. The rub, however, is that the experimenter had configured the room so that the participant was not able to see the computer monitor; rather, she had to rely on the confederate's verbal instructions to guide her through the maze. In the high-maintenance condition, the confederate made a scripted series of errors (e.g., "Wait!" and "Right . . . I mean left") in the directions she gave. In the low-maintenance condition, she followed the same script but without making errors.

Self-regulation was assessed with two different, theoretically derived measures (Gottfredson & Hirschi, 1990): *task motivation*, or whether participants preferred to engage in a challenging task that had the potential to be rewarding or in an easy task that was unlikely to be rewarding, and *task performance*, or how participants performed on a task of intermediate difficulty. Consistent with previous research suggesting that preferring simple tasks to complex ones is a common characteristic of individuals with low self-control (Gottfredson & Hirschi, 1990; Grasmick, Tittle, Bursik, & Arneklev, 1993; see also Flora, Finkel, & Foshee, 2003) and with the observation that depleted people prefer to engage in simple tasks like watching television rather than challenging tasks like doing homework, results revealed that participants who had experienced the high-maintenance interaction were significantly and substantially less likely to choose the challenging task (15%) than were those who had experienced the low-maintenance interaction (62%). After participants selected the easy or the challenging task, the experimenter presented all of them with the identical task of intermediate difficulty. Consistent with the idea that high-maintenance interaction impairs aspects of self-regulation like concentration and motivation, results revealed that participants who had been assigned to interact with the low-maintenance confederate solved 56% more anagrams than did those who had been assigned to interact with the high-maintenance confederate.

The fifth study set out to gather additional evidence for the processes uncovered in the fourth one with a method that employed (1) new coordination and self-regulation tasks and (2) a no-interaction control condition (Finkel et al., 2005, Study 2). Participants once again interacted with a same-sex confederate of the experimenter whose behavior rendered the interaction either high maintenance or low maintenance for them. In this new task, participants were randomly assigned to perform a data entry task (1) with a confederate who made the interaction high maintenance, (2) with a confederate who made the interaction low maintenance, or (3) alone. In the two dyadic conditions, the confederate read a string of numbers to the participant, who entered them into a computer-based spreadsheet. In the high-maintenance condition, the confederate made a scripted series of errors (e.g., "2—I mean 1" and "9, oops, sorry, I meant 4"). To strengthen the manipulation further, the confederate made sure to remain out of sync with the participant: He or she could hear the strokes of the keyboard and deliberately avoided developing a rhythm with the participant. In the low-maintenance condition, he or she followed the same script but without making errors.

After completing this task, participants spent 10 minutes working (alone) on the same GRE task used in the third study. Consistent with expectations, results revealed that participants who had been assigned to experience the high-maintenance interaction subsequently performed worse on the GRE task relative to those who had been assigned to experience the low-maintenance interaction and relative to those who performed the data entry task alone. Similar results emerged for the sixth study (Finkel et al., 2005, Study 3).

The seventh study was inspired by a striking pattern of null findings in the three previous experimental studies: Intensive efforts to find evidence that the effect of high-maintenance interaction on impaired self-regulation was mediated through three plausible conscious processes (subjectively experienced depletion, mood, and self-efficacy) consistently failed to find evidence for mediation. This reliable pattern of findings suggests that high-maintenance interaction may well influence self-regulation without requiring high-level cognitive mediation. Building on the plausible notion that humans are constantly but nonconsciously attuned to their social coordination experiences—particularly to social coordination *failures*—in their everyday lives, the seventh study incorporated a subtle manipulation of high-maintenance interaction in which participants were not consciously aware that social coordination had been inefficient (Finkel et al., 2005, Study 4). This design differed from those employed in the previous studies employing experimental manipulations of high-maintenance interaction because those previous manipulations involved obvious instances of social coordination failure; participants in the high-maintenance interaction conditions, for example, surely recognized that the confederate was making errors when guiding them on how to navigate the maze or on how to enter the data. Unlike these previous studies, the procedure for the seventh study manipulated social coordination without affecting performance on the dyadic task.

In addition, social coordination was manipulated without participants' awareness. To accomplish this, procedures were adapted from the burgeoning literature on nonconscious behavioral mimicry (for a review, see Chartrand, Maddux, & Lakin, 2005). Half of the participants interacted with a confederate who subtly mimicked their mannerisms and gestures (low-maintenance interaction, or *mimicry*, condition) and the other half interacted with a confederate who subtly but deliberately stayed out of sync with their mannerisms and gestures (high-maintenance interaction, or *misalignment*, condition). The reason why this study employed behavioral mimicry and antimimicry procedures to manipulate social coordination nonconsciously is that poorly synchronized behavioral mimicry may well render otherwise efficient social interactions more complex, requiring at a nonconscious level heightened attention to social coordination. The increased vigilance required during interactions characterized by such social misalignment may well transform them into high-maintenance interactions and increase the likelihood of impaired self-regulation on subsequent unrelated tasks.

After participants experienced either the high-maintenance (social misalignment) or low-maintenance (mimicry) interaction, they played the game Operation, a commercial board game for children that involves delicately removing small plastic body parts from a cartoon patient using a tweezer-like device (see Vohs et al., 2005, Study 7). The experimenter explained that the participant's tasks were (1) to remove each of the plastic body parts in a single

smooth motion and (2) to do so as quickly as possible. If participants accidentally failed to remove the piece on a given removal attempt, they were
required to remove the tweezers from the board and initiate a new attempt to
remove that particular piece. Participants were allowed to give up on any particular piece and move on to the next one with the understanding that they
could not go back and attempt to remove that piece again; they knew that
deciding to move on without successfully removing the piece would represent
a failure to perform optimally on the task.

Results revealed that although participants in both conditions successfully removed most of the pieces, participants who had experienced the
high-maintenance (misalignment) interaction experienced 86% more removal
failures relative to those who had experienced the low-maintenance (mimicry) interaction. In addition, relative to participants who were assigned to
the high-maintenance interaction (misalignment) condition, those who were
assigned to the low-maintenance interaction (mimicry) condition were 39%
more likely to remove a piece successfully on any given attempt.

Taken together, these seven studies provide strong support for the
hypothesis that high-maintenance interactions impair personal self-regulation
on subsequent unrelated tasks. We now turn our attention to an independent
line of research suggesting that interracial interactions can serve as high-
maintenance interactions.

Interracial Interactions and Impaired Executive Control

In a series of five studies, Richeson and her colleagues (2003; Richeson &
Shelton, 2003; Richeson & Trawalter, 2005) present evidence that interracial
interactions can impair subsequent executive control (a crucial component of
self-regulation). The logic underlying this line of research is that suppressing
prejudicial behaviors frequently requires that one exert self-regulation (e.g.,
Devine, 1989; Dovidio & Gaertner, 1998; Monteith, 1993). Individuals frequently feel compelled to exert self-regulatory effort to avoid behaving in a
prejudicial manner because there are strong social norms against being prejudiced in modern Western societies (e.g., Crandall, Eshleman, & O'Brien,
2002; Gaertner & Dovidio, 1986). As a result of this self-regulatory exertion,
engaging in an interracial interaction when prejudice concerns are elevated,
we suggest, functions as a high-maintenance interaction.

In the first study, white participants first completed an implicit association test assessing their implicit prejudice against blacks. Subsequently, they
were randomly assigned to talk for 5 minutes to a white or a black confederate
about controversial topics, one of which was racial profiling in light of the Sep-
tember 11th attacks (Richeson & Shelton, 2003). After completing this interaction with the confederate, participants completed the Stroop (1935) color-
naming task. Because effective performance on the Stroop task requires that

individuals override their automatic response tendencies, it is a standard task employed to measure executive control. Results revealed a significant interaction between prejudice and confederate race in predicting Stroop interference: Prejudice was positively associated with Stroop interference for white participants who had interacted with a black confederate but not for those who had interacted with a white confederate. These results suggest that engaging in interracial interaction forced prejudiced participants to exert self-regulatory efforts during the interaction and that these efforts depleted their resources for the subsequent executive control task.

The second study set out to investigate whether individual differences in racial prejudice predict the activation and potential depletion of executive control resources during interracial interactions, which in turn predicts impaired Stroop performance (Richeson et al., 2003). White participants experienced a procedure virtually identical to the one employed in the first study, but this time they also completed a separate and ostensibly unrelated testing session in which their brain activity was recorded using functional magnetic resonance imaging (fMRI) techniques while they looked at pictures of black faces and of white faces. In this fMRI session, the researchers examined differential activation when looking at black faces relative to looking at white faces in two brain areas that have been associated with executive control processes: the dorsolateral prefrontal cortex (DLPFC) and the anterior cingulate cortex (ACC). The fMRI data were matched with the behavioral data to explore the plausibility of the hypothesis that activation in these brain regions might mediate the association of white participants' prejudice scores with impaired Stroop performance after interacting with a black confederate. Results provide preliminary evidence that DLPFC activation does indeed mediate this association, although ACC activation does not. As predicted, results revealed nonsignificant associations of brain activation with Stroop performance for same-race interactions. Taken together, these results are consistent with a resource depletion explanation for the impaired Stroop performance of prejudiced white participants following interracial interaction: Such interactions seem to require that prejudiced white people exert self-regulation (as detected through DLPFC activation), which may well deplete self-regulatory resources and ultimately impair executive control performance.

The goal of the third study was to examine whether elevating white participants' concerns about behaving in a racially prejudicial manner immediately before they experienced an interracial (but not a same-race) interaction would result in especially impaired Stroop performance following the interaction (Richeson & Trawalter, 2005, Study 1). Half of the participants were given feedback suggesting that they were prejudiced; the other half were given negative feedback unrelated to prejudice. After receiving this feedback, the participants (all of whom were white) interacted with a black or a white confederate in a research paradigm similar to that employed in the two previous studies: They talked to the confederate about racially sensitive topics before performing an ostensibly unrelated Stroop task. Results revealed that participants who experienced an interracial interaction after receiving the prejudice feedback exhibited greater interference on the Stroop task relative to those who had received the negative but nonracial feedback. This pattern of findings did not emerge for participants who experienced a same-race interaction. These results suggest that elevated concerns about appearing prejudiced require participants to exert self-regulatory effort in interracial interactions, and that this exertion impairs subsequent efforts at executive control.

Whereas the third study incorporated a manipulation that increased the self-regulatory demands on the participants, the fourth study incorporated a manipulation that decreased such demands (Richeson & Trawalter, 2005, Study 2). White participants again talked to either a black or a white confederate about a racially sensitive topic before completing an ostensibly unrelated Stroop task. To reduce self-regulatory demands, half of the participants read their responses from a standardized script, while the other half were required to generate their own responses during the course of the interaction. The logic underlying this manipulation is that reading racially sensitive information from a standardized script should reduce uncertainty regarding what to say or how to behave during the interracial interaction, thereby reducing the need to exert active self-regulation. In a replication of previous findings, results revealed that participants in the no script condition exhibited greater Stroop interference after interracial interactions than after same-race interactions. Consistent with hypotheses, however, this effect failed to emerge in the script condition. Another way of thinking about these results is that participants in the script condition exhibited less Stroop interference relative to those in the no script condition for interracial interactions, but that the script manipulation failed to influence Stroop interference for same-race interactions. These results suggest that minimizing the self-regulatory demands of interracial interaction can diminish the impairment in subsequent executive control that would otherwise emerge.

Like the fourth study, the fifth study also incorporated a manipulation that decreased the self-regulatory demands on participants. Once again, white participants talked either to a black or a white confederate before engaging in an ostensibly unrelated Stroop task (Richeson & Trawalter, 2005, Study 3). In this study, half of the participants were given the opportunity to misattribute any anxiety they might experience during the interaction to aspects of the testing room rather than to the interaction itself. Specifically, participants in the misattribution condition were told, "Several previous participants have found that this room makes them anxious because of the one-way mirror and the confined feel of the room," whereas participants in the control condition received no information about previous participants' experiences. In a replication of previous findings, results revealed that participants in the control condition exhibited greater Stroop interference after interracial interactions than after same-race interactions. Consistent with hypotheses, this effect failed to emerge in the misattribution condition. Another way of thinking about these results is that participants in the misattribution condition exhibited less Stroop interference relative to those in the control condition for interracial interactions, but the misattribution manipulation failed to influence Stroop interference for same-race interactions. These results further bolster the assertion that minimizing the self-regulatory demands of interracial interaction can diminish the impairment in subsequent executive control that would otherwise emerge.

Taken together, these five studies provide strong support for the hypothesis that interracial interaction can impair performance on subsequent executive control tasks when concerns with appearing prejudiced are elevated. Evidence suggests that this effect is due to depleted self-regulatory strength.

SURFING TOWARD A MODEL OF SELF-REGULATION AND RELATIONSHIP FUNCTIONING

Our principal goal in this chapter has been to present evidence from a slew of recent studies for the hypothesis that high-maintenance interaction impairs self-regulation. In the present section, we strive to expand our thinking about high-maintenance interaction by situating it in a broader model examining the interplay between self-regulation and relationship functioning. Toward this goal, we introduce and briefly discuss a preliminary model called the *self-regulation and relationship functioning model*, abbreviated as the SRRF model (pronounced "surf model").

The SRRF model, as depicted in Figure 15.1, consists of three interrelated constructs: (1) high-maintenance interaction, (2) self-regulatory failure, and (3) interpersonal conflict. A central tenet of the SRRF model is that each of these three constructs influences—and is influenced by—the other two. The research on high-maintenance interaction reviewed above is represented by the directional component of arrow "A" that goes from high-maintenance interaction to self-regulatory failure. We propose, however, that the causal direction also goes in the reverse direction, from self-regulatory failure to high-maintenance interaction. The logic here builds on the idea that it requires psychological exertion to avoid high-maintenance interaction and engender efficient social coordination. For example, coordinating with an unknown cook to prepare a meal for 50 people requires that one attend closely to the other's approach to cooking and modify one's own behavior accordingly. Individuals experiencing impaired self-regulation are likely to lack the requisite ability and/or motivation to get in sync with another person on a dyadic task.

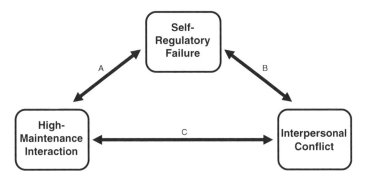

FIGURE 15.1. The self-regulation and relationship functioning (SRRF, or "surf") model.

Other research provides support for the directional component of arrow "B" that goes from self-regulatory failure to interpersonal conflict. This research suggests that diminished self-regulatory ability (both high self-regulatory strength depletion and low dispositional self-control) is associated with less constructive behavior toward a romantic partner in conflictual situations (Finkel & Campbell, 2001; Rawn & Vohs, Chapter 2, this volume). What about the directional component of arrow "B" that goes from interpersonal conflict to self-regulatory failure? Although we are not aware of research directly addressing this question, evidence suggests that interpersonal conflict is associated with, for example, poor mental health (Vinokur & van Ryn, 1993) and immunological down-regulation (Kiecolt-Glaser et al., 1993). It is plausible that interpersonal conflict also impairs the interactants' subsequent self-regulation, as assessed by poor health behaviors (e.g., smoking, unhealthy eating), impaired concentration, and so forth. Future research could fruitfully explore the effects of interpersonal conflict on self-regulation.

Both directional components of arrow "C" are heretofore unexplored empirically. Given that research on high-maintenance interactions is so new, it is perhaps not surprising that none has yet examined the interplay between such interaction and interpersonal conflict. There is, however, reason to believe that these constructs are tightly connected. Consider, for example, the directional component of arrow "C" that goes from high-maintenance interaction to interpersonal conflict. High-maintenance interaction may well engender conflict because people frequently experience frustration and anger when interpersonal coordination is inefficient. In addition, a large fraction of the topics about which people have serious conflict emerges from poor coordination. Imagine a married couple in which the husband, David, is driving the car late at night in search of a campsite. His wife, Delores, reads the map. The map is poor and Delores is not a superb map reader, so she is not 100% certain of where the turnoff is. David suggests that they take the next left, and although Delores has reservations about whether this is the correct turnoff, she does not have any better ideas, so they take a chance. Twenty minutes later they are lost; bickering soon follows. This example illustrates that although David and Delores share the goal of getting to the campsite as efficiently as possible, their coordination is impaired by her map-reading limitations and his faulty intuition. What starts as a coordination problem grows into interpersonal conflict.

What about the directional component of arrow "C" that goes from interpersonal conflict to high-maintenance interaction? A commonly reported aftereffect of interpersonal conflict is the feeling experienced by one or both partners that one must now "walk on eggshells," that is, one must carefully monitor one's words and behaviors to avoid upsetting the partner and rekindling the conflict. The experience of walking on eggshells may well represent a prototypical case of high-maintenance interaction, as it requires that the individual exert effort to get in sync with the partner. What starts as a conflict grows into a coordination problem.

IMPLICATIONS

In addition to advancing the SRRF model as a preliminary model of the interplay between self-regulation and relationship functioning, we also briefly discuss two implications of the high-maintenance interaction research reviewed above (see also Finkel et al., 2005).

Why Does High-Maintenance Interaction Impair Self-Regulation?

The experimental studies in the first line of research summarized above included rigorous attempts to identify aspects of subjective experience that could mediate the effect of experiencing a high-maintenance interaction on subsequent self-regulatory failure (Finkel et al., 2005). These studies revealed a striking lack of support for mediation by subjectively experienced depletion, mood, or self-efficacy. Some evidence emerged from the mimicry study to suggest that this effect may even emerge without the individual's conscious awareness. The research on interracial interactions provided preliminary support for the possibility that brain activity in the DLPFC mediates the effect of interracial versus same-race interaction on subsequent impairment in Stroop performance (Richeson et al., 2003). It also presented evidence that increasing the self-regulatory demands associated with interracial interactions results in greater impairment in subsequent Stroop performance, whereas decreasing such demands reduces it (Richeson & Trawalter, 2005). Taken together, this body of research suggests that (1) the driving mechanism behind the destructive self-regulatory effects of high-maintenance interaction is self-regulatory strength depletion, but (2) individuals may not be consciously aware that the interactions have affected them. We speculate that individuals eventually become aware that they are experiencing depletion as a result of high-maintenance interactions, but that this subjective experience occurs only after cognitive resources are freed up for reflection. We leave this idea as a topic for future research.

Do high-maintenance interactions impair subsequent self-regulation because they render the interactants incapable of performing self-regulatory tasks or because they result in diminished motivation to do so? Two findings provide preliminary evidence to support the motivational explanation. The first is that high-maintenance interaction causes people to prefer to engage in simple tasks that are unlikely to require much effort but also are unlikely to be rewarding (Finkel et al., 2005, Study 1). The second is that high-maintenance interaction causes people to perform subsequent tasks without the care and attention to detail that they would typically apply—that is, they perform the tasks sloppily (Finkel et al., 2005, Study 4).

Emotionally Energizing Interactions?

Although we have focused on interactions that impair self-regulation, we are confident that future research will also identify interpersonal processes that *enhance* self-regulation. We suggest that just as interaction partners can deplete us, they can also replenish us. For example, perhaps a laughter-filled 10-minute conversation with a loved one can replenish depleted self-regulatory resources. Recent evidence suggests that simply thinking about a person with whom one has a close positive relationship increases one's willingness to learn threatening but valuable information about the self (Kumashiro & Sedikides, 2005). Future research could explore when, how, and why close positive relationships can be replenishing or bolstering.

CONCLUSION

Coordinating interaction with others can be challenging, even when the interactants share compatible goals. Emerging evidence suggests that high-maintenance interaction is associated with impaired personal self-regulation on subsequent unrelated tasks. This work (1) serves as one example highlighting the importance of considering the effects of interpersonal processes in understanding self-regulation and (2) advances a preliminary model for investigating the dynamic interplay between high-maintenance interaction, self-regulation, and interpersonal conflict.

REFERENCES

Baumeister, R. F. (1998). The self. In D. T. Gilbert, S. T. Fiske, & G. Lindzey (Eds.), *Handbook of social psychology* (4th ed., Vol. 2, pp. 680–740). New York: McGraw-Hill.

Baumeister, R. F., Bratslavsky, E., Muraven, M., & Tice, D. M. (1998). Ego depletion: Is the active self a limited resource? *Journal of Personality and Social Psychology, 74,* 1252–1265.

Baumeister, R. F., & Heatherton, T. F. (1996). Self-regulation failure: An overview. *Psychological Inquiry, 7,* 1–15.

Baumeister, R. F., & Vohs, K. D. (Eds.). (2004). *Handbook of self-regulation: Research, theory, and applications.* New York: Guilford Press.

Chartrand, T. L., Maddux, W., & Lakin, J. (2005). Beyond the perception–behavior link: The ubiquitous utility and motivational moderators of nonconscious mimicry. In R. Hassin, J. Uleman, & J.A. Bargh (Eds.), *The new unconscious* (pp. 334–361). New York: Oxford University Press.

Crandall, C. S., Eshleman, A., & O'Brien, L. (2002). Social norms and the expression and suppression of prejudice: The struggle for internalization. *Journal of Personality and Social Psychology, 82,* 359–378.

Devine, P. G. (1989). Stereotypes and prejudice: Their automatic and controlled components. *Journal of Personality and Social Psychology, 56,* 5–18.

Dovidio, J. F., & Gaertner, S. L. (1998). On the nature of contemporary prejudice: The causes, consequences, and challenges of aversive racism. In J. L. Eberhardt & S. T. Fiske (Eds.), *Confronting racism: The problem and the response* (pp. 3–32). Thousand Oaks, CA: Sage.

Finkel, E. J., & Campbell, W. K. (2001). Self-control and accommodation in close relationships: An interdependence analysis. *Journal of Personality and Social Psychology, 81,* 263–277.

Finkel, E. J., Campbell, W. K., Brunell, A. B., Dalton, A. N., & Chartrand, T. L. (2005). *High-maintenance interaction: Inefficient social coordination impairs self-regulation.* Manuscript submitted for publication.

Finkel, E. J., Campbell, W. K., & Sands, A. (2004). *High-maintenance interactions in romantic relationships: Implications for self-regulation.* Manuscript in preparation, Northwestern University, Evanston, IL.

Finkel E. J., Rusbult, C. E., Kumashiro, M., & Hannon, P. A. (2002). Dealing with betrayal in close relationships: Does commitment promote forgiveness of betrayal? *Journal of Personality and Social Psychology, 82,* 956–974.

Flora, D. B., Finkel, E. J., & Foshee, V. A. (2003). Higher order factor structure of a self-control test: Evidence from a confirmatory factor analysis with polychoric correlations. *Educational and Psychological Measurement, 63,* 112–127.

Gaertner, S. L., & Dovidio, J. F. (1986). The aversive form of racism. In J. F. Dovidio & S. L. Gaertner (Eds.), *Prejudice, discrimination, and racism* (pp. 61–89). San Diego, CA: Academic Press.

Gottfredson, M. R., & Hirschi, T. (1990). *A general theory of crime.* Stanford, CA: Stanford University Press.

Grasmick, J. F., Tittle, C. R., Bursik, R. J., Jr., & Arneklev, B. J. (1993). Testing the core empirical implications of Gottfredson and Hirschi's general theory of crime. *Journal of Research in Crime and Delinquency, 30*, 5–29.

Hatfield, E., Cacioppo, J. T., & Rapson, R. L. (1994). *Emotional contagion*. Cambridge, UK: Cambridge University Press.

Holmes, J. G., & Rempel, J. K. (1989). Trust in close relationships. In C. Hendrick (Ed.), *Close relationships* (pp. 187–220). Thousand Oaks, CA: Sage.

Kelley, H. H., Holmes, J. G., Kerr, N. L., Reis, H. T., Rusbult, C. E., & Van Lange, P. A. M. (2003). *An atlas of interpersonal situations*. New York: Cambridge University Press.

Kelley, H. H., & Thibaut, J. W. (1978). *Interpersonal relations: A theory of interdependence*. New York: Wiley.

Kiecolt-Glaser, J. K., Malarkey, W. B., Chee, M., Newton, T., Cacioppo, J. T., Mao, H.-Y., & Glaser, R. (1993). Negative behavior during marital conflict is associated with immunological down-regulation. *Psychosomatic Medicine, 55*, 395–409.

Kumashiro, M., & Sedikides, C. (2005). Taking on liability-focused information: Close positive relationships as a self-bolstering resource. *Psychological Science, 16*, 732–739.

Mischel, W. (1974). Processes in delay of gratification. In L. Berkowitz (Ed.), *Advances in experimental social psychology* (Vol. 7, pp. 249–292). New York: Academic Press.

Mischel, W., Shoda, Y., & Rodriquez, M. L. (1989). Delay of gratification in children. *Science, 244*, 933–938.

Monteith, M. J. (1993). Self-regulation of prejudiced responses: Implications for progress in prejudice-reduction efforts. *Journal of Personality and Social Psychology, 65*, 469–485.

Muraven, M., & Baumeister, R. F. (2000). Self-regulation and depletion of limited resources: Does self-control resemble a muscle? *Psychological Bulletin, 74*, 774–789.

Muraven, M., Collins, R. L., & Neinhaus, K. (2002). Self-control and alcohol restraint: An initial application of the self-control strength model. *Psychology of Addictive Behaviors, 16*, 113–120.

Muraven, M., & Slessareva, E. (2003). Mechanisms of self-control failure: Motivation and limited resources. *Personality and Social Psychology Bulletin, 29*, 894–906.

Muraven, M., Tice, D. M., & Baumeister, R. F. (1998). Self-control as limited resource: Regulatory depletion patterns. *Journal of Personality and Social Psychology, 74*, 774–789.

Richeson, J. A., Baird, A. A., Gordon, H. L., Heatherton, T. F., Wyland, C. L., Trawalter, S., & Shelton, J. N. (2003). An fMRI investigation of the impact of interracial contact on executive control. *Nature Neuroscience, 6*, 1323–1328.

Richeson, J. A., & Shelton, J. N. (2003). When prejudice does not pay: Effects of interracial contact on executive control. *Psychological Science, 14*, 287–290.

Richeson, J. A., & Trawalter, S. (2005). Why do interracial interactions impair executive function? A resource depletion account. *Journal of Personality and Social Psychology, 88*, 934–947.

Rusbult, C. E., & Van Lange, P. A. M. (1996). Interdependence processes. In E. T.

Higgins & A. W. Kruglanski (Eds.), *Social psychology: Handbook of basic principles* (pp. 564–596). New York: Guilford Press.

Rusbult, C. E., & Van Lange, P. A. M. (2003). Interdependence, interaction, and relationships. *Annual Review of Psychology, 54*, 351–375.

Rusbult, C. E., Verette, J., Whitney, G. A., Slovik, L. F., & Lipkus, I. (1991). Accommodation processes in close relationships: Theory and preliminary evidence. *Journal of Personality and Social Psychology, 60*, 53–78.

Schmeichel, B. J., & Baumeister, R. F. (2004). Self-regulatory strength. In R. F. Baumeister & K. D. Vohs (Eds.), *Handbook of self-regulation: Research, theory, and applications* (pp. 84–98). New York: Guilford Press.

Schmeichel, B. J., Vohs, K. D., & Baumeister, R. F. (2003). Intellectual performance and ego depletion: Role of the self in logical reasoning and other information processing. *Journal of Personality and Social Psychology, 85*, 33–46.

Stroop, J. R. (1935). Studies of interference in serial verbal reactions. *Journal of Experimental Psychology, 18*, 643–662.

Thibaut, J. W., & Kelley, H. H. (1959). *The social psychology of groups.* New York: Wiley.

Van Lange, P. A. M. (1999). The pursuit of joint outcomes and equality in outcomes: An integrative model of social value orientation. *Journal of Personality and Social Psychology, 77*, 337–349.

Vinokur, A. D., & van Ryn, M. (1993). Social support and undermining in close relationships: Their independent effects on the mental health of unemployed persons. *Journal of Personality and Social Psychology, 65*, 350–359.

Vohs, K. D., & Baumeister, R. F. (2004). Understanding self-regulation: An introduction. In R. F. Baumeister & K. D. Vohs (Eds.), *Handbook of self-regulation: Research, theory, and applications* (pp. 1–9). New York: Guilford Press.

Vohs, K. D., Baumeister, R. F., Twenge, J. M., Schmeichel, B. J., Tice, D. M., & Crocker, J. (2005). *Decision fatigue exhausts self-regulatory resources—but so does accommodating to unchosen alternatives.* Manuscript submitted for publication.

Vohs, K. D., & Heatherton, T. F. (2000). Self-regulatory failure: A resource-depletion approach. *Psychological Science, 11*, 249–254.

Vohs, K. D., & Schmeichel, B. J. (2003). Self-regulation and the extended now: Controlling the self alters the subjective experience of time. *Journal of Personality and Social Psychology, 85*, 217–230.

Wallace, H. M., & Baumeister, R. F. (2002). The effects of success versus failure feedback on further self-control. *Self and Identity, 1*, 35–42.

The Michelangelo Phenomenon

Partner Affirmation and Self-Movement toward One's Ideal

MADOKA KUMASHIRO
CARYL E. RUSBULT
SCOTT T. WOLF
MARIE-JOELLE ESTRADA

I love you for what you are, but I love you yet more for what you are going to be. . . . You are going forward toward something great. I am on the way with you and therefore I love you.
—CARL SANDBURG

I love you not only for what you are, but for what I am when I am with you . . . for what you are making of me. I love you for the part of me that you bring out.
—ELIZABETH BARRETT BROWNING

The love expressed by the poet Carl Sandburg is based partly on the potential that he sees in his partner. The love expressed by the poet Elizabeth Browning is based partly on the potential that her partner sees in her. For a moment, imagine that these poets were lovers, declaring their feelings for one another: Because Carl perceives and celebrates the person Elizabeth aspires to be, she moves ever closer to achieving her ideals. Elizabeth loves Carl in part because she loves herself when she is with him. As Elizabeth moves closer to her ideals, Carl continues to cherish both her actual self and her emerging self.[1] The two continually strengthen one another, thereby enhancing their mutual feelings of love.

Both poets speak of the transformative power of love—a theme that suffuses literature from our earliest exposure to the concept of love. Indeed, the power of love in promoting personal growth is one of the most common themes in children's stories, where we learn that love can transform beasts into princes and cindergirls into princesses. Somewhat surprisingly, this theme has been less frequently addressed in the scientific literature regarding close relationships (for exceptions, see Brunstein, Dangelmayer, & Schultheiss, 1996; Feeney, 2004). Our work regarding the Michelangelo phenomenon seeks to address this deficiency by examining the manner in which close partners "sculpt" one another, thereby moving each person closer to—versus further away from—his or her ideal self (Drigotas, Rusbult, Wieselquist, & Whitton, 1999; Rusbult, Kumashiro, Stocker, & Wolf, 2005).

We begin this chapter with a review of the three theoretical traditions that form the basis for our work. Then we describe the Michelangelo phenomenon and it consequences, introducing the concepts of partner affirmation and movement toward the ideal self, and reviewing the subsequent benefits of these processes to personal well-being and couple well-being. After summarizing empirical findings in support of key model predictions, we explain how this phenomenon differs from other self-relevant processes, such as partner verification and self-expansion. Finally, we discuss specific self processes, partner processes, and relationship processes that are relevant to understanding the Michelangelo phenomenon.

THEORETICAL BACKGROUND

Our analysis of the Michelangelo phenomenon rests on a core proposition regarding human dispositions: the assumption that the self does not spring full blown from a vacuum. We suggest that interpersonal experience plays an integral role in shaping personal traits, values, and behavioral tendencies. Among the many interpersonal forces that shape the self, few if any "sculptors" exert effects as powerful as those of our close partners. Such effects can vary from exceedingly positive to exceedingly negative: Close partners may bring out the best or the worst in one another. In the following paragraphs, we review the three primary research traditions on which our work rests: the behavioral confirmation, interdependence, and self-discrepancy traditions.

Behavioral Confirmation Processes

Our analysis begins with the concept of *behavioral confirmation*, defined as the means by which an interaction partner's expectations about the self become reality by eliciting behaviors from the self that confirm the partner's expectations (Darley & Fazio, 1980; Harris & Rosenthal, 1985). How does this process unfold? Interaction partners tend to act in accord with their preconceived beliefs about the self's strengths and limitations, preferences and disinclinations.[2] In so doing, partners create opportunities for the self to display some behaviors, constrain interaction in such a manner as to inhibit the display of other behaviors, and thereby elicit a subset of the self's full repertoire of possible behaviors (Rosenthal & Jacobson, 1968; Snyder, Tanke, & Berscheid, 1977). As a result, self-perceptions frequently become aligned with others' expectations (Fazio, Effrein, & Falender, 1981; Murray, Holmes, & Griffin, 1996). For example, on their first date, if Mary had heard from friends that John possesses a good sense of humor, then she may laugh at his comments, thereby encouraging John to tell another joke; on the other hand, if Mary had heard that John is somber, she may inadvertently steer the conversation toward serious topics, thereby inhibiting John's display of humor.

Interdependence Processes

Of course, different interaction partners yield differentially robust confirmation effects. The people with whom we are deeply interdependent are likely to exert especially powerful effects, in that strong interdependence entails frequent and powerful influence across diverse types of activity. As such, behavioral confirmation must be understood in the context of specific interactions with specific partners. Interdependence theory analyzes interaction (I) in terms of the goals and motives of the relevant actors (A and B) within the specific interdependence situation (S) in which the two interact ($I = f[S, A, B]$; Kelley et al., 2003). Whereas close partners adjust to one another in the context of specific interactions, over time the adjustments that begin as interaction-specific behavioral adaptations become embodied in stable dispositions and habits (Kelley & Thibaut, 1978; Rusbult & Van Lange, 2003): Both partners selectively develop some aspects of the self and suppress or eliminate others, such that each person's traits, values, and behavioral tendencies come to reflect the particular conditions of interdependence experienced with the partner. For example, in comparison to other interaction partners, Mary may provide greater opportunities for John to display his humorous side, encouraging him to regale their friends with funny stories. Heartened by her reception, John may become more comfortable telling funny stories, and may therefore become increasingly funny. In contrast, if Mary is not particularly fond of John's humor, she may discourage him from telling funny stories, increasing his reluctance to do so even when she is not around. Over time, John may embrace the interdependence reality created by Mary, actually becoming a funnier person (or a more somber and humorless one).

Self-Discrepancy Processes

How should we evaluate the adaptations resulting from behavioral confirmation? What is the preferable outcome for John, becoming a more humorous or a more somber person? Although conventional wisdom may tell us that being funny is preferable to being somber, what if John wants to become a no-nonsense, commanding leader? Our answer to this question begins as a metaphor, and rests on the manner in which sculpting was envisioned by its greatest practitioner: "Michelangelo conceived his figures as lying hidden in the block of marble. . . . The task he set himself as a sculptor was merely to extract the ideal form . . . to remove the stone that covered [the ideal]" (Gombrich, 1995, p. 313). As such, sculpting is a process whereby the artist releases a figure from the block of stone in which it slumbers. The creative process and the artist's tools are thus aspects of salvation. In Michelangelo's vision, the figure hidden in the stone was something heroic, vibrant, and divine—the figure slumbering in the stone was the "ideal form."

Like blocks of stone, humans too possess ideal forms. The human equivalent of Michelangelo's slumbering form is the *ideal self*, a possible self to which the individual aspires (Higgins, 1987, 1996; Markus & Nurius, 1986). The ideal self is defined in terms of the constellation of dispositions, motives, and behavioral tendencies an individual ideally wishes to acquire. Although the ideal self to some degree may slumber, this hidden, internal construct can powerfully influence personal well-being: Individuals experience distress to the extent that they perceive discrepancies between the ideal self and the *actual self*, defined as the dispositions, motives, and behavioral tendencies an individual believes he or she actually possesses. Such distress motivates individuals to bring the actual self into alignment with the ideal self.

Now we return to the question, Is it "better" for Mary to perceive John as humorous or as somber? We suggest that whether behavioral confirmation by a close partner yields positive or negative outcomes depends on the partner's ability to extract the self's ideal form. Like the figure submerged in the block of stone, the ideal self may not yet have been authenticated by any actual social experience, and should therefore be particularly vulnerable to social influence (Markus & Nurius, 1986). Thus the emergence of the ideal self may be particularly susceptible to behavioral confirmation from a close partner. If being funny is part of John's ideal self, Mary's appreciation of his humor is likely to yield positive outcomes, for both John (the self) and the relationship. However, in the event that John does not intend or desire to be funny, Mary's refusal to take him seriously is likely to yield negative outcomes.

THE MICHELANGELO PHENOMENON AND ITS CONSEQUENCES

Partner Affirmation versus Disaffirmation

The Michelangelo metaphor describes a beneficent unfolding of the confirmation process. The concept of partner affirmation describes the manner in which a partner sculpts the self, or the degree to which the partner is an ally (vs. foe) in the self's goal pursuits. *Partner perceptual affirmation* describes the degree to which a partner believes that the self can acquire ideal-congruent qualities: Does John "see the best in what Mary might be?" As illustrated in Figure 16.1, we suggest that partner perceptual affirmation promotes *partner behavioral affirmation*, which describes the degree to which a partner behaves toward the self in such a manner as to elicit ideal-congruent qualities: Does John "draw out the best in Mary?" In turn, partner behavioral affirmation yields *self movement toward the ideal self*: Mary becomes a reflection of that which she ideally wishes to be. For example, because John perceives that Mary wants to be more adventurous, he suggests trips to exotic locations, as a consequence of which Mary indeed begins to feel more adventurous. This three-step process is the Michelangelo phenomenon (Drigotas, Rusbult, Wieselquist, & Whitton, 1999).

Of course, partner sculpting may bring out the best or the worst in the self. Affirmation[3] is a continuum, ranging from high affirmation at the upper end of the continuum, through failure to affirm, to disaffirmation at the lower end of the continuum. There are two ways in which the process may go awry.

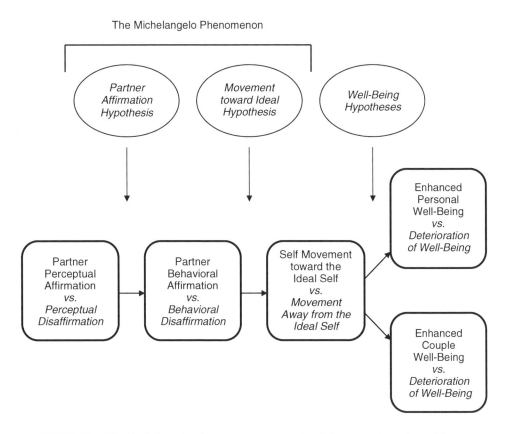

FIGURE 16.1. The Michelangelo phenomenon, personal well-being, and couple well-being.

First, a partner's perceptions and behavior may be antithetical to the self's ideal. For instance, although Mary wants to become more adventurous, John may believe that she is too fastidious about her surroundings to go on a "real" adventure. Based on this belief, he may inadvertently (or deliberately) discourage Mary from vacationing in isolated locations without modern conveniences. After overhearing John explain to a friend that Mary cannot handle the rough outdoors, Mary may become dismayed that his opinion of her is antithetical to her ideals, and that he will not provide opportunities for her to display her adventurous side.

Second, a partner's perceptions and behavior may be oriented toward goals that are irrelevant to the self's ideal. For instance, John may "love Mary for the wrong reasons"—he may love her for her homemaking abilities. John may praise Mary for her cooking and tell her what a great hostess she will become. Even though Mary may value John's admiration and even start cooking more elaborate dishes, if being a homemaker is not a central component of her ideal self, then John's actions—however positive and well intentioned—must be seen as irrelevant to that which she holds most dear. Consequently, John will play no role in promoting her central aspirations, and eventually she may recognize that he has rather thoroughly "missed the boat" about her.

Personal Well-Being and Couple Well-Being

We suggest that partner affirmation and movement toward the ideal self promote enhanced personal well-being and couple well-being (see Figure 16.1). Why might the Michelangelo phenomenon promote personal well-being? Growth striving has been widely postulated as a primary human motive. Freud (1923/1961) argued for such a motive in his discussion of ego ideal, Rogers (1961) and Maslow (1962) described such a motive in terms of self-actualization, and Bowlby (1969) addressed growth striving in his concept of exploration. Contemporary theories of motivation too emphasize the importance of self-determination and personal growth (Deci & Ryan, 2000; Emmons, 2003). To the extent that striving for personal growth is indeed a primary motive, we should find that when individuals move closer to their ideal selves, this motive is gratified. Accordingly, movement toward the ideal self should be associated with a wide range of personal benefits, including enhanced life satisfaction and superior psychological adjustment.

Why might the Michelangelo phenomenon promote couple well-being? First, a partner who perceptually affirms the self demonstrates empathic understanding (Ickes, Stinson, Bissonnette, & Garcia, 1990). Such understanding should enhance feelings of love ("You see me as I ideally want to be."). Second, behavioral affirmation promotes outcome correspondence and ease of coordination in that the behaviors of self and partner are synchronized (rather than at odds) in their pursuit of the self's ideal (Rusbult & Van Lange, 2003; Finkel, Campbell, & Brunell, Chapter 15, this volume). Relationships with greater correspondence should exhibit greater adjustment ("We act in harmony, toward achieving shared goals."). Third, work on attachment processes suggests that close partners may provide a secure base from which the self can engage in exploration (Feeney, 2004), which in turn may strengthen attachment ("I can trust you to be there for me."). And finally, movement toward the ideal self is gratifying in itself (Deci & Ryan, 2000; Emmons, 2003). Partners who play a role in producing such gratifications are likely to be highly valued ("I'm a better person when I'm with you.").

Empirical Evidence Regarding the Michelangelo Phenomenon

We have observed consistent support for model predictions using both experimental and nonexperimental methods, employing both obtrusive and unobtrusive measures, in the context of a wide range of relationships. For example, in several studies of both dating and marital relationships (Drigotas, Rusbult, Wieselquist, & Whitton, 1999; Rusbult, Kumashiro, Finkel, et al., 2005), we employed straightforward self-report measures of key model variables—self-reports of the extent to which the partner perceptually and behaviorally affirms the self (e.g., "My partner behaves in ways that allow me to become who I most want to be.") and the self exhibits movement toward the ideal self (perception of movement toward each of the top five components of the ideal self). To examine whether these findings were attributable to socially desirable response tendencies, we also obtained data from each partner's friends. Analyses of both self-report and friend report data revealed support for our model—for example, friend reports of affirmation and self movement toward ideal predicted breakups 3 months later (Drigotas, Rusbult, Wieselquist, Whitton, 1999).

In other studies we videotaped couples discussing one partner's pursuit of an important personal goal (Rusbult, Coolsen, et al., 2005; Rusbult, Kumashiro, Finkel, et al., 2005). Participants later reviewed their conversation, providing online ratings of both their own and the partner's behavior. In addition, trained coders rated both target and agent behaviors using a coding scheme we developed (e.g., "Partner criticized target's goal pursuits," "Target expressed determination about goal pursuits"). Independent of this conversation, participants completed measures of personal well-being and couple well-being. Analyses examining both types of behavioral measure revealed that when partners were judged to display more affirming behaviors, selves exhibited greater confidence about their ideals and reported greater subjective well-being and couple well-being.

And finally, we have obtained experimental support for model predictions. For example, in a study of potential dating relationships, participants were asked to imagine meeting a hypothetical partner who perceived the self in a certain way (Kumashiro, Wolf, Coolsen, & Rusbult, 2005). This perception centered on qualities that the participant had earlier identified as part of his or her ideal self, indifferent self, or feared self. Participants were asked to predict their interaction experiences with the target. In comparison to the feared self and the indifferent self conditions, in the ideal self condition—where the target thought the participant possessed ideal self attributes—participants anticipated more pleasant interaction and greater liking for the target.

Before moving on, two additional findings should be noted. First, mediation analyses routinely reveal support for hypothesized direct and indirect causal effects, demonstrating that (1) partner behavioral affirmation significantly (and fully) mediates the association of perceptual affirmation with self movement toward ideal, and (2) self movement toward ideal significantly (yet partially) mediates the association of behavioral affirmation with both personal well-being and couple well-being (Drigotas, Rusbult, Wieselquist, & Whitton, 1999; Rusbult, Coolsen, et al., 2005; Rusbult, Kumashiro, Finkel, et al., 2005). (Interestingly, in several studies we have found that [3] in predicting couple well-being, behavioral affirmation may be as important as [or more important than] self movement toward ideal.) Second, analyses of longitudinal data reveal that (1) earlier partner behavioral affirmation predicts change over time in movement toward the ideal self, and (2) earlier behavioral affirmation *and* movement toward ideal self predict change over time in personal well-being and couple well-being (Drigotas, Rusbult, Wieselquist, & Whitton, 1999; Rusbult, Coolsen, et al., 2005; Rusbult, Kumashiro, Finkel, et al., 2005). And importantly, such associations are evident even when we statistically control for a variety of potential confounds, including self-esteem, depression, and socially desirable response tendencies (Drigotas, Rusbult, Wieselquist, & Whitton, 1999; Rusbult, Coolsen, et al., 2005; Rusbult, Kumashiro, Finkel, et al., 2005).

HOW THE MICHELANGELO PHENOMENON DIFFERS FROM OTHER SELF-RELEVANT INTERACTION PROCESSES

Of course, our model is not the only extant theory that addresses self processes in ongoing relationships. In the following paragraphs we distinguish partner affirmation from related interpersonal processes—processes to which it bears some similarity, or with which it may share some common themes. Specifically, we posit that partner affirmation may play a key role in explaining the benefits associated with other self-relevant phenomena.

Partner Affirmation and Partner Enhancement

How does partner affirmation differ from *partner enhancement*, or partner behavior that is exceptionally positive with regard to the self (i.e., idealization, positive illusion)? Many studies have revealed that partner enhancement yields good consequences, demonstrating that selves whose partners view them favorably not only are more satisfied with their relationships, but also develop increasingly positive self-images (e.g., Murray et al., 1996). Do prior findings regarding affirmation merely reflect enhancement effects? We argue that the benefits of partner enhancement stem from positive partner behaviors that are congruent with the self's ideal rather than from a generalized positive perception of the self. To "unconfound" affirmation from enhancement, we define enhancement in terms of *normative desirability*, or the degree to which an elicited trait is "desirable for people of your age and sex." Whereas John's praise of Mary's homemaking skills may be normatively desirable, his behavior will not be beneficial if Mary does not care about homemaking and wishes to be appreciated for her adventurous spirit.

We have conducted empirical work that reveals support for the benefits of partner affirmation over generalized partner enhancement. For example, in the previously described experiment in which participants received false feedback about a target person's first impressions, this information concerned the participant's ideal self, indifferent self, or feared self, *and* was high, medium, or low in normative desirability (Kumashiro et al., 2005). Analyses performed on key criteria—including liking for the target and anticipated pleasantness of interaction—revealed reliable effects of affirmation, along with weak or nonsignificant effects of enhancement. Thus, in the final analysis, people prefer that their partners elicit behaviors that are positive *and* congruent with their ideal selves, rather than elicit behaviors that are merely normatively desirable.[4]

Partner Affirmation and the Pygmalion Phenomenon

Perceiving the self's true ideal form becomes critical in distinguishing the Michelangelo phenomenon from the *Pygmalion phenomenon*, derived from the Greek myth in which the protagonist creates his image of the ideal woman. Whereas the Michelangelo phenomenon describes a partner who sculpts toward the *self's* ideal, the Pygmalion phenomenon describes a partner who sculpts toward the *partner's* ideal. Of course, if the self's and the partner's ideals are compatible, this issue becomes moot. However, in two longitudinal studies, we have found that when self ideals and partner ideals for the self are incompatible, a partner's inclination to "foist his or her own ideals onto the self" yields negative consequences (Rusbult, Coolsen, et al., 2005; Rusbult, Kumashiro, Finkel, et al., 2005). This process is illustrated in Shaw's (1941) play about the Pygmalion myth, in which the sculptor comes to care for his creation only when she rebels against his image of the ideal woman and pursues her own ideals. Thus not all sculpting is beneficial. When partners sculpt one another toward their own ideals rather than the self's ideals—even when the product is masterful and beautiful—the consequences are maladaptive for both selves and couples.

Partner Affirmation and Partner Verification

The preceding review of alternative self-relevant processes illustrates the pitfalls of eliciting (from the self) either normatively desirable qualities or partner-desired qualities. How does partner affirmation relate to *partner verification*, or partner behavior that elicits the actual self (or the self's *beliefs* about the actual self)? Many studies have revealed that people value feedback that confirms their preexisting self-conceptions. For example, positive partner regard is valued and enhances intimacy among people with high self-esteem, whereas positive partner regard is unpleasant for those with low self-esteem (Swann, De la Ronde, & Hixon, 1994). How can we reconcile such findings with work regarding the benefits of affirmation? First, we suggest that to competently affirm the self's ideal, partners must accurately perceive the block of stone they seek to sculpt (e.g., What possibilities are inherent in the block, what flaws must be circumvented?). That is, to affirm John, Mary must possess a reasonably accurate (implicit or explicit) understanding of his actual self. Second, to the extent that the ideal self is a realistic possible self that motivates and guides behavior (Markus & Nurius, 1986), partner affirmation may serve to verify important components of a desired future actual self. Third, although selves may appreciate partners who accurately perceive their strengths *and* limitations, we suggest that they also want to be loved despite their limitations, and hope that the partner will assist in transforming the actual self into the ideal self.

We have conducted several studies to examine the simultaneous effects of affirmation and verification, and have found that (1) partner affirmation consistently accounts for unique variance in key criteria beyond verification, (2) partner verification sometimes accounts for unique variance beyond affirmation, and (3) low self-esteem is not associated with a preference for a disaffirming partner (Drigotas, Rusbult, Wieselquist, & Whitton, 1999; Rusbult, Coolsen, et al., 2005; Rusbult, Kumashiro, Finkel, et al., 2005). Thus it may be good when a partner "lets you be the real you," but, if anything, it is more critical that the partner "help you become the ideal you." Moreover, there is no necessary inconsistency between eliciting another's actual self and eliciting his or her ideal self—these variables sometimes operate in concert, such that both tendencies contribute to growth and vitality.

Partner Affirmation and Self–Other Merger

Finally, how does the Michelangelo phenomenon relate to self–other merger, a process whereby partners experience personal growth through *inclusion of other in the self* (Aron & Aron, 2000; Strong & Aron, Chapter 17, this volume)? Incorporation of a close partner's attributes and resources is argued to be one means of satisfying the need for *self-expansion*, the need to enhance the self's physical and social influence, cognitive complexity, and social identity (Aron & Aron, 2000). However, it is unclear whether the benefits of self–other merger are attributable to the full panoply of acquired partner attributes, or whether such benefits are mainly attributable to the acquisition of desirable partner attributes. We suggest that it is not straightforward self-expansion per se, but expansion toward the ideal self that promotes personal well-being and couple vitality. That is, inclusion of the partner's less desirable characteristics is unlikely to lead to positive outcomes.

Moreover, ideal self-expansion should be facilitated to the extent that a partner possesses key components of the self's ideal. When a partner possesses qualities that are important aspects of one's ideal, the partner is better able to affirm the self's ideal (e.g., understand what the self hopes to become, make useful suggestions) and the self is better able to use the partner as a model for achieving the ideal. In two studies examining this reasoning, mediation analyses demonstrated that (1) Michelangelo model variables partially to wholly mediate the associations of self–other merger with key criteria; (2) partner possession of the self's ideal partially mediates the associations of Michelangelo model variables with key criteria; and (3) partner possession of the self's ideal partially to wholly accounts for the associations of self-other merger with key criteria (Rusbult, Coolsen, et al., 2005; Rusbult, Kumashiro, Finkel, et al., 2005). Thus self–other merger is particularly beneficial when it entails acquiring partner qualities that are components of one's ideal self.

SELF PROCESSES AND THE MICHELANGELO PHENOMENON

Self Ideals: The Block of Stone and the Slumbering Figure

Our work rests on the assumption that there is a slumbering form inside the block of stone. That is, we assume that people possess ideal selves, and that the ideal self serves to frame and guide cognition and behavior (Higgins, 1987, 1996). Our work emphasizes internally defined ideals, the goals the self genuinely wishes to achieve, not the goals that parents, friends, or lovers think the self *ought* to achieve. In short, our work concerns the *ideal* self, not the *ought* self. Paralleling prior conceptualizations, we suggest that (1) pursuit of the ideal self centers on aspirations, whereas pursuit of the ought self centers on obligations; (2) movement toward the ideal self yields exhilaration, whereas movement toward the ought self yields comfort and safety; and (3) disparities from the ideal self induce dejection, whereas disparities from the ought self induce anxiety. As such, pursuit of the ideal self is at the core of personal growth strivings.[5]

Nature of the Ideal Self

We examine the ideal self in an idiographic, person-specific manner, and define this construct broadly and abstractly, as the general type of person that the self aspires to become, specific to each individual. The ideal self can be further delineated in terms of more diverse and specific goals and aspirations. For example, among young adults, important components of the ideal self tend to involve career goals (e.g., education, professional excellence), social goals (e.g., relations with partners, friends, parents), personal traits (e.g., becoming more generous, spontaneous, spiritual), accomplishments (e.g., traveling in Europe, developing musical abilities), material goals (e.g., wealth, wardrobe), and health goals (e.g., diet, exercise). Moreover, the ideal self is likely to include relational components that require the presence and involvement of others (e.g., to become a more loving husband, a good parent).

As self-complexity theory posits (Linville, 1987), possessing a complex ideal self may benefit individuals to the extent that with greater complexity, personal well-being does not rest wholly on achieving one specific goal. Moreover, applying the principle of equifinality, the same goal is posited to be attainable through different, substitutable means (Heider, 1958). To the extent that individuals become fixated on one means of achieving the ideal self—rather than pursuing the ideal self in a flexible manner—failure may exert more detrimental consequences on personal well-being. In addition, to the extent that a constellation of ideals represents a diverse array of possible selves, it may not be possible to simultaneously fulfill all components of the ideal—that is, the pursuit of one ideal may conflict with the pursuit of others. Thus movement toward the ideal self rests on achieving a suitable balance among diverse goals, or adopting strategies that involve sequential goal pursuits over a given time period or across life stages.

Origins and Evolution of the Ideal Self

Where does the ideal self come from? We employ an incremental model, suggesting that (1) ideals typically develop in a step-by-step manner (rather than emerging full blown in a flash of insight), (2) the emergence and modification of ideals may entail systematic or automatic processes, and (3) the ideal self may change over time (Higgins, 1987; Markus & Nurius, 1986). For example, whereas Mary's love of books may initially cause her to pursue an academic career, the incidental fact that she is involved in volunteer work may inspire special proficiency in the area of poverty. At the same time, "turning points" may also precipitate recognition or adoption of an ideal self. Such insights may accompany traumatic events or loss, in that trauma often serves as a catalyst for the quest for purpose (Emmons, Colby, & Kaiser, 1998), thereby promoting examination and reassessment of the ideal self (King & Raspin, 2004). For example, after being fired from his job, John may realize that he had dedicated only moderate effort to his lucrative but ultimately unsatisfying career. Being fired may induce reexamination of the ideal self, thereby promoting increasing dedication to volunteer work and other worthy causes.

Does the desire to realize one's ideals vary as a function of life stage? Lay construals of growth frequently assume that such strivings are confined to young adulthood, at which time people are particularly oriented toward achievement. Although we have not examined this issue empirically, our theoretical analysis suggests that we will not observe significant moderation of key findings as a function of age or life stage. Granted, the character of the ideal self may vary over the course of development. Important components of ideals may center on industry or professional achievement at one life stage, intimacy concerns at another stage, and generativity at yet other stages (Erikson, 1950). Moreover, during childhood and adolescence individuals are likely to try on many "hats" and identities to discover what they wish to become. But at the same time, we assume that the desire to realize one's ideals—whatever their character—is a relatively abiding human concern. Striving toward an ideal self is posited to be a dynamic, evolving process that is unlikely to ever be experienced as "complete"—success in achieving one set of goals may motivate individuals to establish new goals or to dedicate increasing effort to existing, but as yet unachieved, goals (e.g., Scheier & Carver, 1988; Wood & Bandura, 1989).

Thus far we have represented the emergence of ideals as a self-driven process. But just as movement toward the ideal self is partially governed by interpersonal forces, the character of the ideal self may be at least partially interpersonal. Parents, colleagues, friends, and lovers may play a role in shaping our ideals. For example, through the process of self-expansion, romantic partners invariably expose one another to new activities and values, which the self may internalize. This process too is incremental, and may entail systematic or automatic processes. For example, parents may dedicate extensive thought to the nature of their children's aspirations, actively contemplating what the child ideally would like to become and encouraging certain sorts of goals. Alternatively, parents may foster particular ideals in a relatively unthinking, unsystematic, and incidental manner. Parents may even unintentionally sculpt the self by serving as positive or negative role models. For example, John's desire to become a victims' advocate may stem from the fact that his parents were socially involved and enlightened, or alternatively (and reactively) from growing up with abusive parents.

Role of the Self in the Sculpting Process

What qualities of the self are relevant to understanding movement toward one's ideal? Many social scientists have explored self-regulation, goal pursuit, and growth processes (Bandura, 2000; Carver & Scheier, 1998; Emmons, 2003; Mischel, Cantor, & Feldman, 1996). We limit our discussion to three classes of variable that are relevant to understanding the Michelangelo phenomenon: variables resting on the self's insight, ability, and motivation.

First, movement toward the ideal self should be more probable to the extent that individuals possess greater *insight*, or greater clarity in their construal of the actual and the ideal selves (Campbell, 1990; Swann, 1990). When John possesses insightful and accurate knowledge of "where he stands" and "where he wishes to go," he is more likely to accurately gauge the required effort and develop effective strategies for closing the gap.[6] Also, awareness of vast and insurmountable actual–ideal discrepancies may cause John to abandon some goals and dedicate himself to alternative, more attainable components of the ideal self. Insight also requires recognizing when a given component of the ideal self has lost it luster, such that it is time to turn to new ideals. Sometimes reconceptualized ideals entail pursuit of an existing goal through alternative means (e.g., an actor may turn to directing); sometimes reconceptualized ideals entail pursuit of preexisting goals that have been set aside or neglected (e.g., following significant professional success, Mary may seek adventure). Indeed, self- and partner reports of the self's movement toward the ideal self are positively associated with the self's level of self-clarity (Rusbult, Coolsen, et al., 2005).

Second, movement toward the ideal self should be more probable to the extent that an individual possesses adequate *ability*, or to the extent that the potential for achieving a given ideal realistically is greater. To begin with, we state the obvious: if Mary lacks the native ability or the specific skills that are needed to achieve her ideal, little movement toward that ideal is probable. An equally obvious point is that individuals are more likely to achieve a given ideal to the extent that they are closer to the ideal, or that there is less disparity between the actual and the ideal selves. But beyond this, John must perceive that the resources relevant to attaining his goals are under his control, he must experience efficacy with respect to his goals and ideals, and he must develop good strategies for goal attainment (Bandura, 2000; Deci & Ryan, 2000; Mischel et al., 1996). Indeed, self- and partner reports of self movement toward the ideal self are positively associated with self attributes such as competence, mastery, self-control, and perceived likelihood of attaining a goal (Rusbult, Coolsen, et al., 2005). Moreover, given the difficulties associated with pursuit of the ideal self, in understanding moment-to-moment effort expenditure, it may be important to take into account self-regulatory resources, including both dispositional self-control and situation-specific depletion of regulatory resources (Baumeister & Vohs, 2003).

Third, movement toward the ideal self should be more probable to the extent that *motivation* is greater. On average, John may be most likely to attain those components of his ideal self that are most important to him, in that he is more likely to assiduously dedicate himself to those goals. For challenging ideals or temporally extended goals, movement toward the ideal may rest not only on importance of the goal, but also on qualities such as commitment to the goal, centrality of the goal to achieving the overall ideal self, and dispositional orientation toward pursuing the ideal self (Higgins, 1987). Moreover, we speculate that innate striving toward the ideal self may be thwarted by factors such as internalization of another's values (Rogers, 1961), extrinsic motivation (Deci & Ryan, 2000), preoccupation with security of attachment (e.g., Hazan & Shaver, 1987), a preference for fantasy over actual goal pursuit activities (Oettingen, Pak, & Schnetter, 2001), or the necessity of fulfilling basic, lower level needs (Maslow, 1962). For example, rather than initiating a quest for the perfect career, an unemployed, single parent may worry about simply finding a job (any job) to pay the bills.

We suggest that all three classes of variable are critical to understanding movement toward the ideal self: People with enormous insight cannot achieve their ideals in the absence of adequate ability and sustained motivation. People with exceptional ability cannot achieve their ideals in the absence of keen insight and strong motivation. And people with powerful motivation cannot achieve their ideals in the absence of good insight and plenty of ability. Moreover, we suggest that these three classes of variables operate in concert and may exert causal effects on one another. For example, clear insight may promote effective goal pursuit strategies or may increase motivation to achieve the ideal. Possessing high ability may allow for greater resilience in the face of setbacks (Block & Kremen, 1996) or yield clearer insights into the ideal self. Likewise, high motivation may induce thinking about the ideal self or diligence at attempts to increase ability. In addition, it may be difficult to clearly categorize some attributes as components of insight, ability, or motivation in that some attributes may contribute to all three classes of variable. Indeed, self movement toward ideals is positively associated with self attributes such as self-esteem, self-respect, and self-control, which may operate by contributing to increased self-efficacy and the inclination to delay gratification (Bandura, 2000; Mischel et al., 1996).

Whereas some ideals may be pursued and attained chiefly as a result of the self's actions, selves clearly benefit from the backing of insightful, able, and motivated sculptors. In fact, effective partner affirmation may work in part through promoting self's insight, ability, and motivation regarding the ideal self. Before turning to the partner per se, it is important to address a final class of self variable: qualities that *elicit* partner affirmation. Affirmation is facilitated to the extent that an individual (1) *elicits partner insight*, or clear understanding of the self's ideals (by sharing her dreams, Mary makes her ideals visible to John); (2) *elicits partner ability*, or calls forth the skills that are relevant to promoting the self's ideals (John must signal his needs and convey what types of assistance would be helpful); and (3) *elicits partner motivation*, or genuine desire to promote the self's ideals (John must be willing to make himself dependent upon Mary, inspire her commitment to his goals, and express gratitude for her efforts on his behalf).

PARTNER PROCESSES AND THE MICHELANGELO PHENOMENON

Partner Affirmation: The Sculptor and the Slumbering Figure

To understand how partner affirmation promotes self movement toward the ideal self, we must also address the partner's role in the sculpting process. By what mechanisms might partners "select" certain of the self's behaviors, motives, or dispositions? First, partners may engage in *retroactive selection* (selective reinforcement), wherein they reward (or punish) certain of the self's preferences, motives, and behaviors. For example, John may enthusiastically attend to Mary's review of her dissertation ideas, but turn away when she complains about the workload. Second, partners may engage in *preemptive selection* (selective instigation), wherein they enact specific behaviors that elicit (or inhibit) certain preferences, motives, and behaviors on the part of the self. For example, in a situation wherein Mary would normally become upset by a critical review of her work, John may point out the positive implications of Reviewer B's comments, thereby promoting her sense of self-efficacy. And third, partners may engage in *situation selection* (manipulation of interdependence situations), wherein they create situations in which certain of the self's preferences, motives, and behaviors become more probable (or less probable). For example, during a particularly stressful period for Mary, John may offer to do the housework and cooking so that Mary can concentrate on her work.

Thus affirmation does not entail treating the actual and the ideal selves as one and the same. Rather, effective affirmation entails perceiving the self's *potential* to move closer to his or her ideal, and behaving in such a manner as to elicit that ideal. Some forms of affirmation are active (steering the self toward situations in which the self will excel), whereas others are passive (providing unconditional support, a secure emotional environment); some forms are deliberate (offering information or instrumental support), whereas others are inadvertent (projecting one's own ideals onto the self; unconsciously serving as a model for the self). And importantly, affirmation is not necessarily warm and gentle; sometimes affirming behavior is "tough." When Mary enumerates the many tasks she must complete before beginning to write her dissertation, John may tell her to quit procrastinating and simply write.

Effective affirmation is not necessarily consciously controlled (Bargh & Chartrand, 1999): On some occasions partners may consciously promote the self's ideals; on other occasions, this process may be unconscious and automatic. For example, when Mary feels discouraged about her work, John may make it a point to highlight her accomplishments; at other times, he may not consciously recognize that his actions or values have inspired Mary's goal pursuits. Such unconscious and automatic compatibility of self goals and partner goals for the self might result from any of several causes, including congruence of personal values, compatible implicit personality theories, or similarity of actual selves or ideal selves (Byrne, 1971; Schneider, 1973; Wetzel & Insko, 1982).[7] Moreover, an affirming partner need not necessarily be physically present for sculpting to transpire, in that priming thoughts of a close partner may activate the partner's expectations regarding the self's goal attainment (Shah, 2003; Shah, Chapter 19, this volume).

Role of the Partner in the Sculpting Process

Just as the "self variables" that are relevant to understanding movement toward an ideal can be characterized in terms of insight, ability, and motivation, so too can relevant "partner variables." First, effective affirmation is facilitated—and self movement toward the ideal self is promoted—by *partner insight*, or a clear understanding of the self's actual and ideal selves. For example, Mary is more likely to achieve her ideals when John intuits precisely when and how she needs his support, as well as when he engages in perspective taking and achieves a deeper understanding of her ideal self.[8] In cases wherein the actual and the ideal selves are highly discrepant, special insight is required to see through the unpromising exterior to the inner potential, and to perceive the possibilities for making that potential "real." Moreover, effective sculpting involves recognizing changes in the content or priorities attached to various components of the ideal self. If Mary stubbornly clings to the belief that John wishes to be a successful (and perhaps ruthless) entrepreneur, she may not recognize that he hopes to build his business in an enlightened and compassionate manner. Indeed, partner affirmation and self movement toward the ideal self are positively associated with the partner's empathy and perspective taking, perceptual and behavioral attentiveness to the actual self, and accurate understanding of the self's goals and ideals (Rusbult, Coolsen, et al., 2005; Rusbult, Kumashiro, Finkel, et al., 2005).

Second, the Michelangelo phenomenon is enhanced by *partner ability*, or possession of the skills and resources that are relevant to promoting the self's ideals—for example, by proposing effective strategies, delivering the precise type of assistance that is needed (instrumental *and* social-emotional support), directly assisting the self, actively participating in the self's goal pursuits, and challenging the self to work toward his or her ideal. For example, Mary may use her writing skills to help John draft a compassionate corporate mission statement. Indeed, partner affirmation and self movement toward the ideal are greater to the extent that partners exhibit competence and self-control, provide direct assistance or actively participate in the self's goal pursuits, are perceived as being naturally more talented at eliciting other people's ideals, provide autonomy support, and actually possess key components of the self's ideal (Rusbult, Coolsen, et al., 2005; Rusbult, Kumashiro, Finkel, et al., 2005).

And third, the Michelangelo phenomenon is facilitated by *partner motivation*, or genuine desire to promote the self's ideal, including unconditional support, sincere enthusiasm for the self's goal pursuits, and willingness to sacrifice personal interests to promote the self's goals (e.g., by exerting effort, enduring costs). Motivation is particularly important when the partner feels ambivalent about the self's goal pursuits or those pursuits are costly for the partner. For example, Mary's motivation to support John's compassionate corporate strategy may be strained if such a policy would seriously reduce company profits. Motivation may exert direct effects on affirmation, or may exert indirect effects, via its impact on insight or ability. For example, strong motivation may cause Mary to seek greater insight into John's ideals or to develop more effective strategies for his goal pursuits. And, of course, partners may be motivated to affirm one another for self-oriented reasons: partners may directly benefit from the self's goal pursuits, affirmation may increase the self's dependence on the relationship, or affirmation may be a central component of the partner's identity. Factors that have been shown to promote motivation include properties of relationships as well as individual differences, such as commitment, promotion orientation, and security of attachment (Rusbult, Coolsen, et al., 2005; Rusbult, Kumashiro, Finkel, et al., 2005).

Finally, we postulate that insight, ability, and motivation may most powerfully promote self movement toward the ideal to the extent that they enhance the perception of partner responsiveness. *Responsiveness* is central to understanding what constitutes effective affirmation, and entails behaving toward the self in such a manner as to communicate (1) understanding, or accurate knowledge of the self's goals and needs; (2) validation, or approval of the self's goals and needs; and (3) caring, or genuine commitment to the self's goals and needs (Reis & Shaver, 1988). Importantly, responsiveness does not necessarily require wholehearted endorsement of the self's ideal. Partners can be responsive even when their own ideals are not aligned with the self's ideals, and even when they do not believe that the self's goals constitute the "best" constellation for the self. In addition, responsive behavior is characterized by contingencies: Some of Mary's needs may be well defined and clearly attainable as a result of her own efforts, such that she simply needs approval and encouragement. Other needs may require active support, such as advice or assistance. In short, *responsive* partner affirmation is (1) contingent on the self's resources, circumstances, and signals of need; (2) affectively attuned to the self's emotional state; (3) geared toward matching the self's needs in both type of support and timing of support; and (4) encouraging of autonomy rather than dependence.

INTERDEPENDENCE AND THE MICHELANGELO PHENOMENON

Of course, our description of the Michelangelo phenomenon would be neither complete nor satisfying if we concentrated solely on how one partner brought out the best in the other, and vice versa. We end this chapter with a brief discussion of how the Michelangelo phenomenon relates to broader interdependence processes.

Affirmation and Dependence

When partners make important contributions to one another's goal strivings, their lives become intertwined. Indeed, to the extent that an individual relies uniquely on a partner for the gratification of important needs, he or she becomes increasingly *dependent* on that person (Drigotas & Rusbult, 1992). Thus, if John provides affirmation of superior quality or quantity than Mary receives from friends or kin, she quite literally needs her relationship with him.[9] Increasing dependence tends to yield several important consequences: (1) greater voluntary persistence ("through thick and thin"); (2) increasing commitment, along with increasingly prosocial motivation and behavior (e.g., accommodation, sacrifice, forgiveness; Rusbult, Olsen, Davis, & Hannon, 2001); (3) enhanced subjective "we-ness," or a sense of being part of a team (e.g., if John relies on friends rather than Mary for affirmation, she may feel inadequate or isolated); and (4) more consequential relationship termination, whether through separation, divorce, or death (e.g., greater depression, more impaired functioning).

All forms of dependence entail vulnerability, in that as we become dependent, we increasingly rely on our partners' goodwill and benevolence. At the same time, three special properties of affirmation-based dependence are noteworthy: First, the ideal self is a possible self that is not yet grounded in reality, which means that it is especially vulnerable to the social environment (Markus & Nurius, 1986). Thus, when John confides to Mary that he dreams of becoming a great novelist, he exhibits trust that she will not react with derision. If his conviction is already shaky (e.g., his short story was recently rejected for publication), the stakes are even higher, in that rejection by Mary might destroy an important dream (e.g., he might become despondent and give up writing altogether). Second, the intense vulnerability characterizing affirmation-based dependence may ultimately promote effective partner affirmation, in that to the extent that John is "wide open" with Mary about his ideal self, she is likely to achieve a more insightful and nuanced understanding of his goals and needs. And third, to the extent that Mary is vital in the process by which John achieves personal growth, losing her will be doubly devastating, in that it entails not only loss of an important relationship, but also very real "loss of John's self" (he will not be the same person without her).

Mutual Cyclical Growth

We have advanced a model of *mutual cyclical growth* to describe the process by which each person's dependence, commitment, and prosocial acts are perceived by the other and feed off the other in such a manner as to sustain mutuality of dependence and promote relational vitality (Wieselquist, Rusbult, Foster, & Agnew, 1999). In the context of our work on the Michelangelo phenomenon, the model operates as follows: (1) because John relies on Mary for affirmation, he becomes increasingly dependent on their relationship; (2) his dependence promotes strengthened commitment; (3) his strengthened commitment motivates affirming acts, even when such acts may be costly or effortful; (4) when Mary perceives such acts of affirmation, she develops increased trust in John; and (5) her strengthened trust promotes enhanced dependence—she is not only more satisfied, but also more increasingly willing to drive away or derogate alternative partners and to invest in her relationship (materially and nonmaterially—e.g., by confiding in John about her ideal self). This brings us full circle, in that Mary's enhanced dependence strengthens her commitment, as well as her inclination to affirm John's ideal self; when John perceives such acts, he develops increased trust in Mary, and so on. This cyclical process ultimately yields high mutuality: the partners achieve roughly mutual levels of trust, dependence, commitment, and inclinations to affirm the other. And as in other groups and dyads, mutuality is a stable, congenial pattern, yielding reduced vulnerability, more positive emotional experiences, and increased personal well-being and couple well-being (Drigotas, Rusbult, & Verette, 1999).

CONCLUSIONS

Our goal in this chapter was to review theory and research regarding the Michelangelo phenomenon. This work incorporates concepts from the behavioral confirmation, interdependence, and self-discrepancy traditions to identify processes that are central to understanding the self in its relational context. To date, empirical evidence suggests that the three components of the Michelangelo phenomenon—partner perceptual affirmation, partner behavioral affirmation, and self movement toward the ideal self—relate to one another in predicted ways. Moreover, partner affirmation and self movement toward the ideal self play strong and reliable roles in shaping both personal well-being and couple well-being. Recent findings also begin to identify the processes and mechanisms that underlie the Michelangelo phenomenon, including a variety of self and partner dispositions, motives, and behavioral tendencies.

Research on this phenomenon is still in its infancy, and, as such, holds the promise of future growth. Two fruitful directions for future work should be noted. First, research regarding the Michelangelo phenomenon has thus far examined highly educated young adults residing in the United States—a culture that advocates individuality, pursuit of the ideal self, and the American dream (e.g., all things are possible given sufficient determination). In future work, it will be important to determine whether our findings generalize to other cultures—for example, to cultures that downplay or discourage individuality, or to cultures in which rigid class- or sex-based roles may rather thoroughly shape aspirations and beliefs about the self. And second, assuming that humans seek lifelong pursuit of their ideals *and* lifelong involvement with their closest partners, it becomes important to study the affirmation process over extended periods of time. In this regard, it might be particularly fruitful to examine issues such as (1) changes over time in the ideal self—for example, do partners provide opportunities for and encourage (vs. inhibit and discourage) such change, and what are the consequence of such events?; how do couples adjust to one another's evolving goals and ideals?; (2) conflicting interests, or circumstances wherein the self's goal pursuits require effort or yield costs for the partner—for example, what motives yield affirmation despite such costs?; what are the causes and consequences of sacrifice, on the part of self (foregoing goals) and/or partner (affirming despite costs)?; and (3) power dynamics in relationships—for example, is one partner's ideal self a more abiding and "important" concern?; what sorts of negotiation and coordination problems accompany the process?

Is there a kernel of truth to the adage "Behind every great man [woman] is a great woman [man]"? Of course, we do not wish to claim that great things cannot be accomplished through individual effort. However, we *do* wish to emphasize the powerful role that close partners can play (and do play) in helping one another achieve each person's goals and ideals. Thus, to understand the metamorphosis of the self into its ideal form, it is important to examine the self not as an independent entity —separate from others—but rather to examine the self as it operates in conjunction with close partners. We hope that our work on the Michelangelo phenomenon may extend our scientific understanding of the social nature of the self, highlighting one important means by which adaptation to interdependence partners shapes everyday experience.

ACKNOWLEDGMENTS

The research reviewed in this chapter was supported by grants to Caryl E. Rusbult from the National Science Foundation (No. BCS-0132398), the Fetzer Institute, and the Templeton Foundation.

NOTES

1. And, of course, one hopes that Elizabeth, in turn, would love Carl not only for "the part of her that he brings out," but also because he too is "moving forward toward something great" and because she can help him achieve that emerging self.
2. The two members of a dyad may act as both target and observer: as (a) self, or the target of another's perception and behavior, and as (b) partner, or the observer who perceives the target and directs behavior toward the target. We use "self" to

describe the target, and use "partner" to describe the observer; we speak of "self perceptions of the self" (target perceptions of target), "partner perceptions of the self" (observer perceptions of target), and "partner perceptions of him- or herself" (observer perceptions of observer). Parallel structure is used to describe behavior ("self behavior," "partner behavior toward self," and "partner behavior").

3. Unless otherwise specified, the term "affirmation" is used to denote both partner perceptual affirmation and partner behavioral affirmation.

4. Of course, this issue frequently boils down to terminology, in that when researchers operationally define enhancement in terms of *what the self regards as positive* (e.g., as in Murray et al., 1996), enhancement is tantamount to affirmation (and, perhaps, should be described as such).

5. Moreover, our work concerns the ideal self, not the feared or the undesired self. Although individuals may be motivated to remove themselves from undesired states (Carver, Lawrence, & Scheier, 1999), they are unlikely to effectively work toward personal growth in the absence of an ideal self to guide behavior. For example, John's despondency about his unfulfilling job is unlikely in itself to yield successful career strategies, in the absence of self-knowledge of the type of career that he would find gratifying.

6. Of course, success may not wholly rest on precise and clearly articulated ideals. Sometimes individuals may simply intuit that they are "moving in the right direction." People may possess an innate ability to recognize and shift toward what is important for them to lead fulfilling lives, moving away from extrinsic goal pursuits, adopting intrinsic goals, and enjoying increasing subjective well-being as a consequence (Sheldon, Arndt, & Houser, 2003).

7. In our ongoing research, we use diverse procedures to determine whether partners are consciously aware of one another's ideals, whether they reach active decisions to affirm one another, and whether affirmation is an automatic or a controlled process (e.g., using indirect measures to assess the accuracy with which partners perceive one another's ideals; determining whether selves perceive acts of affirmation that their partners do not apprehend).

8. But granted, to the extent that a partner shares the self's ideals or actually possesses the self's ideals, the partner may be an effective sculptor as a simple consequence of projecting his or her own ideals onto the self.

9. Of course, even if John is a poor sculptor, Mary may nevertheless be dependent on their relationship—and may opt to remain in it—if other people in her social environment offer even lower levels of affirmation than John. Mary might also remain involved with a poor sculptor because she cannot imagine that alternative partners might have more to offer, or because she believes she is confronting such enormous actual–ideal self disparities that she may not be capable of achieving her ideals even with a talented sculptor.

REFERENCES

Aron, A., & Aron, E. (2000). Self-expansion motivation and including other in the self. In W. Ickes & S. Duck (Eds.), *The social psychology of personal relationships* (pp. 109–128). New York: Wiley.

Bandura, A. (2000). Social cognitive theory: An agentic perspective. *Annual Review of Psychology, 52*, 1–26.

Bargh, J. A., & Chartrand, T. L. (1999). The unbearable automaticity of being. *American Psychologist, 54*, 462–479.

Baumeister, R. F., & Vohs, K. D. (2003). Willpower, choice, and self-control. In G. Loewenstein & D. Read (Eds.), *Time and decision: Economic and psychological perspectives on intertemporal choice* (pp. 201–216). New York: Russell Sage Foundation.

Block, J., & Kremen, A. M. (1996). IQ and ego resiliency: Conceptual and empirical connections and separateness. *Journal of Personality and Social Psychology, 70*, 349–361.

Bowlby, J. (1969). *Attachment and loss: Vol. 1. Attachment.* New York: Basic Books.

Brunstein, J. C., Dangelmayer, G., & Schultheiss, O. C. (1996). Personal goals and social support in close relationships: Effects on relationship mood and marital satisfaction. *Journal of Personality and Social Psychology, 71*, 1006–1019.

Byrne, D. (1971). *The attraction paradigm.* New York: Academic Press.

Campbell, J. D. (1990). Self-esteem and clarity of self-concept. *Journal of Personality and Social Psychology, 59*, 538–549.

Carver, C. S., Lawrence, J. W., & Scheier, M. F. (1999). Self-discrepancies and affect: Incorporating the role of feared selves. *Personality and Social Psychology Bulletin, 25*, 783–792.

Carver, C. S., & Scheier, M. F. (1998). *On the self-regulation of behavior.* New York: Cambridge University Press.

Darley, J. M., & Fazio, R. H. (1980). Expectancy confirmation processes arising in the social interaction sequence. *American Psychologist, 35*, 867–881.

Deci, E. L., & Ryan, R. M. (2000). The "what" and "why" of goal pursuits: Human needs and the self-determination of behavior. *Psychological Inquiry, 11*, 227–268.

Drigotas, S. M., & Rusbult, C. E. (1992). Should I stay or should I go?: A dependence model of breakups. *Journal of Personality and Social Psychology, 62*, 62–87.

Drigotas, S. M., Rusbult, C. E., & Verette, J. (1999). Level of commitment, mutuality of commitment, and couple well-being. *Personal Relationships, 6*, 389–409.

Drigotas, S. M., Rusbult, C. E., Wieselquist, J., & Whitton, S. (1999). Close partner as sculptor of the ideal self: Behavioral affirmation and the Michelangelo phenomenon. *Journal of Personality and Social Psychology, 77*, 293–323.

Emmons, R. A. (2003). Personal goals, life meaning, and virtue: Wellsprings of a positive life. In C. L. Keyes & J. Haidt (Eds.), *Flourishing: Positive psychology and the life well-lived* (pp. 105–128). Washington, DC: American Psychological Association.

Emmons, R. A., Colby, P. M., & Kaiser, H. A. (1998). When losses lead to gains: Personal goals and the recovery of meaning. In P. S. Fry & P. T. P. Wong (Eds.), *The human quest for meaning: A handbook of psychological research and clinical applications* (pp. 163–178). Mahwah, NJ: Erlbaum.

Erikson, E. (1950). *Childhood and society* (2nd ed., pp. 247–269). New York: Norton.

Fazio, R. H., Effrein, E. A., & Falender, V. J. (1981). Self-perceptions following social interactions. *Journal of Personality and Social Psychology, 41*, 232–242.

Feeney, B. C. (2004). A secure base: Responsive support of goal strivings and exploration in adult intimate relationships. *Journal of Personality and Social Psychology, 87*, 631–648.

Freud, S. (1961). The ego and the id. In J. Strachey (Ed. & Trans.), *The standard edition of the complete psychological works of Sigmund Freud* (Vol. 19, pp. 3–66). London: Hogarth Press. (Original work published 1923)

Gombrich, E. H. (1995). *The story of art* (16th ed.). London: Phaidon.

Harris, M. J., & Rosenthal, R. (1985). Mediation of interpersonal expectancy effects: 31 meta-analyses. *Psychological Bulletin, 97*, 363–386.

Hazan, C., & Shaver, P. (1987). Romantic love conceptualized as an attachment process. *Journal of Personality and Social Psychology, 52*, 511–524.

Heider, F. (1958). *The psychology of interpersonal relations*. New York: Wiley.

Higgins, E. T. (1987). Self-discrepancy: A theory relating self and affect. *Psychological Review, 94*, 319–340.

Higgins, E. T. (1996). The "self digest": Self-knowledge serving self-regulatory functions. *Journal of Personality and Social Psychology, 71*, 1062–1083.

Ickes, W., Stinson, L., Bissonnette, V., & Garcia, S. (1990). Naturalistic social cognition: Empathic accuracy in mixed-sex dyads. *Journal of Personality and Social Psychology, 59*, 730–742.

Kelley, H. H., Holmes, J. G., Kerr, N. L., Reis, H. T., Rusbult, C. E., & Van Lange, P. A. M. (2003). *An atlas of interpersonal situations*. New York: Cambridge University Press.

Kelley, H. H., & Thibaut, J. W. (1978). *Interpersonal relations: A theory of interdependence*. New York: Wiley.

King, L. A., & Raspin, C. (2004). Lost and found possible selves, subjective well-being, and ego development in divorced women. *Journal of Personality, 72*, 603–632.

Kumashiro, M., Wolf, S., Coolsen, M., & Rusbult, C. E. (2005). *Partner affirmation, verification, and enhancement as determinants of attraction to potential dates: Experimental evidence of the unique effect of affirmation*. Unpublished manuscript, Free University at Amsterdam.

Linville, P. W. (1987). Self-complexity as a cognitive buffer against stress-related illness and depression. *Journal of Personality and Social Psychology, 52*, 663–676.

Markus, H., & Nurius, P. (1986). Possible selves. *American Psychologist, 41*, 954–969.

Maslow, A. H. (1962). *Toward a psychology of being*. Princeton, NJ: Van Nostrand.

Mischel, W., Cantor, N., & Feldman, S. (1996). Principles of self-regulation: The nature of willpower and self-control. In E. T. Higgins & A. W. Kruglanski (Eds.), *Social psychology: Handbook of basic principles* (pp. 329–360). New York: Guilford Press.

Murray, S. L., Holmes, J. G., & Griffin, D. W. (1996). The self-fulfilling nature of positive illusions in romantic relationships: Love is not blind, but prescient. *Journal of Personality and Social Psychology, 71*, 1155–1180.

Oettingen, G., Pak. H., & Schnetter, K. (2001). Self-regulation of goal setting: Turning free fantasies about the future into binding goals. *Journal of Personality and Social Psychology, 80*, 736–753.

Reis, H. T., & Shaver, P. (1988). Intimacy as an interpersonal process. In S. Duck (Ed.), *Handbook of personal relationships* (pp. 367–389). Chichester, UK: Wiley.

Rogers, C. R. (1961). *On becoming a person*. Boston: Houghton Mifflin.

Rosenthal, R., & Jacobson, L. (1968). *Pygmalion in the classroom*. New York: Holt, Rinehart, & Winston.

Rusbult, C. E., Coolsen, M., Kirchner, J., Stocker, S., Kumashiro, M., Wolf, S., et al.

(2005). *Partner affirmation and self movement toward ideal in newly-committed relationships*. Unpublished manuscript, Free University at Amsterdam.

Rusbult, C. E., Kumashiro, M., Finkel, E., Kirchner, J., Coolsen, M., Stocker, S., & Clarke, J. (2005). *A longitudinal study of the Michelangelo phenomenon in marital relationships*. Unpublished manuscript, Free University at Amsterdam.

Rusbult, C. E., Kumashiro, M., Stocker, S. L., & Wolf, S. T. (2005). The Michelangelo phenomenon in close relationships. In A. Tesser, J. Wood, & D. A. Stapel (Eds.), *On building, defending, and regulating the self: A psychological perspective* (pp. 1–29). New York: Psychology Press.

Rusbult, C. E., Olsen, N., Davis, J. L., & Hannon, P. (2001). Commitment and relationship maintenance mechanisms. In J. H. Harvey & A. Wenzel (Eds.), *Close romantic relationships: Maintenance and enhancement* (pp. 87–113). Mahwah, NJ: Erlbaum.

Rusbult, C. E., & Van Lange, P. A. M. (2003). Interdependence, interaction, and relationships. *Annual Review of Psychology, 54*, 351–375.

Scheier, M. F., & Carver, C. S. (1988). A model of behavioral self-regulation: Translating intention into action. In L. Berkowitz (Ed.), *Advances in experimental social psychology: Vol. 21. Social psychological studies of the self: Perspectives and programs* (pp. 303–346). San Diego, CA: Academic Press.

Schneider, D. J. (1973). Implicit personality theory: A review. *Psychological Bulletin, 79*, 294–309.

Shah, J. (2003). The motivational looking glass: How significant others implicitly affect goal appraisals. *Journal of Personality and Social Psychology, 85*, 424–439.

Shaw, B. (1941). *Pygmalion*. New York: Dodd, Mead.

Sheldon, K. M., Arndt, J., & Houser, M. L. (2003). In search of the organismic valuing process: The human tendency to move towards beneficial goal choices. *Journal of Personality, 71*, 835–869.

Snyder, M., Tanke, E., & Berscheid, E. (1977). Social perception and interpersonal behavior: On the self-fulfilling nature of social stereotypes. *Journal of Personality and Social Psychology, 35*, 656–666.

Swann, W. B. Jr. (1990). To be adored or to be known? The interplay of self-enhancement and self-verification. In E. T. Higgins & R. M. Sorrentino (Eds.), *Handbook of motivation and cognition: Vol. 2. Foundations of social behavior* (pp. 408–448). New York: Guilford Press.

Swann, W. B. Jr., De la Ronde, C., & Hixon, J. G. (1994). Authenticity and positivity strivings in marriage and courtship. *Journal of Personality and Social Psychology, 66*, 857–869.

Wetzel, C. G., & Insko, C. A. (1982). The similarity–attraction relationship: Is there an ideal one? *Journal of Experimental Social Psychology, 18*, 253–276.

Wieselquist, J., Rusbult, C. E., Foster, C. A., & Agnew, C. R. (1999). Commitment, pro-relationship behavior, and trust in close relationships. *Journal of Personality and Social Psychology, 77*, 942–966.

Wood, R., & Bandura, A. (1989). Impact of conceptions of ability on self-regulatory mechanisms and complex decision making. *Journal of Personality and Social Psychology, 56*, 407–415.

CHAPTER 17

The Effect of Shared Participation in Novel and Challenging Activities on Experienced Relationship Quality

Is It Mediated by High Positive Affect?

GREG STRONG
ARTHUR ARON

A number of studies by others and ourselves (e.g., Aron, Norman, Aron, McKenna, & Heyman, 2000) suggests that shared participation in novel and challenging activities, an interpersonal process, enhances each partner's positive affect, an intrapersonal process. In turn, the positive affect generated in each person through the shared activities with the partner generates an increase in his or her subjectively experienced relationship quality, also an intrapersonal process. In this chapter, we briefly review this research and its theoretical foundation and then consider the hypothesis that this effect is mediated specifically by increased positive affect (and only minimally by decreased negative affect). We conclude with a brief discussion of theoretical and practical implications of this mediation.

THE EFFECT OF SHARED PARTICIPATION IN NOVEL AND CHALLENGING ACTIVITIES ON EXPERIENCED RELATIONSHIP QUALITY

Brief Review

Several survey studies of U.S. married couples (Holman & Jacquart, 1988; Kingston & Nock, 1987; Orden & Bradburn, 1968; Orthner, 1975) have reported substantially stronger correlations with relationship quality for activities that are intensely interactive between partners versus those that are passive, parallel, or merely in the company of others. Hill (1988), in finding a strong overall link between shared activities and marital stability, reported the strongest effects for shared "recreational activities," all of which were somewhat active and challenging (such as "outdoor activities, active sports, card games, and travel" [p. 447]). Focusing specifically on shared participation in "exciting" activities, and using both newspaper and door-to-door surveys, Aron and colleagues (2000, Studies 1 and 2) reported strong correlations with relationship quality.

Several experiments have examined the causal direction of the association of novel and challenging activities and relationship quality. Reissman, Aron, and Bergen (1993) presented members of married couples with a long list of activities and instructed them to indicate for each how "exciting" and how "pleasant" it would be to do with the partner. Activities typically rated as potentially *highly* exciting, but not also rated as *highly* pleasant, included skiing, hiking, and attending concerts and plays—activities that for most couples are novel and challenging but may be experienced as less than optimally "pleasant" perhaps just because of their novelty and challenge, which may create some tension, or just concentration. Activities typically rated as potentially *highly* pleasant, but not also rated as *highly* exciting, included seeing friends, going to movies, and eating out—activities that for most couples are enjoyable but mundane. After they had completed the activity listings, couples were randomly assigned to one of three conditions: an exciting activity condition, a pleasant activity condition, or a waiting list control condition. Couples assigned to the exciting or pleasant condition were instructed to engage in an activity from an individually constructed list appropriate to their condition for at least 1.5 hours each week for 10 weeks. (For example, the exciting activity condition list consisted of activities each of which both members of the couple had independently rated as highly exciting but only moderately pleasant.) Compliance was monitored weekly. Nearly all couples carried out the tasks as instructed. Prior to the activity listing and again at the end of 10 weeks all couples completed a standard measure of relationship quality. The results revealed that couples in the exciting activities condition had significantly greater increases in relationship quality when compared to couples in the pleasant activity or no activity control conditions. (The pleasant activity and control condition couples were not significantly different.)

To test these encouraging results in a more controlled setting, Aron and colleagues (2000, Studies 3–5) conducted three laboratory experiments with couples recruited from the community. In these experiments, couples were tested on standard measures of experienced relationship quality before and after participating in structured activities designed to be either novel and challenging or enjoyable but mundane (i.e., less novel and challenging). In the novel and challenging activity task, couples were joined at the wrists and ankles and required to jointly push a cylindrical cushion (similar to a large, round sofa pillow) over a roughly 2-foot-high barrier made of gymnasium mats under a tight time limit. In the mundane activity, one member of the couple slowly pushed the cushion over flattened gym mats into the center of the room, and then returned, without the cushion, to the corner he or she had started from. Following this part of the activity, the other member of the couple crawled to the cushion and pushed it to the other end of the room, then back to the center again. In all three experiments, there was a significantly greater increase in reported relationship quality from before to after the task for those in the novel and challenging condition than for those in the mundane condition. Furthermore, these results seem to be due specifically to the novel and challenging condition; in one of the experiments there was also a no activity control, which showed results similar to those for the mundane activity condition. Also, in one of the experiments, Aron et al. showed the same pattern of results using observers' systematic ratings of couples' conversations before and after the tasks as their measure of relationship quality.

Two further experiments have examined this effect. In the first of these, Aron and Norman (2005) employed a version of the same novel and challenging activity, but each member of the couple carried out the activity *individually*. In this experiment, what was manipulated was whether or not the partner was salient while doing the activity. The procedure was arranged so that when each participant did the task alone across the mat, he or she had to look at a directional signal located just below a TV screen. For half the participants, the screen was showing the participant's partner filling out questionnaires; for the other half, the TV was off. Thus, in one condition, the partner was salient to the participant while doing the novel and challenging task; in the other condition, the partner was not particularly salient. Participants were not aware (as confirmed in debriefing) that whether the TV was on or off had anything whatsoever to do with the study. Results revealed a greater increase in relationship quality for those who did the activity while their partner was on the screen, compared to those in the control condition. This result suggests that what is important about the novel and challenging activities being shared in the previous studies is that by sharing the activity, the partner is made salient. (Notice also that this result undermines a cooperation interpretation of the results of the earlier studies.)

In the other follow-up experiment, Lewandowski and Aron (2005) investigated the importance of arousal versus novel activities for increasing experienced relationship quality. This is an important issue because a number of studies have shown that arousal can lead to romantic attraction in the context of meeting a stranger (for a review, see Foster, Witcher, Campbell, & Green, 1998); also, novel and challenging activities (including those used in the experiments described above) are typically physiologically arousing. In the Lewandowski and Aron study, couples were assigned to engage in either a novel, challenging, and arousing activity (bouncing an unevenly weighted ball to each other while running short distances with ankle weights attached to each person individually [in order to make running more difficult, and thereby increasing physiological arousal]), a novel and challenging but nonarousing activity (bouncing the ball and walking without weights), an arousing but not novel and challenging activity (running with the weights but without ball bouncing), or a nonarousing and not novel and challenging activity (walking with no weights and no ball bouncing). Results revealed a significant main effect for novel and challenging versus not novel and challenging, and no significant main effect for arousal (or for the interaction). That is, relationship quality increased for couples in the novel and challenging group versus the mundane group regardless of whether they were doing the arousing or the nonarousing activity. (Interestingly, a replication of this same study with stranger couples showed the usual arousal–attraction effect, but no significant effect for novelty and challenge [Lewandowski & Aron, 2004].)

In sum, several survey and experimental studies lend consistent support to the notion that shared participation in novel and challenging activities enhances experienced relationship quality for couples, and they also suggest that the crucial elements may be the novelty and challenge (vs. the cooperative nature of or the arousal often associated with such activities) and the salience of the partner while carrying out the activities.

Theoretical Foundation: The Self-Expansion Model

Most of the above research was conducted specifically in the context of the self-expansion model of motivation and cognition in close relationships (Aron, Aron, & Norman, 2001), which predicts that shared participation in novel and challenging activities leads to increased relationship quality. According to the model, when two people begin a relationship, each begins to include the other in the self (Aron, Mashek, & Aron, 2004). Inclusion of the other in the self describes a process by which an individual begins to identify his or her self-image as a new combination with the other's self. The partner's identity, that is, his or her beliefs, feelings, ideology, resources, and personality, begin to become associated with one's own self (e.g., Aron, Aron, Tudor, & Nelson, 1991). Shared outcomes may also increase inclusion of the other in the self (e.g., Aron et al., 2004). For instance, two people trapped in an elevator when the power fails or two people who share an amusing predicament may feel they now have more in common with each other as a result of the mutual experience (e.g., Fraley & Aron, 2004). Even potential, unrealized factors may contribute to greater inclusion of the other in the self. For example, vacations planned for the future or common goals may help to merge the two people into a "couple." This process takes place through mutual self-disclosure, time spent with the partner, shared activities, and common ideas and interests.

Because these unique aspects of the partner are added to one's already defined self, the self expands to include these new aspects. Likewise, the partner's self is expanded. Indeed, when forming a new romantic relationship ("falling in love"), there is a literal increase in the diversity of the spontaneous self-concept. Aron, Paris, and Aron (1995) tested 325 students five times, once every 2½ weeks over a 10-week period. At each testing, the participants listed as many self-descriptive words or phrases as came to mind during a 3-minute period in response to the question "Who are you today?" and answered a number of other questions that included items indicating whether the participant had fallen in love since the last testing. As predicted, there was a significantly greater increase in diversity of self-content domains in the self-descriptions from before to after falling in love, as compared to the average changes from before to after other testing sessions for those who fell in love or as compared to typical testing-to-testing changes for participants who did not fall in love. In a sense, there was a literal expansion of self. A new sample of 529 participants was recruited and administered scales measuring self-efficacy and self-esteem every 2½ weeks. As predicted, there was a significantly greater increase in these variables from before to after falling in love, as compared to the average changes from before to after other testing sessions, for those who fell in love or as compared to typical testing-to-testing changes for those who did not fall in love. In both of these studies, the effects on the self were maintained when measures of mood change were controlled statistically.

Based on this same line of thinking, Lewandowski and Aron (2005) hypothesized that the more expansion provided by a relationship before its dissolution, the greater the contraction of the working self-concept after its dissolution, and further hypothesized that this pattern would remain when controlling for predissolution closeness. These hypotheses were supported in two questionnaire studies and a priming experiment. In the questionnaire studies, individuals who had recently experienced a breakup were asked to recall relationship qualities for their recently dissolved relationships. In both studies, degree of predissolution self-expansion predicted degree of postdissolution diminished self-concept as assessed either by a direct self-report or by an implicit measure, a result that remained after controlling for recalled predissolution closeness. Self-expansion was measured using the Self-Expansion Questionnaire (SEQ; Lewandowski & Aron, 2005), comprised of 14 items measured on a 7-point, Likert-type scale. Sample items include "How much does being with your partner result in your having new experiences?" and "How much do you feel you have a larger perspective on things because of your partner?" Low scores indicate the participant experiences less self-expansion; high scores indicate the participant's higher self-expansion. In the priming experiment, individuals completed a task that increased the salience of either highly self-expanding or non-self-expanding aspects of their current relationships and then were led through a guided imagery task in which they imagined breaking up with their partner. At the start and the end of the study, all participants completed the measure of spontaneous self-concept used in the Aron and colleagues (1995) falling in love study described above. The result was a significant decline in the diversity of the content of the self-concept. This result is exactly parallel (in the opposite direction) to what was found in Aron and colleagues for individuals falling in love.

Self-expansion is not necessarily limited to romantic relationships; friends, parents and children, and teachers and students, to name a few examples, are capable of including each other in the self and consequently expanding their own self (e.g., Aron, Aron, & Smollan, 1992; Mashek, Aron, & Boncimino, 2003). Still, romantic relationships appear to offer a greater opportunity for the necessary self-disclosure and sharing of ideas and resources that instigate rapid expansion of the self. Thus the self-expansion model offers a unique perspective regarding the formation and maintenance of romantic relationships.

The self-expansion model also bears on change in relationship experience as a relationship progresses. During the beginning stages of a relationship (e.g., within the first year), this expansion of the self is often quite rapid. The early relationship formation period is typically a time when couples engage in large amounts of self-disclosure (e.g., talking on the telephone for hours, spending extensive time with each other, continually thinking about the partner, etc.). Rapid expansion of the self, so long as it is not overwhelming, is associated with feelings of great pleasure, arousal, and excitement (Aron, Aron, & Norman, 2001; Aron, Norman, & Aron, 1998, 2001). Because this rapid expansion is pleasurable, in addition to a desire to be expanded (to possess high levels of potential efficacy), a key motivator is the desire to experience the process of expanding, to feel one's self increasing rapidly in potential self-efficacy. This notion is similar to Carver and Scheier's (1990) self-regulatory process in which people monitor the rate at which they are making progress toward goals and experience positive affect when the perceived rate exceeds an expected rate. Indeed, they argue further that accelerations in the rate cause feelings of exhilaration. Our notion of being motivated to experience the expanding process is also similar to Pyszczynski, Greenberg, and Solomon's (1997) "growth-expansion system" (the source of one of their two major hypothesized motivations). According to the growth-expansion system, it is the process, rather than the end product, of expanding one's skills and understanding that produces a sense of exhilaration.

When considering the implications for relationship development, what happens after the initial rush of high positive affect from the rapid expansion of self associated with relationship formation? Couples typically become more accustomed to one another as time passes. Self-disclosure slows as each person runs out of new things to disclose to the partner. The two people, once new and exciting to each other, become less and less novel to each other and self-expansion slows or ceases. As a result of the decline of rapid self-expansion, some couples may experience distress or boredom (Aron & Aron, 1986). The couple may not feel as happy or passionate about the relationship now that the newness and excitement begins to disappear into feelings of predictability and complacency. The decline of satisfaction over time in close relationships is well documented (see Bradbury, Fincham, & Beach, 2000, for a review). Loss of excitement due to this type of habituation and slowing of expansion is likely to lead to boredom with the partner and with the relationship in general. (As a matter of fact, boredom with the relationship was assessed in the Aron et al. [2000] survey studies, and the relationship of exciting activities with relationship quality was strongly mediated by low relationship boredom.)

Dissatisfaction with one's partner and relationship due to decreased self-expansion may cause larger problems to begin appearing (e.g., arguing, avoidance of one's partner, infidelity). Indeed, many couples experiencing distress and problems in their relationship and who seek professional help to alleviate these problems may only be exhibiting symptoms of an underlying boredom and disenchantment with the relationship and partner. Thus simply becoming bored and uninterested in the relationship, and perhaps experiencing a lack of any positive or negative affect, are potentially substantial predictors of subsequent relationship distress and dissolution (e.g., Aron & Aron, 1986; Fincham & Linfield, 1997; Gigy & Kelly, 1992).

In terms of the focus of the present chapter, the self-expansion model predicts that associating the partner with rapid expansion of the self impacts relationship quality. In new relationships, as just discussed, this typically occurs by the usual process of relationship formation in which the self-expansion arises from including the partner in the self. In long-term relationships, however, the model theorizes that relationship quality is likely to be enhanced primarily when individuals experience rapid self-expansion in some other way than through relationship formation, such as by engaging in novel and challenging activities that are associated with the partner (as when the activities are shared) (e.g., Aron, Norman, Aron, & Lewandowski, 2002).

What is missing in this analysis, however, is a precise description of the causal chain from novel and challenging activities being self-expanding to enhanced relationship quality. For that analysis we turn to the role of positive affect.

POSITIVE AFFECT AS A MEDIATOR OF THE IMPACT OF SHARED NOVEL AND CHALLENGING ACTIVITIES ON EXPERIENCED RELATIONSHIP QUALITY

What Is Positive Affect and What Is Its Role in Relationships?

Before turning to the role of positive affect as a mediator, we need to briefly clarify some key terms and distinctions.

Independence of Positive and Negative Affect

Affect can manifest itself as positive (e.g., happy, joyous, elated) or negative (e.g., angry, sad, frightened). Positive and negative affects have traditionally been depicted as opposing ends of a single dimension. However, the model that appears to have the most consistent support in the contemporary research literature posits two separate dimensions, one representing positive affect, and the other representing negative affect (see Figure 17.1). The positive and negative dimensions are generally independent of (orthogonal to) each other (e.g., Carver & Scheier, 1990, 1998; Diener & Emmons, 1984; Fincham & Linfield, 1997; Watson, Clark, & Tellegen, 1988). In this model, one end of each dimension or axis represents a high presence (high positive or high negative) of that affect and the other end represents an absence (low positive or low negative) of that affect. For example, elation, exhilaration, and excitement are at the high end of the positive axis and boredom, unhappiness, and loneliness lie on the low end of the positive axis. Similarly, anger, anxiety, and fear are at the high end of the negative axis and peacefulness, contentment, and security lie at the low end. One implication of this model is that a person could feel both exhilaration (positive affect) and fear (negative affect) simultaneously (or nearly simultaneously), as when riding a roller coaster.

The model of relationship-related affect (Figure 17.1) builds upon Higgins's (1997) regulatory focus theory. That is, success (or failure) in an approach-related goal (a goal in which one is seeking to gain something, e.g., being promoted at work) results in a different affective outcome than success (or failure) in an avoidance-related goal (a goal in which one is seeking to avoid something, e.g., being fired; see also Carver & Scheier, 1990, 1998). For example, when a person is doing well in approaching a desired goal, the result is an increase in highly positive affect, such as joy or happiness. When a person is doing poorly at reaching the same goal, the result is an increase in low positive affect, such as unhappiness or boredom. When a person is doing well at avoiding a particular undesired goal, the result is an increase in low negative affect (in other words, a removal of negative affect), such as relief and security, not joy and excitement, whereas when a person is doing poorly at this task, the result is an increase in highly negative affect, such as fear, anger,

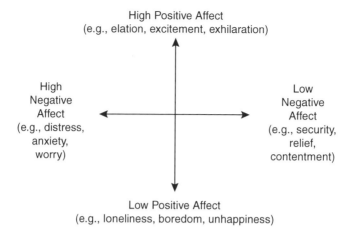

FIGURE 17.1. Two-dimensional model of relationship-related affect represented as independent positive and negative axes. Data from Carver and Scheier (1999) and Laurenceau and Troy (2002).

or sadness, not low positive affect like boredom. Successfully avoiding a conflict with your spouse is rewarding; nevertheless, it is not the same as successfully receiving praise from your spouse. Avoiding an argument is not the same thing as receiving a gift, even though in both cases goals are being achieved (avoidance goals for the former and approach goals for the latter—avoiding pain vs. pursuing pleasure).

Implications for Relationships

The main point of all this is that distinguishing positive from negative affect represents a very different way than has been typical of understanding the role of affect in relationships. Indeed, for as long as psychologists have been studying close relationships, the role of affect in those relationships has received much consideration. Berscheid and Ammazzalorso (2001) remarked, "Close interpersonal relationships are the setting in which people most frequently experience intense emotions, both the positive emotions, such as joy and love, and the negative emotions, such as anger and fear" (p. 308). However, most of this consideration has been with regard to negative affect, with much less consideration of positive affect (Reis & Gable, 2003). There has been some research examining positive affect in relationships (e.g., Gottman, Coan, Carrere, & Swanson, 1998). For example, Birchler, Weiss, and Vincent (1975) asked couples to list things that both pleased and displeased them about their partners and found a greater "pleases" to "displeases" ratio in happy couples. Nevertheless, most investigators consistently focus only on negative affect. In the present context, a largely overlooked but likely cause of marital dissatisfaction is that couples become bored with each other due to habituation (e.g., Aron & Aron, 1986; Aron, Norman, & Aron, 1998). Affection and positive affect decline as a result of this, and, in turn, negative affect either increases or simply surpasses the ratio of positive to negative affect, in essence, becoming more salient to the couple. It would seem more likely for people to reduce positive affect to a more baseline rate after the initial "honeymoon period" and subsequently notice all the negative affect as a result rather than for negative affect to somehow increase for no reason, especially since these same effects are not seen in close friendships (e.g., Reis & Gable, 2003).

In any case, the heavy focus on negative affect and conflict in relationships has left research on positive affect in relationships behind. Most important for present purposes, however, these distinctions bear importantly on how we can understand the relation of novel and challenging activities to experienced relationship quality.

Positive Affect as a Mediator

Participating in novel and challenging activities with one's partner presumably creates relationship satisfaction by a standard associational process in which the activity serves as a reward that becomes linked with the partner. But what is rewarding about these activities? One possibility is that the activities create strong positive affect, which becomes associated with the partner through positive reinforcement. Simply satisfying the basic need for self-expansion should be rewarding and should create a positive association with the partner. But ordinary self-expansion from new learning and experiences is likely to be relatively weakly rewarding, just as eating an enjoyable ordinary meal is only weakly rewarding. However, when the expansion is rapid, then an additional element arises. As noted earlier, we hypothesize that rapid self-expansion creates high levels of positive affect (an idea we also noted that is consistent with work by Carver and Scheier [1990] and other motivational theorists regarding the effect of rapid progress toward goals). Thus we hypothesize that it is not just self-expansion, but rapid self-expansion of the kind associated with novelty and overcoming challenge, that is associated with highly positive affect. Furthermore, we hypothesize that this highly positive affect is the primary mediator in the effect of shared participation in novel and challenging activities leading to greater experienced relationship quality.

An alternative explanation, however, is that the activities are rewarding because they reduce strong negative feelings, and this reduction is associated with the partner through negative reinforcement.

In this section, we offer several arguments for the former interpretation (positive reinforcement through rapid self-expansion creates increases in strong positive affect) rather than the latter (negative reinforcement through reduction of strong negative affect).

First, in light of the issues just considered, recall that decreased boredom was observed as a mediator of the association of exciting activities and relationship satisfaction in the two Aron and colleagues (2000, Studies 1 and 2) survey studies mentioned briefly above. Note that what is reduced here, boredom, is low on the positive affect dimension but *not* on the negative affect dimension. Interestingly, reducing negative affect in a relationship (such as conflict or distress) may actually *increase* boredom! (If fighting with each other was the only interaction a couple had, once the fighting is gone, what do they do with each other now?)

Second, the key idea of the self-expansion model applied in this context is that the novel and challenging activities reinstate a situation similar to that at the onset of relationships. In that context, it seems clear that initial attraction is driven more by positive reward opportunities than by relief from punishment. That is, people seem to begin romantic relationships, to "fall in love," because the other person offers something an individual desires or needs. Indeed, a number of lines of research suggest that early relationship stages and falling in love are associated with passion (Passionate Love Scale [PLS]; Hatfield & Sprecher, 1986), positive idealization (Murray, Holmes, & Griffin, 2004), seeing the partner as perfect (Aron, Aron, & Allen, 1998), and high levels of positive reward of a sort similar to that of taking cocaine (Aron et al., 2005).

It seems less likely that people often begin relationships because the other person lacks some unwanted or undesirable qualities (e.g., Gable & Reis, 2001; Reis & Gable, 2003). Of course, in some cases, people may seek partners for social support or distraction when faced with troubles or when a loved one has rejected them. However, even in such cases, it seems likely that the result at best will be reduction of low negative affect, and thus not likely as strong an effect as would be the case for a reduction of high negative affect. Furthermore, while such cases no doubt occur, individuals' descriptions of initial falling in love rarely mention such factors (Aron, Dutton, & Aron, 1989).

Third, we think the positive reinforcement scenario is more likely because in the various studies we have cited participants consistently report the novel and challenging activities to be highly enjoyable. Indeed, the manipulation check in the various experiments cited consisted of the following items: exciting, interesting, fun, dull, and boring (with the last two items reverse-scored). It is nevertheless possible that what was driving the effect of shared participation in novel and challenging activities leading to greater relationship quality was that the activity distracted couples from whatever distress and conflict may have been characterizing their relationship. If this were the case, however, the effect would be stronger for more distressed couples. In fact, in the various studies in which this possibility was assessed, there was no such effect and in two of the studies a near significant trend in the opposite direction emerged (in which less distressed couples benefited most from the activities).

Fourth, novel and challenging activities seem to fit well the situation described by Carver and Scheier (1999) in which strong positive affect is induced by rapid progress toward a desired goal. That is, novel and challenging activities (at least when they are successfully negotiated, as they have been in the various studies to date) represent situations of rapid progress toward achieving the desired goal. This creates positive affect, which (in association with the partner) creates the increase in experienced relationship quality.

Finally, Strong (2004) correlated measures of positive and negative affect with experienced relationship quality in a sample of 123 dating individuals. Experienced relationship quality was assessed with the Marital Opinion Scale (Huston, McHale, & Crouter, 1986; e.g., "All things considered, how satisfied or dissatisfied have you been with your relationship over the past two months?") and the PLS (Hatfield & Sprecher, 1986; e.g., "Sometimes I feel I can't control my thoughts; they are obsessively on my partner"). Results showed significantly higher experienced relationship quality for people in a highly positive affective state but not for those in a low positive or a low negative affective state; these results held up when controlling statistically for the other valence in each analysis. This suggests that high positive affect, such as elation and exhilaration, may be uniquely important for increased relationship quality (see also Laurenceau, Troy, & Carver, 2004). This supports the key second link of the proposed mediation, from enhanced positive affect to increased relationship quality (see Figure 17.2).

In sum, there are several lines of argument and findings that support the hypothesis that increased positive affect (and only minimally reduced negative affect) mediates the relation between shared participation in novel and challenging activities and increased experienced relationship quality.

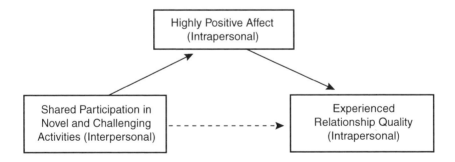

FIGURE 17.2. Proposed mediational model of shared novel and challenging activities (an interpersonal process) leading to greater experienced relationship quality (an intrapersonal process) through increasing highly positive affect.

IMPLICATIONS

A major implication of the mediation of the focal effect specifically by positive affect is that it supports the idea that there is something special about novel and challenging activities that cannot be attributed to reinforcement in general. That is, simple reinforcement seems insufficient for explaining the association of shared participation in novel and challenging activities and experienced relationship quality. Perhaps more important, it suggests the importance of focusing specifically on positive affect in relationship research overall, as well as pointing to the need to look at many related issues, such as the potential interaction of positive and negative affect.

There are also considerable applied implications. For example, the potential special role of positive emotion should encourage couple therapists to adopt a style of treatment with the intention of increasing highly positive affect instead of relying exclusively on reducing conflict. Obviously, if a couple is on the verge of divorce (or worse) due to violence or extremely negative affect and behavior, the necessity to protect the couple's, and possibly their children's, safety is of utmost importance. However, if the couple is simply bored with the relationship and the boredom has resulted in general conflict, then removing conflict without addressing the issue of disenchantment with the partner and the relationship may not be accomplishing anything lasting.

Gottman (1998) reports that, among couples who receive marital therapy, approximately three-fourths report immediate improvement in marital satisfaction. Unfortunately, half to two-thirds of these eventually return to their state of conflict and discontent; he even speculates that the number of them who relapse may be greater if long-term follow-ups were conducted. Gottman's explanation focuses on the man's inability to soothe himself or otherwise reduce his physiological arousal without the presence of the therapist (see also Gottman et al., 1998). However, there is an alternative explanation. Perhaps the very act of going to a marital therapist is, in itself, a novel and challenging activity. After all, it is unlikely the couple has experienced anything quite like a therapy session together and the demands of marital therapy are deeply challenging. Engaging in this activity may increase positive affect in a context that is associated with the partner (e.g., Greenberg, Paul, & Conry, 1988; Helmeke & Sprinkle, 2000), which in turn increases relationship satisfaction. Then, when therapy is over and the couple is no longer engaging in a novel and challenging activity, positive affect is reduced and conflict returns.

More generally, perhaps couples experiencing a lack of excitement and joy in their relationship may need to be instructed to engage in new activities and events with their partner, events that increase the amount of highly positive affect. Some clinicians have, in fact, endorsed increasing positive activities in relationship assessment (e.g., Inventory of Rewarding Activities;

Birchler & Weiss, 1977) and treatment (e.g., Baucom & Epstein, 1990; Jacobson & Margolin, 1979; Stuart, 1980). Unfortunately, one of the major problems with therapy, as noted by Bradbury and Fincham (1990), is that few couples on the verge of separation or divorce actually seek out therapy. Because of this, Christensen and Heavey (1999) suggest that prevention of conflict may be more important or more useful than trying to fix an already troubled relationship, especially if it is unlikely that the distressed couple will ever appear in the therapist's office. It is also worth noting that Christensen and Heavey reviewed the literature on marital therapy outcomes and found that what they consider the most effective couple therapy (the Prevention and Relationship Enhancement Program [PREP]; Renick, Blumberg, & Markman, 1992) is also the only one of those they reviewed that increased positive affect in couples.

In sum, there are both theoretical and applied implications of the present hypothesis that positive affect mediates the link of novel and challenging activities on experienced relationship quality.

CONCLUSION

In this chapter, we reviewed studies suggesting that shared participation in novel and challenging activities, an interpersonal process, enhances experienced relationship quality, an intrapersonal process. We then summarized the self-expansion model explanation for this effect, that novel and challenging activities create a rapid self-expansion which, when associated with the partner (as happens when relations form as well as when partners do exciting activities together), leads to enhanced relationship quality. However, we also put forward the hypothesis that high levels of positive affect mediate this effect. In this light, we briefly examined the relevant research on affect, noting the widely accepted contemporary view that positive and negative affect represent independent dimensions, with high levels representing excited states of affect. Based on this model, we argued that specifically increased levels of high positive affect (and not decreased levels of negative affect) are the primary mediator of the effect of novel and challenging activities on relationship quality and we noted some theoretical and practical implications. Specifically, treating positive affect as the opposite of negative affect (and negative as the opposite of positive), placing them on opposite ends of a single dimension, results in concluding that relieving negative affect will necessarily lead to an increase in positive affect. But the opposite of bad is not always good, and the opposite of good is not always bad. In fact, relieving negative affect may, as we have noted above, lead instead to boredom or something more akin to the absence of positive or negative affect entirely. This, in turn, may directly impact the way marital and couple therapy is approached. Therapists might consider encouraging distressed couples to engage in activities that induce positive affect because reducing negative affect, while beneficial, may only provide part of what is necessary for couples to be happy with each other and with the relationship overall.

REFERENCES

Aron, A., & Aron, E. (1986). *Love and the expansion of self: Understanding attraction and satisfaction*. New York: Hemisphere.

Aron, A., Aron, E., & Allen, J. (1998). Motivations for unreciprocated love. *Personality and Social Psychology Bulletin, 24,* 787-796.

Aron, A., Aron, E., & Norman, C. C. (2001). Self-expansion model of motivation and cognition in close relationships and beyond. In G. J. O. Fletcher & M. Clark (Eds.), *Blackwell handbook of social psychology: Interpersonal processes* (pp. 478–501). Malden, MA: Blackwell.

Aron, A., Aron, E., & Smollan, D. (1992). Inclusion of Other in the Self Scale and the structure of interpersonal closeness. *Journal of Personality and Social Psychology, 63,* 596–612.

Aron, A., Aron, E., Tudor, M., & Nelson, G. (1991). Close relationships as including other in the self. *Journal of Personality and Social Psychology, 60,* 241–253.

Aron, A., Dutton, D. G., & Aron, E. (1989). Experiences of falling in love. *Journal of Social and Personal Relationships, 6,* 243–257.

Aron, A., Fisher, H. E., Mashek, D. J., Strong, G., Li, H., & Brown, L. L. (2005). Reward, motivation, and emotion systems associated with early-stage intense romantic love. *Journal of Neurophysiology, 94,* 327–337.

Aron, A., Mashek, D. J., & Aron, E. (2004). Closeness as including other in the self. In D. Mashek & A. Aron (Eds.), *Handbook of closeness and intimacy* (pp. 27–41). Mahwah, NJ: Erlbaum.

Aron, A., & Norman, C. C. (2005). *Couple participation in self-expanding activities and relationship quality: Is* shared *participation necessary?* Manuscript in preparation.

Aron, A., Norman, C. C., & Aron, E. (1998). The self-expansion model and motivation. *Representative Research in Social Psychology, 22,* 1–13.

Aron, A., Norman, C. C., & Aron, E. (2001). Shared self-expanding activities as a means of maintaining and enhancing close romantic relationships. In J. Harvey & A. Wenzel (Eds.), *Close romantic relationships: Maintenance and enhancement* (pp. 47–66). Mahwah, NJ: Erlbaum.

Aron, A., Norman, C. C., Aron, E. N., & Lewandowski, G. Jr. (2002). Shared participation in self-expanding activities: Positive effects on experienced marital quality. In P. Noller & J. Feeney (Eds.), *Understanding marriage: Developments in the study of couple interaction* (pp. 177–194). New York: Cambridge University Press.

Aron, A., Norman, C. C., Aron, E. N., McKenna, C., & Heyman, R. (2000). Couple's shared participation in novel and arousing activities and experienced relationship quality. *Journal of Personality and Social Psychology, 78,* 273–283.

Aron, A., Paris, M., & Aron, E. (1995). Falling in love: Prospective studies of self-concept change. *Journal of Personality and Social Psychology, 69,* 1102–1112.

Baucom, D. H., & Epstein, N. (1990). *Cognitive-behavioral marital therapy.* New York: Brunner/Mazel.

Berscheid, E., & Ammazzalorso, H. (2001). Emotional experience in close relationships. In G. J. O. Fletcher & M. Clark (Eds.), *Blackwell handbook of social psychology: Interpersonal processes* (pp. 308–330). Malden, MA: Blackwell.

Birchler, G. R., & Weiss, R. L. (1997). *Inventory of Rewarding Activities. Unpublished measure.* (Available from Dr. Robert L. Weiss, Department of Psychology, University of Oregon, Eugene, OR).

Birchler, G. R., Weiss, R. L., & Vincent, J. P. (1975). Multimethod analysis of social reinforcement exchange between martially distressed and nondistressed spouse and stranger dyads. *Journal of Personality and Social Psychology, 59,* 73–82.

Bradbury, T. N., & Fincham, F. D. (1990). Preventing marital dysfunction: Review and analysis. In F. D. Fincham & T. N. Bradbury (Eds.), *Psychology of marriage* (pp. 375–401). New York: Guilford Press.

Bradbury, T. N., Fincham, F. D., & Beach, S. R. (2000). Research on the nature and determinants of marital satisfaction: A decade in review. *Journal of Marriage and the Family, 62,* 964–980.

Carver, C. S., & Scheier, M. F. (1990). Origins and functions of positive and negative affect: A control–process view. *Psychological Review, 97,* 19–35.

Carver, C. S., & Scheier, M. F. (1998). *On the self-regulation of behavior.* New York: Cambridge University Press.

Carver, C. S., & Scheier, M. F. (1999). Themes and issues in the self-regulation of behavior. In R. S. Wyer Jr. (Ed.), *Perspectives on behavioral self-regulation* (pp. 1–106). Mahwah, NJ: Erlbaum.

Christensen, A., & Heavey, C. L. (1999). Interventions for couples. *Annual Review of Psychology, 50,* 165–190.

Diener, E., & Emmons, R. A. (1984). The independence of positive and negative affect. *Journal of Personality and Social Psychology, 47,* 1105–1117.

Fincham, F. D., & Linfield, K. J. (1997). A new look at marital quality: Can spouses feel positive and negative about their marriage? *Journal of Family Psychology, 11,* 489–502.

Foster, C. A., Witcher, B. S., Campbell, W. K., & Green, J. D. (1998). Arousal and attraction: Evidence for automatic and controlled processes. *Journal of Personality and Social Psychology, 74,* 86–101.

Fraley, B., & Aron, A. (2004). The effect of a shared humorous experience on closeness in initial encounters. *Personal Relationships, 11,* 61–78.

Gable, S. L., & Reis, H. T. (2001). Appetitive and aversive social interaction. In J. Harvey & A. Wenzel (Eds.), *Close romantic relationships: Maintenance and enhancement* (pp. 169–194). Mahwah, NJ: Erlbaum.

Gigy, L., & Kelly, J. B. (1992). Reasons for divorce: Perspectives of divorcing men and women. *Journal of Divorce and Remarriage, 18,* 169–187.

Gottman, J. M. (1998). Psychology and the study of marital processes. *Annual Review of Psychology, 49,* 169–197.

Gottman, J. M., Coan, J., Carrere, S., & Swanson, C. (1998). Predicting marital happiness and stability from newlywed interactions. *Journal of Marriage and the Family, 60,* 5–22.

Greenberg, L. S., Paul, J. S., & Conry, R. F. (1988). Perceived change processes in emotionally focused couples therapy. *Journal of Family Psychology, 2*, 5–23.

Hatfield, E., & Sprecher, S. (1986). Measuring passionate love in intimate relationships. *Journal of Adolescence, 9*, 383–410.

Helmeke, K. B., & Sprinkle, D. H. (2000). Clients' perceptions of pivotal moments in couples therapy: A qualitative study of change in therapy. *Journal of Marital and Family Therapy, 26*, 469–483.

Higgins, E. T. (1997). Beyond pleasure and pain. *American Psychologist, 52*, 1280–1300.

Hill, M.S. (1988). Marital stability and spouses' shared time: A multidisciplinary hypothesis. *Journal of Family Issues, 9*, 427–451.

Holman, T. B., & Jacquart, M. (1988). Leisure-activity patterns and marital satisfaction: A further test. *Journal of Marriage and the Family, 50*, 69–77.

Huston, T., McHale, S., & Crouter, A. (1986). When the honeymoon's over: Changes in the marriage relationship over the first year. In R. Gilmour & S. W. Duck (Eds.), *The emerging field of personal relationships* (pp. 109–132). Hillsdale, NJ: Erlbaum.

Jacobson, N. S., & Margolin, G. (1979). *Marital therapy: Strategies based on social learning and behavior exchange principles.* New York: Brunner/Mazel.

Kingston, P. W., & Nock, S. L. (1987). Time together among dual-earner couples. *American Sociological Review, 52*, 391–400.

Laurenceau, J. -P., & Troy, A. B. (2002, July). Positive and appetitive processes in close relationships: Towards a regulation model of close relationship functioning. In S. Gable & J.-P. Laurenceau (Cochairs), *Flourishing relationships: Positive and adaptive processes in relationship maintenance and health.* Symposium conducted at the 11th International Conference on Personal Relationships, Halifax, NS, Canada.

Laurenceau, J. -P., Troy, A. B., & Carver, C. S. (2004, July). Daily emotional experience in romantic relationships as a function of perceived progress regarding relational approach and avoidance goals. In G. Strong (Chair), *Emotion and close relationships.* Symposium conducted at the meeting of the International Association for Relationship Research, Madison, WI.

Lewandowski, G. W. Jr., & Aron, A. (2004). Distinguishing arousal from novelty and challenge in initial romantic attraction between strangers. *Social Behavior and Personality, 32*, 361–372.

Lewandowski, G. W. Jr., & Aron, A. (2005). *The effects of novel/challenging versus arousing activities on couples' experienced relationship quality.* Manuscript submitted for publication.

Mashek, D. J., Aron, A., & Boncimino, M. (2003). Confusions of self with close others. *Personality and Social Psychology Bulletin, 29*, 382–392.

Murray, S. L., Holmes, J. G., & Griffin, D. W. (2004). The benefits of positive illusions: Idealization and the construction of satisfaction in close relationships. In H. T. Reis & C. E. Rusbult (Eds.), *Close relationships: Key readings* (pp. 317–338). Philadelphia: Taylor & Francis.

Orden, S. R., & Bradburn, N. M. (1968). Dimensions of marriage happiness. *American Journal of Sociology, 73*, 715–731.

Orthner, D. K. (1975). Leisure activity patterns and marital satisfaction over the marital career. *Journal of Marriage and the Family, 37,* 91–102.

Pyszczynski, T., Greenberg, J., & Solomon, S. (1997). Why do we need what we need?: A terror management perspective on the roots of human social motivation. *Psychological Inquiry, 8,* 1–20.

Reis, H. T., & Gable, S. L. (2003). Toward a positive psychology of relationships. In C. L. M. Keyes & J. Haidt (Eds.), *Flourishing: Positive psychology and the life well-lived* (pp. 129–159). Washington, DC: American Psychological Association.

Reissman, C., Aron, A., & Bergen, M. R. (1993). Shared activities and marital satisfaction: Causal direction and self-expansion versus boredom. *Journal of Social and Personal Relationships, 10,* 243–254.

Renick, M. J., Blumberg, S. L., & Markman, H. J. (1992). The Prevention and Relationship Enhancement Program (PREP): An empirically based preventive intervention program for couples. *Family Relations, 41,* 141–147.

Strong, G. (2004). *Positive and negative affect and experienced relationship quality.* Unpublished master's thesis, State University of New York at Stony Brook.

Stuart, R. B. (1980). *Helping couples change: A social learning approach to marital therapy.* New York: Guilford Press.

Watson, D. W., Clark, L. A., & Tellegen, A. (1988). Development and validation of brief measures of positive and negative affect: The PANAS scales. *Journal of Personality and Social Psychology, 54,* 1063–1070.

CHAPTER 18

Self-Regulation in Interpersonal Relationships

The Case of Action versus State Orientation

SANDER L. KOOLE
JULIUS KUHL
NILS B. JOSTMANN
CATRIN FINKENAUER

$Self\text{-}regulation$ can be defined as the set of psychological processes through which people bring their thoughts, feelings, and behaviors in line with abstract standards, goals, or values (Baumeister, Heatherton, & Tice, 1993; Kuhl & Koole, 2004). In recent years, psychologists have developed a variety of different models and metaphors to try to explain how self-regulation works. Among other things, self-regulation has been conceived as a cybernetic control process (Carver & Scheier, 1981), a limited resource (Vohs & Baumeister, 2004), a synthesis (Ryan & Deci, 2004), a dynamic system (Vallacher & Nowak, 1999), and an interaction between psychological systems (Kuhl & Koole, 2004). Metaphorically, self-regulation has been likened to a thermostat (Carver & Scheier, 1981), a muscle (Muraven & Baumeister, 2000), a baseball team (Gray, 2004), a political system (Kuhl & Koole, 2004), and a society of interacting automata (Nowak, Vallacher, Tesser, & Borkowksi, 2000).

Prevailing models and metaphors of self-regulation, despite their differences, have at least one thing in common: They portray self-regulation as a private process that predominantly takes place within the individual psyche.

In everyday life, however, complete privacy is the exception rather than the rule. Self-regulation therefore often serves important interpersonal functions. For instance, people frequently engage in self-regulation to respond constructively in close relationships (Finkel & Campbell, 2001) or to meet the goals and expectations of the social environment (Baumann & Kuhl, 2003). The idea that self-regulation and interpersonal relationships are interdependent is not exactly new. For instance, decades ago Freud (1949) speculated that the development of the superego derived from an internalization of parental norms and values (cf. Moretti & Higgins, 1999). Nevertheless, the interface between self-regulation and interpersonal relationships did not receive much research attention until fairly recently. Currently, a growing number of studies have found that interpersonal relationships shape the person's capacity for self-regulation (Diamond & Aspinwall, 2003; Finkenauer, Engels, & Baumeister, 2005; Kuhl, 2000; Mikulincer, Shaver, & Pereg, 2003; Wegner & Erber, 1993). Conversely, it is becoming increasingly apparent that self-regulation is a key moderator of people's behavior in interpersonal relationships (Finkel & Campbell, 2001).

In the present chapter, we aim to shed more light on the interface between self-regulation and interpersonal relationships. Our discussion focuses particularly on the notion of *action* versus *state orientation* (Kuhl, 1981, 1984). Action orientation refers to a *meta-static*, or change-promoting, mode of control during which self-regulation is facilitated. State orientation refers to a *cata-static*, or change-preventing, mode of control, during which self-regulation is inhibited. The notion of action versus state orientation has inspired considerable theory and research over the last few decades. In the present chapter, we build on this work to analyze the mutual dependence between self-regulation and interpersonal relationships. In what follows, we start by considering the notion of action versus state orientation in more detail. We then discuss how dispositions toward action versus state orientation are shaped, triggered, and manifested in the context of interpersonal relationships. We end with our main conclusions and possibilities for future research and applications on the crossroads between self-regulation and interpersonal relationships.

SHIELDING EFFECTS OF ACTION VERSUS STATE ORIENTATION

The concept of action versus state orientation was originally developed to explain the dynamics of human action (Kuhl, 1984; cf. Atkinson & Birch, 1970). After committing to a particular course of action, people are typically exposed to multiple conflicting action tendencies. For instance, consider a woman who has decided to spend more time with her partner. At the same time, this woman wants to spend time with her friends and family, to exercise regularly, to learn Spanish, and to work overtime to get a promotion. In situations like this, the person faces conflicting action tendencies that are all highly feasible and desirable. Consequently, considerations about feasibility and desirability, the traditional province of motivation theory, are often insufficient to resolve the conflict between different action tendencies (Atkinson & Birch, 1970). Therefore, people need psychological mechanisms that can shield their commitment to a chosen course of action against competing action tendencies. Such *action control* mechanisms (Kuhl, 1984) allow people to remain steady in their goal pursuits even under demanding or threatening circumstances.

Action control facilitates goal achievement, and thus will often be adaptive. Nevertheless, action control can sometimes yield adverse outcomes (Koole, Kuhl, Jostmann, & Vohs, 2005). In complex or uncertain situations, it is often prudent to keep an open mind instead of committing to a losing course of action (De Dreu, Koole, & Steinel, 2000; Simonson & Staw, 1992). Likewise, during uncontrollable situations, even the most sophisticated action plans are unlikely to produce desired outcomes. Thus it may be better to rely on simple but robust behavior routines that require a minimum of resources (McIntosh, Sedek, Fojas, Brzezicka-Rotkiewicz, & Kofta, in press). In view of these considerations, it would be adaptive if people could suspend action control from time to time. Consistent with this idea, Kuhl (1984) proposed that people vary in the degree to which they are oriented toward action control. People may be strongly oriented toward action control, and thus become action-oriented. *Action orientation* is defined as a control mode that promotes the enactment of change-oriented intentions. Alternatively, people may suspend action control, and become state-oriented. *State orientation* is defined as a control mode that inhibits the enactment of change-oriented intentions.

Under extremely demanding or threatening conditions, most people are bound to become state-oriented. This is because even the most powerful forms of action control may be insufficient when people are faced with extreme difficulties. Under extremely demanding conditions, for instance, even very efficient action plans may not keep people from being overloaded by their duties and responsibilities. Likewise, in the face of an immediate threat like an attacking bear or an approaching tsunami, people may have insufficient time to plan the quickest escape route. Under these circumstances, the only way to save one's skin may be to act on one's first impulses, without premeditation. In line with the normative functionality of state orientation under extreme conditions, research indicates that most people opt for more primitive forms of behavior control when they are confronted with uncontrollable situations (Maier & Seligman, 1976; McIntosh et al., in press).

But in more moderate situations, individual differences in action versus state orientation are likely to emerge. Some individuals may remain action-oriented even under highly demanding and threatening circumstances; other individuals may become state-oriented at relatively mild levels of demand or threat. Kuhl (1981, 1994) has developed a self-report instrument to measure individual differences in action versus state orientation, the ACS90 (for psychometric validation, see Diefendorff et al., 2000, and Kuhl & Beckmann, 1994b). Illustrative items are presented in Table 18.1. The ACS90 distinguishes between *demand-related action orientation* (AOD), which relates to action control in demanding situations, and *threat-related action orientation* (AOT), which relates to action control in threatening situations. Each ACS90 item presents individuals with a description of a stressful situation and two different ways of responding to the situation, an action- or a state-oriented response. The number of action-oriented responses across the scale is taken as an indicator of the individual's action orientation. If the individual responds to the majority of situations in an action-oriented manner, we infer that the individual is inclined toward action orientation. If the individual responds to the majority of situations in an state-oriented manner, we infer that the individual is inclined toward state orientation.

Individual differences in action versus state orientation have been extensively investigated in more than 60 published studies (for reviews, see Diefendorff et al., 2000; Koole & Kuhl, in press; Kuhl & Beckmann, 1994b).

TABLE 18.1. Illustrative Items of the ACS90

Threat-related action orientation (AOT) versus preoccupation
- When I have lost something that is very valuable to me and I can't find it anywhere:
  A. I have a hard time concentrating on anything else
  B. I put it out of my mind after a little while*
- If I've worked for weeks on a project and then everything goes completely wrong with the project:
  A. It takes me a long time to adjust myself to it
  B. It bothers me for a while, but then I don't think about it anymore*
- When I am being told that my work is completely unsatisfactory:
  A. I don't let it bother me for too long*
  B. I feel paralyzed

Demand-related action orientation (AOD) versus hesitation
- When I know I must finish something soon:
  A. I have to push myself to get started
  B. I find it easy to get it over and done with*
- When I am getting ready to tackle a difficult problem
  A. It feels like I am facing a big mountain I don't think I can climb
  B. I look for a way to approach the problem in a suitable manner*
- When I have a boring assignment:
  A. I usually don't have a problem getting through it*
  B. I sometimes just can't get moving on it

Note. Action-oriented responses are marked with an asterisk.

Throughout this work, consistent differences between action- versus state-oriented individuals have emerged across cognitive, emotional, behavioral, neurobiological, and psychophysiological responses. Moreover, predictable differences between action- versus state-oriented individuals have been found across a broad range of different tasks and contexts, ranging from well-controlled laboratory tasks to behavior in real-life situations such as job success, academic achievement, and athletic performance. Finally, the effects of action versus state orientation could not be explained by achievement motivation (Heckhausen & Strang, 1988), self-esteem (Koole & Jostmann, 2004), or emotion suppression and reappraisal strategies (Koole, 2004), and occurred over and above the effects of the Big Five personality dimensions (Baumann & Kuhl, 2002; Diefendorff et al., 2000; Palfai, 2002).

The effects of action orientation can be summarized into three main mechanisms: *affect shielding*, *intention shielding*, and *self shielding*. Affect shielding refers to the person's ability to inhibit unwanted affective states. Action orientation is a strong predictor of down-regulation of negative affect in response to real-life stressors (Kuhl, 1983) and reduced depression (Rholes, Michas, & Shroff, 1989). In response to threatening or demanding laboratory manipulations, action orientation is associated with fewer spontaneous expressions of negative affect (Brunstein & Olbrich, 1985), tension reduction (Koole & Jostmann, 2004), and reduced physiological arousal (Heckhausen & Strang, 1988). Especially under demanding conditions, action orientation correlates with down-regulation of implicit negative affect, for instance, as assessed by an interference task (Koole & Jostmann, 2004) or a lexical decision task (Koole & Van den Berg, in press). Recent studies found that action orientation even predicts down-regulation of negative affect on subliminal levels (Jostmann, Koole, van der Wulp, & Fockenberg, 2005; Koole & Van den Berg, 2005).

Both forms of action orientation, AOT and AOD, are related to affect shielding (e.g., Koole & Jostmann, 2004; Koole & Van den Berg, 2005). Intention shielding and self shielding, however, relate specifically to either AOT or AOD. AOD is associated with *intention shielding*, that is, efficiency at forming, maintaining, and executing difficult intentions under demanding circumstances. Compared with individuals low on AOD, individuals high on AOD are faster at decision making (Stiensmeier-Pelster & Schürmann, 1994) and are better able to commit themselves to their own decisions (Beckmann & Kuhl, 1984). AOD further predicts efficient implementation of difficult intentions (Heckhausen & Strang, 1988; Kuhl, 1985; Kuhl & Beckmann, 1994a). The intention-shielding effects of AOD have been documented for well-controlled laboratory tasks, such as the Stroop color-naming task, the control of automatically activated gender stereotypes, and working memory tests (Jostmann & Koole, 2005a, 2005b). Notably, AOD also predicts intention shielding in real-life settings, as indicated by superior work performance (Diefendorff et al., 2000) and more effective health change behavior (Palfai, 2002; Palfai, McNally, & Roy, 2002).

AOT is associated with *self shielding*, that is, efficiency at forming and maintaining coherent self-representations. Self shielding is often accompanied by the experience of autonomy, or a subjective sense of "self-determination" (Deci & Ryan, 2000). From a functional perspective, effective shielding of the self requires that aspects of the self are cognitively accessible. Consistent with this idea, AOT is associated with improved memory for decisions made by the self (Kuhl & Kazén, 1994). This improved cognitive access to the self emerges especially under aversive conditions (Baumann & Kuhl, 2003). A sense of self-determination can also be achieved by integrating new experiences that are initially not part of the self's intrinsic needs and preferences (Deci & Ryan, 2000). Several studies support the idea that AOT is linked with cognitive integration abilities, particularly under aversive conditions. AOT is associated with improved ability to form coherence among different cognitive elements, especially when negative affect is high (Baumann & Kuhl, 2002). Cognitive integration abilities should also help the individual to integrate implicit and explicit personality aspects. Consistent with this idea, AOT is associated with greater congruence between explicit goals and implicit needs, as assessed by the Thematic Apperception Test (Brunstein, 2001; cf. McClelland, Koestner, & Weinberger, 1989).

ACTION VERSUS STATE ORIENTATION IN INTERPERSONAL RELATIONSHIPS

To date, most studies on action versus state orientation were not designed to link this disposition to interpersonal relationships. Nevertheless, over the years, more and more findings have accumulated that seem relevant to the interpersonal dimension of action versus state orientation. It thus seems timely to consider how action versus state orientation can be situated within the context of interpersonal relationships. There are at least three basic ways in which action versus state orientation and interpersonal relations are mutually intertwined. First, interpersonal relations may be critical *antecedents* of chronic dispositions toward action versus state orientation. Second, interpersonal relations can provide the proximal *triggers* that cause individual dispositions toward action versus state orientation to become manifest. Third, many of the *consequences* of action versus state orientation become manifest in the context of interpersonal relationships. In the next paragraphs, we discuss each of these three interfaces between interpersonal relations and action versus state orientation.

INTERPERSONAL ANTECEDENTS OF ACTION VERSUS STATE ORIENTATION

The development of self-regulation skills through socialization processes is endorsed both by classic theories (Bowlby, 1969; Freud, 1949) and by contemporary accounts of self-regulation (Finkenauer et al., 2005; Mikulincer et al., 2003; Moretti & Higgins, 1999; Wegner & Erber, 1993). In line with these various approaches, Kuhl (2000) suggested that chronic dispositions toward action versus state orientation may be shaped more by socialization processes than by genetic factors. This proposal was tested empirically by Kästele (1988, cited in Kuhl, 2000), who examined individual differences in action versus state orientation among mono- and dizygotic twins. Kästele also examined individual differences in extraversion and neuroticism, two traditional personality traits that are known to possess a sizable genetic component (e.g., Jang, Livesley, & Vernon, 1996). Consistent with prior research, extraversion and neuroticism were more similar among monozygotic twins than among dizygotic twins. Action versus state orientation, however, was no more similar among monozygotic than among dizygotic twins. The genetic component in action versus state orientation thus appears to be modest, and indeed significantly smaller compared to the genetic component of more traditional personality traits.

Socialization conditions that impair children's ability to disengage from unwanted affective or motivational states may increase dispositions toward state orientation in adulthood (Kuhl, 1994). Examples of such conditions include authoritarian educational styles, overemphasis of duties and responsibilities, achievement, or behavioral consistency. Some initial studies suggest that these socialization conditions are indeed important in shaping dispositions toward action versus state orientation. One relevant study found that mothers' socialization practices during early childhood were correlated with their children's action versus state orientation scores (Humbert, 1981). Mothers who were controlling, for instance, who reported that they frequently interrupted their children when they were playing, had children with significantly increased state orientation scores. Another, more recent, study found that an inconsistent educational attitude of mothers was associated with more state orientation among their daughters (Marszal-Wisniewska, 2001).

Severe life stressors may also promote state orientation, especially to the extent that they lead to chronic negative affect. One such severe stressor may be parental divorce. Children whose parents are divorced tend to have more difficulty in school, more behavior problems, more negative self-concepts, more problems with peers, and more trouble getting along with their parents (Amato & Keith, 1991). Accordingly, parental divorce may increase children's dispositions toward state orientation. This notion was recently tested by Koole (2005) in an empirical study involving a group of 142 university students (41 men and 101 women, average age 21). In this study, male participants' orientations were not affected by parental divorce, F's < 1. However, parental divorce did affect female participants' AOT scores. As shown in Figure 18.1, female participants from divorced families displayed significantly lower AOT than female participants from intact families (p < .05). Parental divorce had no effect on female participants' AOD scores (F < 1). Parental divorce thus appeared to increase children's proneness to become state-oriented, at least for female children. The more pronounced effects of parental divorce on female children might be due to women's greater tendency to ruminate over negative events (Nolen-Hoeksema, 1987). Moreover, parental divorce appears to primarily influence women's ability to cope with threatening situations, while parental divorce may have little influence on women's ability to cope with demanding situations.

How might socialization factors influence the person's disposition toward action versus state orientation? A systematic approach to this question is provided by the *systems-conditioning model* (Kuhl, 2000). According to the model, the pathway between two psychological systems becomes strengthened each time the systems are activated within a brief time window. Based on this conditioning process, the person's self (i.e., central executive systems) can develop links with other psychological subsystems, and thereby acquire the capacity to regulate the activation of these subsystems. This developmental process can be illustrated in the context of a mother's interactions with her children. The child is genetically predisposed to respond with positive affect to the mother's encouraging vocalizations and her initiation of eye contact (Schore, 1996). The child's ensuing expression of positive affect is presumably mediated by the child's rudimentary self system. Thus, over time, the positive affect that the mother generates will gradually become associated with the child's self. As a result of this conditioned association, merely activating the

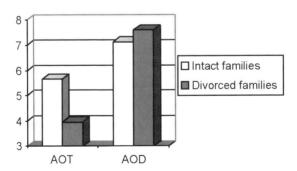

FIGURE 18.1. Parental divorce and female children's action orientation. Action orientation scores ranged from 1 (= very low) to 12 (= very high). From Koole (2005). Reprinted by permission of the author.

child's self can be sufficient to activate positive affect. Ultimately, the child's self has acquired the capacity to activate positive affect without external help (from, in this case, the mother).

The systems-conditioning model remains to be subjected to systematic empirical testing. Even so, available evidence is supportive of the model. More specifically, the systems-conditioning model is consistent with evidence that autonomy-supporting education styles promote intrinsic motivation and emotional well-being (Deci & Ryan, 2000) and numerous studies showing that harsh and chaotic parenting leads to deficits in emotion regulation skills (Repetti, Taylor, & Seeman, 2002; Taylor, Lerner, Sage, Lehman, & Seeman, 2004). The notion of responsivity in attachment research (Bowlby, 1969) is also relevant to systems-conditioning processes. Based on the systems-conditioning model, autonomy-supportive conditions and responsivity can be interpreted as temporally contingent and behaviorally adequate responding to the self-expressions of the child (Keller, 2000; Keller et al., 1999). As such, autonomy-supportive conditions and responsivity may function as catalysts of systems-conditioning processes. Conversely, harsh and chaotic styles of interpersonal interaction interfere with systems-conditioning processes, and thereby inhibit the development of self-regulation skills.

To date, the most direct test of the systems-conditioning model has been conducted by Schulte, Hartung, and associates. These researchers analyzed 192 videotaped interactions between 17 therapists and 48 phobic patients (Schulte, Hartung, & Wilke, 1997). Their findings indicated that a specific interaction sequence was indicative of the therapists' efforts to guide their clients' self-regulation processes. During this interaction sequence, the client started with an action-oriented expression (e.g., "I know I can make it happen!"). The therapist then responded with an action-oriented statement (e.g., "How do you intend to make it happen?"). This interaction sequence maps onto the systems-conditioning model, in that the therapist provides matching responses to the self-expressions of the client. The matching sequence was a frequent type of interaction, occurring during 25.3% of all interactions. Importantly, the frequency of the matching sequence during therapy was an important predictor of therapeutic success, especially when the sequence occurred during early therapy sessions.

Alternatively, a state-oriented mode expressed by the client ("I simply feel awful") may be counterregulated by a therapist's action-oriented mode ("What thought might help you overcome this feeling?"). Another study found this counterregulation to be another efficient method of facilitating self-regulation of affect through systems conditioning (Hartung & Schulte, 1994). Based on the systems-conditioning model, we speculate that counterregulation by the therapist helps the client to access the self system, which is a necessary precondition for building up the clients' own affect regulation skills. Accordingly, the counterregulation strategy may be particularly helpful when clients' cognitive access to the self is chronically inhibited (i.e.. the client has difficulty with self-expression). Taken together, there is growing evidence that interpersonal interactions that support the self can strengthen dispositions toward action orientation. Conversely, threatening interpersonal interactions appear to strengthen dispositions toward state orientation.

INTERPERSONAL TRIGGERS OF ACTION VERSUS STATE ORIENTATION

Having a predisposition toward action or state orientation does not mean that one is constantly driven to respond in line with this orientation. Rather, a predisposition toward action or state orientation refers to the person's *potential* for becoming either action- or state-oriented in situations that call for active self-regulation. Predispositions toward action or state orientation may often remain latent and thus invisible in the person's overt behavior. Indeed, research indicates that functional differences between action- versus state-oriented individuals are minimal under low-stress conditions (i.e., situations that are characterized by low levels of demand and low levels of threat). When conditions are sufficiently relaxing, state-oriented individuals may even outperform action-oriented individuals on self-regulation measures (Koole et al., 2005).

Dispositions toward action or state orientation tend to manifest themselves especially when situational cues indicate an immediate need for active self-regulation. These situational cues can be thought of as *proximal triggers* that activate the person's latent potential for action- versus state-oriented coping. In some cases, these proximal triggers may be self-generated. For instance, a person may suddenly realize that she has missed an important opportunity and has to redouble her efforts to meet her goals. This dawning realization may then trigger a latent predisposition toward action versus state orientation. If the person has a predisposition toward action orientation, an awareness of upcoming difficulties may lead that person to engage in proactive planning and to mobilize her resources to rise to the occasion (Aspinwall & Taylor, 1997). By contrast, if the person has a predisposition toward state orientation, an awareness of upcoming difficulties may lead the person to feel overwhelmed and to ruminate incessantly (Kuhl, 1994).

Proximal triggers of action versus state orientation may also originate from the social environment. Indeed, there are reasons to believe that the social environment is very important in triggering latent predispositions toward action versus state orientation. First, social cues are closely associated with the learning conditions that give rise to dispositions toward action or state orientation. It thus seems plausible that social cues can be powerful stimuli for reinstating those learning conditions, and thereby trigger latent dispositions toward action or state orientation. Second, the need for self-regulation often arises in the context of interpersonal relations (Finkel & Campbell, 2001). After all, interpersonal relations are replete with demands, difficulties, negative feedback, miscommunication, conflict, and other conditions that require individuals to exert extra effort to remain calm, motivated, and ready to act.

The interpersonal nature of triggering conditions of action versus state orientation has often remained somewhat implicit in the literature. Nevertheless, a close examination of the literature reveals that researchers have often capitalized on interpersonal settings to examine individual differences in action versus state orientation. First, it is noteworthy that many effects of action versus state orientation have emerged in settings in which there existed powerful achievement norms, such as educational settings (Boekaerts, 1994), businesses (Dieffendorf et al., 2000; Kuhl & Kazén, 2003), or competitive sports (Beckmann & Kazén, 1994; Heckhausen & Strang, 1988). Second, experimental procedures that have been used to study differences between action- versus state-oriented individuals often contain important interpersonal cues. Consider the self-discrimination task, a task that has consistently yielded differences between action- and state-oriented individuals (Baumann & Kuhl, 2002; Kazén, Baumann, & Kuhl, 2003; Kuhl & Kazén, 1994). During the self-discrimination task, researchers compare participants' memory for self- versus other-assigned activities. Although the self-discrimination task might appear to be primarily a cognitive task, the task has a significant interpersonal dimension. In particular, the task requires that the experimenter assumes the role of the "boss" who assigns activities, whereas participants assume the role of a "secretary" who executes activities. It seems plausible that the interpersonal power dynamics that are implied by this scenario serve as proximal triggers of the effects of action versus state orientation.

Notably, recent research has used procedures that explicitly involve interpersonal dynamics in triggering effects of action versus state orientation. In particular, recent experiments manipulated performance-contingent versus noncontingent rewards to trigger effects of action versus state orientation (Jostmann & Koole, 2005a; Koole, 2004; Koole & Jostmann, 2004). Performance-contingent rewards are a much studied form of social control, which is used pervasively in modern society (Deci, Koestner, & Ryan, 1999). Research indicates that action- versus state-oriented individuals function very differently in response to performance-contingent rewards. Performance-contingent rewards enhance self-regulation among action-oriented individuals, whereas performance-contingent rewards undermine self-regulation among state-oriented individuals (Koole, 2004). By contrast, differences between action- versus state-oriented individuals are much smaller or even reversed in response to noncontingent rewards. Similar to the self-discrimination task, social control appears to be a powerful proximal trigger of individual differences in action versus state orientation.

Other recent experiments have used *relationship schema priming* (Baldwin, 1992) to trigger effects of action versus state orientation (Koole, 2004; Koole & Jostmann, 2004). In this paradigm, participants are asked to visualize a demanding versus an accepting relationship partner. The underlying idea here is that visualizing a relationship partner implicitly activates the interaction patterns and psychological responses that individuals experienced within a specific relationship context. Consistent with this, research indicates that action- versus state-oriented individuals function differently after visualizing a demanding person (Koole, 2004; Koole & Jostmann, 2004). Visualizing a demanding person appears to enhance self-regulation among action-oriented individuals, whereas visualizing a demanding person appears to undermine self-regulation among state-oriented individuals. By contrast, differences between action- versus state-oriented individuals tend to be much smaller or even reversed after visualizing an accepting person. Taken together, relationship schemas appear to act as important triggers of individual differences in action versus state orientation.

INTERPERSONAL CONSEQUENCES OF ACTION VERSUS STATE ORIENTATION

As we have seen, chronic differences in action versus state orientation are shaped and triggered by interpersonal relations. It thus seems intuitively plausible that action versus state orientation will moderate at least some interpersonal behaviors. To date, however, the interpersonal consequences of action versus state orientation have not received much research attention. Nevertheless, we consider some theoretical conjectures and preliminary findings on how action versus state orientation influences interpersonal relations.

Theoretically, the influence of action versus state orientation on interpersonal relations is likely to depend on the nature of the relationship. In particular, it is important to take into account the degree to which the relationship is freely chosen and congruent with the totality of the person's self, psychological needs, motives, and desires. For *self-congruent relationships*, action orientation can be expected to facilitate relationship maintenance mechanisms. Among the various relationships that people maintain, romantic relationships seem especially likely to be self-congruent. Thus one would expect action orientation to be associated with positive outcomes in romantic relationships. Consistent with this expectation, a recent study of 45 couples found that couples with high scores on the AOT scale reported greater relationship satisfaction and commitment than couples with low scores on the AOT scale (r's = .33

and .34, respectively; Jostmann & Finkenauer, 2004). In the same study, correlations between relationship satisfaction and commitment and couples' scores on the AOD scale were positive but not statistically reliable (both r's = .15).

Though suggestive, the aforementioned association between action orientation and relationship outcomes should be regarded as preliminary. First, because the result is purely correlational, it is conceivable that couples' action orientation was the *outcome* rather than the *cause* of relationship satisfaction and commitment. Second, more work is needed to understand the mechanisms through which action versus state orientation may affect relationship outcomes. For instance, it is possible that action-oriented individuals are better able to perform the cognitive work that is required to manage empathic accuracy (Ickes & Simpson, 2001). In a previous study, participants scoring high on AOD were better able than those scoring low to guess their partner's preferred leisure activities on an imaginary vacation trip (Gunsch, 1996; Kuhl & Kazén, 1997). Moreover, AOD was significantly associated with participants' inclination to change their own preferences by thinking about their partner's preferences. Thus some initial work suggests that action orientation promotes empathic accuracy.

Alternative relationship maintenance mechanisms are suggested by the literature on close relationships. For instance, efficient affect shielding might allow action-oriented individuals to maintain a more favorable image of the relationship (Van Lange & Rusbult, 1995). In a related vein, action-oriented individuals (especially those of the AOT type) might be more capable of doing the cognitive work that is needed to see virtues in their partners' faults (Murray & Holmes, 1993). Finally, action-oriented individuals (especially those of the AOD type) can be expected to initiate more new and arousing activities that are needed to keep a relationship fresh over time (Aron, Norman, Aron, McKenna, & Heyman, 2000). These respective mechanisms may be addressed in future research.

Not all interpersonal relationships are likely to be congruent with the person's self. Indeed, most people have at least occasionally experienced interaction partners who were overly demanding of or threatening to the self. For such *self-incongruent relationships*, action orientation can be expected to promote active resistance against interpersonal relationships that are overly demanding or threatening to the self. Conversely, it can be expected that state orientation promotes succumbing or giving in to overly demanding or threatening interpersonal relationships. Initial evidence is consistent with this notion. Specifically, an investigation using the classic Asch conformity paradigm found that state-oriented individuals were especially likely to comply with unreasonable group demands (Beckmann, 1994). Action-oriented individuals, by contrast, showed no evidence of conforming as the result of group pressures. In a related vein, another study showed that state-oriented children are more inclined than their action-oriented counterparts to engage in effortful self-control (i.e., delay of gratification) in response to controlling instructions by an authority figure (Baumann & Kuhl, 2005).

Research has further shown that state-oriented individuals (especially those scoring low on the AOT scale) are prone to *self-infiltration*, that is, mistaking assigned activities for self-chosen activities (Kuhl & Kazén, 1994). By contrast, action-oriented individuals typically show no evidence of a tendency toward self-infiltration. Ironically, state-oriented individuals are especially susceptible to self-infiltration when they are experiencing negative affect (Baumann & Kuhl, 2002) and when the assigned activities are aversive (Kazén et al., 2003). Thus it seems that state-oriented individuals are most vulnerable to self-infiltration under conditions that are likely to predominate within the context of overly demanding or threatening interpersonal relationships. Notably, self-infiltration may not only relate to concrete activities, but also to more abstract evaluations of the self. Indeed, we have recently found evidence that demanding relationship partners may activate negative self-evaluations in state-oriented individuals, both explicitly (Koole & Jostmann, 2004, Study 3) and implicitly (Koole, 2004, Study 1).

The self-infiltration tendencies of state-oriented individuals may be part of a more general pattern among these individuals to gravitate toward relationships in which self–other boundaries are not clearly defined (Kuhl, 2000). In the psychoanalytic literature, the latter type of relationships is referred to as *symbiotic relationships* (Halberstadt-Freud, 1993; Silverman, 2003; Silverman & Weinberger, 1985). Indeed, state orientation is positively correlated with self-reported tendency toward self–other blurring in romantic relationships (Gunsch, 1996). Symbiotic tendencies are characterized by an unwillingness to grant the partner personal and emotional autonomy. The need to have another person regulating one's emotions may be one factor that underlies state-oriented individuals' preference for symbiotic relationships.

Does state orientation always constitute a liability in interpersonal relations? Perhaps not. First, the positive effects of action orientation on interpersonal relations may be confined to the Western cultures. Indeed, recent research suggests that state orientation may have positive interpersonal effects in interdependent cultures. In these cultures, action-oriented individuals' emotional autonomy may be regarded as an impediment to social integration (Olvermann, Metz-Göckel, Hannover, & Pöhlmann, 2004).

Even within independent cultures, action- and state-oriented individuals may achieve synergistic benefits whenever they manage to combine their efforts (Koole et al., 2005). For instance, action-oriented individuals may provide emotional support to state-oriented individuals under acute stress. In turn, state-oriented individuals may contribute their sensitivity for potential risks (as a remedy against excessive optimism), and their willingness to compromise even on issues that are important to themselves. Initial support for this reasoning has been observed among airbus crews, where crews consisting of an action-oriented pilot and a state-oriented copilot were found to be more effective than fully action-oriented or fully state-oriented crews (Haschke & Kuhl, 1995). In a similar vein, a recent study found that dyads consisting of both types of individuals were more effective at a complex problem-solving task than dyads consisting of one type alone (Witte & Von Pablocki, 1999). Notably, the latter findings were statistically weak and the study's design suffered from some important methodological shortcomings (e.g., lack of statistical power, neglect of moderating variables). Even so, there are some initial grounds for believing that action- and state-oriented individuals may achieve synergistic benefits by working together as a team.

SUMMARY AND FUTURE DIRECTIONS

In the present chapter, we have sought to ground the construct of action versus state orientation within the context of interpersonal relations. We distinguished three basic ways in which action versus state orientation and interpersonal relations are intertwined, which are summarized in Table 18.2. First, interpersonal relations are antecedents of individual dispositions toward action versus state orientation. The genetic component of action versus state orientation appears rather modest, leaving much room for the social environment to shape people's dispositions toward either orientation. Childhood socialization experiences appear to be critical, as indicated by evidence that state orientation is fostered by frequent interruptions by caregivers, inconsistent or unresponsive educational attitudes, and parental divorce. Nevertheless, dispositions toward action versus state orientation may continue to change throughout adulthood, as studies show that therapists may increase their clients' action orientation by affirming clients' action-oriented responses.

After a disposition toward action or state orientation becomes engrained in the individual's repertoire, interpersonal relations can provide proximal cues that trigger action- or state-oriented coping responses. Many studies that have found effects of individual differences in action versus state orientation were conducted in the presence of salient achievement norms or authority figures. Thus the latter two conditions may trigger latent dispositions toward action versus state orientation. There is also evidence that performance-contingent rewards and demanding relationship schemas can serve as interpersonal triggers of action versus state orientation. Given that achievement norms, power differences, and performance pressures are very common aspects of interpersonal relationships, interpersonal settings may frequently trigger differences between action- and state-oriented individuals.

Once triggered, individual dispositions toward action versus state orientation may influence the outcomes of interpersonal relationships. At present,

TABLE 18.2. Interpersonal Antecedents, Triggers, and Consequences of Chronic Dispositions toward Action versus State Orientation

Antecedents	Triggers	Consequences
Environmental influences seem to outweigh genetic influences in shaping chronic dispositions toward action versus state orientation (Kästele, 1988).	Latent disposition toward action versus state orientation can be triggered by strong *achievement norms* (e.g., Diefendorff et al., 2000); *interpersonal power dynamics* (e.g., Kuhl & Kazén, 1994); *performance-contingent rewards* (e.g., Koole & Jostmann, 2004); and *activated relationship schemas* (e.g., Koole, 2004).	Action orientation is associated with *relationship satisfaction and commitment* (Jostmann & Finkenauer, 2004).
In childhood, chronic disposition toward state orientation is fostered by *frequent interruptions by caregivers* (Humbert, 1981); *inconsistent educational attitude of caregivers* (Marszal-Wisniewska, 2001); and *parental divorce* (Koole, 2004).		State orientation is associated with *conformity* (Beckmann, 1994); *self-infiltration* (Kuhl & Kazén, 1994); *impaired knowledge of partner's preferences* (Gunsch, 1996); and *preference for symbiotic relationships* (Gunsch, 1996).
In adulthood, chronic disposition toward action orientation is fostered by *social affirmation of action-oriented responses* (Schulte, Hartung, & Wilke, 1997).		Team of action- and state-oriented individuals may achieve synergy (Haschke & Kuhl, 1995; Witte & Von Pablocki, 1999).

research on action versus state orientation and relationship outcomes has been exclusively correlational. Thus it is not possible to draw firm conclusions about the causal role of action versus state orientation in interpersonal relationships. Nevertheless, research has uncovered some suggestive findings. First, action orientation is associated with greater relationship satisfaction and commitment. Second, state orientation is associated with conformity and self-infiltration (i.e., internalization of social expectations that are negative and alien to the self). Third, state orientation is associated with a preference for symbiotic relationships, that is, relationships in which the boundaries between self and other are blurred. Although the observed associations are preliminary, the available evidence suggests that action versus state orientation may exert an important influence on interpersonal behavior.

The present chapter highlights the need for more empirical research on the role of action versus state orientation in interpersonal relations. In particular, more research is needed on the interpersonal origins of dispositions toward action versus state orientation. Some groundbreaking research has been done in clinical settings (Schulte et al., 1997). However, additional longitudinal research is necessary to chart how children's interactions with caregivers influence the development of chronic dispositions toward action versus state orientation.

Future research should also do well to track the development of action versus state orientation within romantic relationships. Recent work on the "Michelangelo phenomenon" suggests that romantic partners can foster each other's personal growth (see Kumashiro, Rusbult, Wolf, & Estrada, Chapter 16, this volume). Accordingly, it would be worthwhile to examine how secure romantic relationships influence the development of dispositions toward action versus state orientation. In particular, secure relationships are likely to foster the development of chronic action orientation. Furthermore, promoting *flexibility* in action versus state orientation might be a particularly beneficial way for relationship partners to affect the self. Future work would also benefit from a greater process-oriented focus. In this regard, the systems-conditioning model (Kuhl, 2000) may stimulate more fine-grained analyses of the social–affective dynamics that underlie the development of action versus state orientation.

Further research is also needed to understand precisely how interpersonal interactions can trigger latent dispositions toward action versus state orientation. Here, the notion of relationship schemas (Baldwin, 1992) may be useful. Dispositions toward action versus state orientation may be regarded as a sediment of the person's prior experiences in relationships with significant others, which to some extent have developed into "habitualized" and "generalized" coping styles. This conceptualization raises the intriguing possibility that action versus state orientation may not only vary between individuals, but also between relationship partners. Conceivably, some relationship contexts lead individuals to be more action-oriented, whereas other relationship contexts lead individuals to be more state-oriented. Such a contextualized approach to action versus state orientation remains to be tested in future research. The process through which specific relationship experiences become generalized coping responses also merits further investigation. This generalization process may be facilitated by interpersonal transference (Chen & Andersen, 1999), so that experiences that are specific to a particular relationship come to influence responses to new relationship partners. Accordingly, future research may examine the role of transference in triggering action- versus state-oriented coping styles.

Finally, the interpersonal consequences of action versus state orientation should be given more systematic empirical attention. It is important to know if action orientation can indeed promote relationship satisfaction and commitment. To establish whether action versus state orientation plays a causal role in determining these relationship outcomes, future research should incorporate longitudinal designs (sec Cooper & Skaggs Sheldon, 2002, for methodological recommendations for research on personality and close relationships). Future research should also examine the influence of experimental manipulations of action orientation and test for variables that mediate the effects of action orientation on relationship outcomes. Finally, future research should explore the potential synergistic benefits of action and state orientation. Although initial work is suggestive of such benefits, there likely exist important moderators and boundary conditions to a synergy between action- and state-oriented individuals. Given the great theoretical and applied interest in this topic, the potential synergistic benefits of action and state orientation constitute an important avenue for further research.

CONCLUDING REMARKS

In the present chapter, we have emphasized the close interdependence between individual dispositions toward action versus state orientation and interpersonal relationships. Dispositions toward action versus state orientation become shaped and triggered by interpersonal relationships. In turn, the maintenance of interpersonal relationships may be significantly influenced by dispositions toward action versus state orientation. More generally, the present analysis has important implications for the scientific understanding of self-regulation processes. Self-regulation appears to function as an integral part of a *social system*, in which there is a continual, dynamic, and reciprocal influence between individuals and their social networks. Any comprehensive analysis of self-regulation should therefore consider how self-regulation unfolds within the context of interpersonal relationships.

ACKNOWLEDGMENT

This research was facilitated by an Innovation Grant from the Netherlands Organization for Scientific Research (NWO) to Sander L. Koole.

REFERENCES

Amato, P. R., & Keith, B. (1991). Parental divorce and the well-being of children: A meta-analysis. *Psychological Bulletin, 110,* 26–46.
Aron, A., Norman, C. C., Aron, E. N., McKenna, C., & Heyman, R. E. (2000). Couples' shared participation in novel and arousing activities and experienced relationship quality. *Journal of Personality and Social Psychology, 78,* 273–284.
Aspinwall, L. G., & Taylor, S. E. (1997). A stitch in time: Self-regulation and proactive coping. *Psychological Review, 121,* 417–436.

Atkinson, J. W., & Birch, D. (1970). *The dynamics of action.* New York: Wiley.

Baldwin, M. W. (1992). Relational schemas and the processing of social information. *Psychological Review, 112,* 461–484.

Baumann, N., & Kuhl, J. (2002). Intuition, affect and personality: Unconscious coherence judgments and self-regulation of negative affect. *Journal of Personality and Social Psychology, 83,* 1213–1223.

Baumann, N., & Kuhl, J. (2003). Self-infiltration: Confusing assigned tasks as self-selected in memory. *Personality and Social Psychology Bulletin, 29,* 487–498.

Baumann, N., & Kuhl, J. (2005). How to resist temptation: The effects of external control versus autonomy support on self-regulatory dynamics. *Journal of Personality Psychology, 73,* 443–470.

Baumeister, R. F., Heatherton, T. F., & Tice, D. M. (1994). *Losing control: How and why people fail at self-regulation.* New York: Academic Press.

Beckmann, J. (1994). *Alienation and conformity.* Unpublished manuscript, Max Planck Institute for Psychological Research, Munich, Germany.

Beckmann, J., & Kazén, M. (1994). Action and state orientation and the performance of top athletes. In J. Kuhl & J. Beckmann (Eds.), *Volition and personality: Action versus state orientation* (pp. 439–451). Göttingen, Germany: Hogrefe & Huber.

Beckmann, J., & Kuhl, J. (1984). Altering information to gain action control: Functional aspects of human information processing in decision making. *Journal of Research in Personality, 18,* 223–279.

Boekaerts, M. (1994). Action control: How relevant is it for classroom learning? In J. Kuhl & J. Beckmann (Eds.), *Volition and personality: Action versus state orientation* (pp. 427–435). Göttingen, Germany: Hogrefe & Huber.

Bowlby, J. (1969). *Attachment and loss* (Vol. 1). New York: Basic Books.

Brunstein, J. C. (2001). Persönliche Ziele und Handlungs- versus Lageorientierung: Wer bindet sich an realistische und bedürfniskongruente Ziele? [Personal goals and action versus state orientation: Who builds a commitment to realistic and need-congruent goals?]. *Zeitschrift für Differentielle und Diagnostische Psychologie, 22,* 1–12.

Brunstein, J. C., & Olbrich, E. (1985). Personal helplessness and action control: Analysis of achievement-related cognitions, self-assessments, and performance. *Journal of Personality and Social Psychology, 48,* 1540–1551.

Carver, C. S., & Scheier, M. F. (1981). *Attention and self-regulation: A control-theory approach to human behavior.* New York: Springer-Verlag.

Chen, S., & Andersen, S. M. (1999). Relationships from the past in the present: Significant-other representations and transference in interpersonal life. In M. P. Zanna (Ed.), *Advances in experimental social psychology* (Vol. 31, pp. 123–190). New York: Academic Press.

Cooper, M. L., & Skaggs Sheldon, M. (2002). Seventy years of research on personality and close relationships: Substantive and methodological trends over time. *Journal of Personality, 70,* 783–812.

Deci, E. L., Koestner, R., & Ryan, R. M. (1999). A meta-analytic review of experiments examining the effects of extrinsic rewards on intrinsic motivation. *Psychological Bulletin, 125,* 627–668.

Deci, E. L., & Ryan, R. M. (2000). The "what" and "why" of goal pursuits: Human needs and the self-determination perspective. *Psychological Inquiry, 11,* 227–268.

De Dreu, C. K., Koole, S. L., & Steinel, W. (2000). Unfixing the fixed pie: A motivated information processing approach to integrative negotiation. *Journal of Personality and Social Psychology, 79,* 975–987.

Diamond, L. M., & Aspinwall, L. G. (2003). Emotion regulation across the life span: An integrative perspective emphasizing self-regulation, positive affect, and dyadic processes. *Motivation and Emotion, 27,* 125–156.

Diefendorff, J. M., Hall, R. J., Lord, R. G., & Strean, M. L. (2000). Action-state orientation: Construct validity of a revised measure and its relationship to work-related variables. *Journal of Applied Psychology, 85,* 250–263.

Finkel, E. J., & Campbell, W. K. (2001). Self-control and accommodation in close relationships: An interdependence analysis. *Journal of Personality and Social Psychology, 81,* 265–277.

Finkenauer, C., Engels, R. C., & Baumeister, R. F. (2005). Parenting and adolescent externalizing and internalizing problems: The role of self-control. *International Journal of Behavioral Development, 1,* 58–69.

Freud, S. (1949). *An outline of psychoanalysis.* New York: Norton.

Gray, J. R. (2004). Integration of emotion and cognitive control. *Current Directions in Psychological Science, 13,* 46–48.

Gunsch, D. (1996). *Self-determination and personality styles in intimate relationships.* Unpublished thesis, University of Osnabrück, Osnabrück, Germany

Halberstadt-Freud, H. C. (1993). Postpartum depression and symbiotic illusion. *Psychoanalytic Psychology, 10,* 407–423.

Hartung, J., & Schulte, D. (1994). Action and state orientation during therapy of phobic disorders. In J. Kuhl & J. Beckmann (Eds.), *Volition and personality: Action versus state orientation* (pp. 217–231). Seattle, WA: Hogrefe.

Haschke, R., & Kuhl, J. (1995). Frust und Fliegen [Frustration and flying]. *Aeromed Info, 6,* 1–2.

Heckhausen, H., & Strang, H. (1988). Efficiency under record performance demands: Exertion control—An individual difference variable? *Journal of Personality and Social Psychology, 55,* 489–498.

Humbert, C. (1981). *Choice of difficulty and performance after success and failure as a function of state orientation and standard setting.* Unpublished diploma thesis, Ruhr-University Bochum, Bochum, Germany.

Ickes, W., & Simpson, J. A. (2001). Motivational aspects of empathic accuracy. In G. J. O. Fletcher & M. Clark (Eds.), *The Blackwell handbook of social psychology: Interpersonal processes* (pp. 229–249). Oxford, UK: Blackwell.

Jang, K. L., Livesley, W. J., & Vernon, P. A. (1996). Heritability of the Big Five personality dimensions and their facets: A twin study. *Journal of Personality, 64,* 577–591.

Jostmann, N. B., & Finkenauer, C. (2004). *Action versus state orientation and relationship outcomes.* Unpublished data, Free University, Amsterdam.

Jostmann, N. B., & Koole, S. L. (2005a). *On the regulation of cognitive control: Effects of action orientation and external demands in Stroop-like tasks.* Unpublished manuscript, Free University, Amsterdam.

Jostmann, N. B., & Koole, S. L. (2005b). *Working memory under pressure: The moderating role of action versus orientation.* Unpublished manuscript, Free University, Amsterdam.

Jostmann, N. B., Koole, S. L., Van der Wulp, N., & Fockenberg, D. (2005). Subliminal affect regulation: The moderating role of action versus state orientation. *European Psychologist, 10,* 209–217.

Kazén, M., Baumann, N., & Kuhl, J. (2003). Self-infiltration versus self-compatibility checking in dealing with unattractive tasks: The moderating influence of state versus action orientation. *Motivation and Emotion, 27,* 157–197.

Keller, H. (2000). Human parent–child relationships from an evolutionary perspective. *American Behavioral Scientist, 43,* 957–969.

Keller, H., Lohaus, A., Völker, S., Cappenberg, M., & Chasiotis, A. (1999). Temporal contingency as a measure of interactional quality. *Child Development, 70,* 474–485.

Koole, S. L. (2004). Volitional shielding of the self: Effects of action orientation and external demands on implicit self-evaluation. *Social Cognition, 22,* 117–146.

Koole, S. L. (2005). *Effects of parental divorce on action versus state orientation among male and female university students.* Unpublished data set, Free University, Amsterdam.

Koole, S. L. , & Jostmann, N. B. (2004). Getting a grip on your feelings: Effects of action orientation and external demands on intuitive affect regulation. *Journal of Personality and Social Psychology, 87,* 974–990.

Koole, S. L., & Kuhl, J. (in press). Dealing with unwanted feelings: The role of affect regulation in volitional action control. In J. Shah & W. Gardner (Eds.), *Handbook of motivation science.* New York: Guilford Press.

Koole, S. L., Kuhl, J., Jostmann, N., & Vohs, K. D. (2005). On the hidden benefits of state orientation: Can people prosper without efficient affect regulation skills? In A. Tesser, J. Wood, & D. A. Stapel (Eds.), *On building, defending, and regulating the self: A psychological perspective* (pp. 217–243). London: Taylor & Francis.

Koole, S. L., & Van den Berg, A. E. (2005). Lost in the wilderness: Terror management, action orientation, and evaluations of nature. *Journal of Personality and Social Psychology, 88,* 1014–1028.

Kuhl, J. (1981). Motivational and functional helplessness: The moderating effect of state versus action orientation. *Journal of Personality and Social Psychology, 40,* 155–170.

Kuhl, J. (1983). Motivationstheoretische Aspekte der Depressionsgenese: Der Einfluss von Lageorientierung auf Schmerzempfinden, Medikamentenkonsum und Handlungskontrolle [Motivation-theoretical aspects of the development of depression: The influence of state orientation on the experience of pain, drug consumption and action control]. In M. Wolfersdorf, R. Staub, & G. Hole (Eds.), *Der depressiv Kranke in der psychiatrischen Klinik: Theorie und Praxis der Diagnostik und Therapie.* Weinheim: Beltz Verlag.

Kuhl, J. (1984). Volitional aspects of achievement motivation and learned helplessness: Toward a comprehensive theory of action-control. In B.A. Maher (Ed.), *Progress in experimental personality research* (Vol. 13, pp. 99–171). New York: Academic Press.

Kuhl, J. (1985). Volitional mediators of cognition–behavior consistency: Self-regulatory processes and action versus state orientation. In J. Kuhl & J. Beckmann (Eds.), *Action control: From cognition to behavior* (pp. 101–128). New York: Springer.

Kuhl, J. (1994). Action versus state orientation: Psychometric properties of the Action Control Scale (ACS-90). In J. Kuhl & J. Beckmann (Eds.), *Volition and personality: Action versus state orientation* (pp. 47–59). Göttingen, Germany: Hogrefe & Huber.

Kuhl, J. (2000). A functional-design approach to motivation and self-regulation: The dynamics of personality systems interactions. In M. Boekaerts, P. R. Pintrich, & M. Zeidner (Eds.), *Handbook of self-regulation* (pp. 111–169). San Diego, CA: Academic Press.

Kuhl, J., & Beckmann, J. (1994a). Alienation: Ignoring one's preferences. In J. Kuhl & J. Beckmann (Eds.), *Volition and personality: Action versus state orientation* (pp. 375–390). Göttingen, Germany: Hogrefe & Huber.

Kuhl, J., & Beckmann, J. (1994b). *Volition and personality: Action versus state orientation*. Göttingen, Germany: Hogrefe & Huber.

Kuhl, J., & Kazén, M. (1994). Self-discrimination and memory: State orientation and false self-ascription of assigned activities. *Journal of Personality and Social Psychology, 66,* 1103–1115.

Kuhl, J., & Kazén, M. (1997). *Das Persönlichkeits-Stil-und-Störungs-Inventar (PSSI): Manual* [Personality Styles and Disorders Inventory: Manual]. Göttingen, Germany: Hogrefe.

Kuhl, J., & Kazén, M. (2003). *Impress them or convince them?: Sales performance, social needs, and psychological well-being as a function of histrionic vs. action-oriented personality.* Unpublished manuscript, University of Osnabrück, Osnabrück, Germany.

Kuhl, J., & Koole, S. L. (2004). Workings of the will: A functional approach. In J. Greenberg, S. L. Koole, & T. Pyszczynski (Eds.), *Handbook of experimental existential psychology* (pp. 411–430). New York: Guilford Press.

Maier, S. F., & Seligman, M. E. P. (1976). Learned helplessness: Theory and evidence. *Journal of Experimental Psychology: General, 105,* 3–46.

Marszal-Wisniewska, M. (2001). Wychowawcze uwarunkowania orientacji na stan: Jak mozna nie wykstalcic silnej woli? [Educational antecedents of state orientation: How is it possible not to develop strong will?]. *Przeglad Psychologiczny, 44,* 479–494.

McClelland, D. C., Koestner, R., & Weinberger, J. (1989). How do self-attributed and implicit motives differ? *Psychological Review, 96,* 690–702.

McIntosh, D. N., Sedek, G., Fojas, S., Brzezicka-Rotkiewicz, A., & Kofta, M. (2005). Cognitive performance after pre-exposure to uncontrollability and in a depressive state: Going with a simpler "plan B". In R. Engle, G. Sedek, U. von Hecker, & D. N. McIntosh (Eds.), *Cognitive limitations in aging and psychopathology: Attention, working memory, and executive functions.* Cambridge, UK: Cambridge University Press.

Mikulincer, M., Shaver, P. R., & Pereg, D. (2003). Attachment theory and affect regulation: The dynamics, development, and cognitive consequences of attachment-related strategies. *Motivation and Emotion, 27,* 77–102.

Moretti, M. M., & Higgins, E. T. (1999). Internal representations of others in self-regulation: A new look at a classic issue. *Social Cognition, 17,* 186–208.

Muraven, M., & Baumeister, R. F. (2000). Self-regulation and depletion of limited resources: Does self-control resemble a muscle? *Pychological Bulletin, 126,* 247–259.

Murray, S. L., & Holmes, J. G. (1993). Seeing virtues in faults: Negativity and the transformation of interpersonal narratives in close relationships. *Journal of Personality and Social Psychology, 65,* 707–722.

Nolen-Hoeksema, S. (1987). Sex differences in unipolar depression: Evidence and theory. *Psychological Bulletin, 101,* 259–282.

Nowak, A., Vallacher, R. R., Tesser, A., & Borkowski, W. (2000). Society of self: The emergence of collective properties in self-structure. *Psychological Review, 107,* 39–61.

Olvermann, R., Metz-Göckel, H., Hannover, B., & Pöhlmann, C. (2004). Motivinhalte und Handlungs- versus Lageorientierung bei independenten oder interdependenten Personen [Motive contents and action versus state orientation among independent versus interdependent individuals]. *Zeitschrift für Differentielle und Diagnostische Psychologie, 25,* 87–103.

Palfai, T. P. (2002). Action-state orientation and the self-regulation of eating behavior. *Eating Behavior, 3,* 249–259.

Palfai, T. P., McNally, A. M., & Roy, M. (2002). Volition and alcohol-risk reduction: The role of action orientation in the reduction of alcohol-related harm among college student drinkers. *Addictive Behaviors, 27,* 309–317.

Repetti, R. L., Taylor, S. E., & Seeman, T. E. (2002). Risky families: Family social environments and the mental and physical health of offspring. *Psychological Bulletin, 128,* 330–366.

Rholes, W. S., Michas, L., & Shroff, J. (1989). Action control as a vulnerability factor in dysphoria. *Cognitive Therapy and Research, 13,* 263–274.

Ryan, R. M. & Deci, E. L. (2004). Autonomy is no illusion: Self-determination theory and the empirical study of authenticity, awareness, and will. In J. Greenberg, S. L. Koole, & T. Pyszczynski (Eds.), *Handbook of experimental existential psychology* (pp. 449–479). New York: Guilford Press.

Schore, A. N. (1996). *Affect regulation and the origin of the self: The neurobiology of emotional development.* Hillsdale, NJ: Erlbaum.

Schulte, D., Hartung, J., & Wilke, F. (1997). Handlungskontrolle der Angstbewältigung: Was macht Reizkonfrontationsverfahren so effektiv? [Action control in coping with anxiety: What makes exposure so effective?]. *Zeitschrift für Klinische Psychologie, 26,* 118–128.

Silverman, D. K. (2003). Mommy nearest: Revisiting the idea of infantile symbiosis and its implications for females. *Psychoanalytic Psychology, 20,* 261–270.

Silverman, L. H., & Weinberger, J. (1985). Mommy and I are one: Implications for psychotherapy. *American Psychologist, 40,* 1296–1308.

Simonson, I., & Staw, B. M. (1992). Deescalation strategies: A comparison of techniques for reducing commitment to losing courses of action. *Journal of Applied Psychology, 77,* 419–426.

Stiensmeier-Pelster, J., & Schürmann, M. (1994). Antecedents and consequences of action versus state orientation: Theoretical and empirical remarks. In J. Kuhl &

J. Beckmann (Eds.), *Volition and personality: Action versus state orientation* (pp. 329–340). Göttingen, Germany: Hogrefe & Huber.

Taylor, S. E., Lerner, J. S., Sage, R. M., Lehman, B. J., & Seeman, T. E. (2004). Early environment, emotions, responses to stress, and health. *Journal of Personality, 72,* 1365–1393.

Vallacher, R. R., & Nowak, A. (1999). The dynamics of self-regulation. In R. S. Wyer, Jr. (Ed.), *Advances in social cognition* (Vol. 12, pp. 241–259). Mahwah, NJ: Erlbaum.

Van Lange, P. A. M., & Rusbult, C. E. (1995). My relationship is better than—and not as bad as—yours is: The perception of superiority in close relationships. *Personality and Social Psychology Bulletin, 21,* 32–44.

Vohs, K. D., & Baumeister, R. F. (2004). Ego depletion, self-control, and choice. In J. Greenberg, S. L. Koole, & T. Pyszczynski (Eds.), *Handbook of experimental existential psychology* (pp. 398–410). New York: Guilford Press.

Wegner, D. M., & Erber, R. E. (1993). Social foundations of mental control. In D. M. Wegner & J. W. Pennebaker (Eds.), *Handbook of mental control* (pp. 36–56). Englewood Cliffs, NJ: Prentice-Hall.

Witte, E. H., & Von Pablocki, F. (1999). Differences in styles of behavior: State- and action-orientation in problem-solving dyads. *Psychologische Beiträge, 41,* 308–319.

INTERPERSONAL COGNITIVE PROCESSES

CHAPTER 19

When Your Wish Is My Desire

A Triangular Model of Self-Regulatory Relationships

JAMES SHAH

Since its very beginnings, social psychology has focused on how others affect our own pursuits and strivings (see Triplett, 1898). It has often been assumed that the scope of such social influence extends to the "psychological presence" of significant others in that we are influenced not only by the actual company of these individuals, but by how we mentally *represent* them, whether they be family, friends, colleagues, or even general "reference groups" (see, e.g., Bowlby, 1969; Kelley, 1952; Sherif, 1948). Indeed, there has been a long-standing emphasis in psychology on how such internal representations may come to influence our sense of self and efforts at self-regulation through, for instance, role taking (Mead, 1934), reflected self-appraisals (Cooley, 1902/ 1964), identification (Freud, 1912/1958), or the process of internalization (Schaffer, 1968). Surprisingly, however, there has been relatively little empirical exploration of how such "inner audiences" (see Horney, 1946; Moretti & Higgins, 1999b) are invoked and the cognitive mechanisms that may underlie their self-regulatory influence (but see Andersen & Glassman, 1996). Such influence may be quite strong given evidence suggesting that our self-representations are often associated with both our representations of close significant others and the goals, values, and expectations that these others have for us (whether these goals are to be pursued in the moment or over a lifetime) and come to influence our everyday behavior and subjective experiences (e.g., Hinkley & Andersen, 1996; Moretti & Higgins, 1999b).

Our mental construal of others, then, may impact our everyday behavior because of our relationship to significant others and their close association with various goals. Moreover, as with other cognitive associations, such associative effects may occur quite spontaneously. The mere activation of one's internal representation of a close other may be enough to invoke the goals with which this individual is associated. Unlike other goal associations, however, goal associations through significant others may depend on the nature of one's relationship to the significant other in question. The present chapter seeks to articulate the nature and consequences of such interpersonal goal associations by considering the different reasons why significant others may be associated with our goal pursuits, the different factors that may moderate such associations, and the various consequences of such activation for goal pursuit and self-regulation.

Moreover, in examining the implicit link between significant others and goals, the present chapter also seeks to explore another route through which goals may be linked to significant others that may have important implications for social relations and social behavior. Thus, just as an individual's significant others may invoke goals, so might an individual's goal pursuits automatically invoke significant others and affect how one feels about and behaves toward these individuals. When pursuing a goal, for instance, individuals may come to link this goal to significant others who would facilitate the goal's attainment or even to significant others who would likely provide feedback about the success of a pursuit. Such associations may serve to "prime" these significant others, affecting how they are perceived and acted toward.

A TRIANGLE OF SELF-REGULATORY RELATIONSHIPS

With both of the above possibilities in mind, then, the present chapter seeks to examine how and why we associate significant others with our goal pursuits and the implications of such associations not only for our social relationships but for our efforts at self-regulation. In doing so, this chapter presents a model of "self-regulatory relationships" that seeks to articulate how our representations of goals, significant others, and the self may be triangularly associated with each other, as illustrated in Figure 19.1. This model articulates three separate self-regulatory relationships: how individuals perceive themselves in relation to a goal, how they perceive themselves in relation to a significant other, and how the goal and the significant other in question are perceived to relate to each other. In highlighting the interdependence of our mental construals of self, goals, and significant others, this model specifies at least two routes through which our mental associations of our significant others may come to be associated with our goal pursuits. One route depends on the nature and strength of our relationship to significant others, while the other route

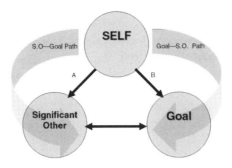

FIGURE 19.1. A triangular model of self-regulatory relationships.

depends on the nature and strength of our "relationship" to the goal in question. As discussed in greater detail below, each direction of association between significant other and goal (or goal and significant other) may not only have distinct determinants but also unique social and self-regulatory consequences.

WHEN SIGNIFICANT OTHERS ARE LINKED TO GOALS

Psychology has long noted the psychological relevance of our interpersonal construals (see Freud, 1912/1958; Sullivan, 1940, 1953). Indeed, recent research on the classic phenomenon of transference has offered ample evidence that the qualities, emotions, and motivations associated with close significant others may frequently be conferred on ourselves and those around us (e.g., Andersen & Berk, 1998; Andersen, Reznik, & Chen, 1997; Andersen, Reznik, & Manzella, 1996). Moreover, as originally noted by Freud (1912/1958), such transference may often occur quite automatically, requiring little, if any, conscious intent or awareness (see Glassman & Andersen, 1999). Baldwin, Carrell, and Lopez (1990), for instance, found that psychology graduate students assessed their own research ideas more negatively when they were primed with a scowling picture of their department chair than when they were primed with a smiling picture of a postdoctoral student. Similarly, practicing Catholic students were found to rate themselves more harshly when first subliminally presented with a scowling picture of the pope than when presented with the scowling picture of an unknown other. Interestingly, this effect was not found for "nonpracticing" Catholics whose identification with the pope was presumably weaker (see also Baldwin, 1992, 1994).

In line with these findings, the present analysis assumes that, in addition to affecting our evaluations of others and ourselves, our complex representations of significant others may also come to influence what we desire and pursue (see Kruglanski, 1996). Indeed, models of intrinsic motivation have long recognized that although everyday goals, such as those involving one's grades or athletic pursuits, may often arise from "internal" sources (involving needs for autonomy, competence, and relatedness), they may also result from external pressures, such as those originating from parents, friends, or authority figures (e.g., Deci & Ryan, 2000; Ryan & Deci, 2000). Similarly, self-discrepancy theory (see Higgins, 1999) assumes that in addition to pursuing our own ideals and obligations, we often pursue the ideals and obligations that significant others have for us. Moretti and Higgins (1999a), for example, demonstrated that the pursuit of these "external" goals may significantly influence psychological well-being and interpersonal functioning when these goals match one's own "internal" ideals and obligations. While these latter results suggest that significant others may influence our goal pursuits as we gradually come to internalize the goals that others have for us, the effects of significant others may often be more spontaneous: representations of important individuals may automatically trigger goal pursuit by increasing the salience of the goals that these individuals have for us.

Why might significant others become strongly associated with specific goals? The present analysis assumes that an important factor is the nature and strength of one's relationship to a significant other. The quality of one's relationship to a significant other may moderate the degree to which one understands and accepts the goals this individual has for him or her, and the goals this individual has for him- or herself. Moreover, one's relationship to significant others may also determine the degree to which these individuals come to "embody" a goal, as when an individual is a role model or a romantic interest. Each possibility is considered in some detail below.

The Goals That Significant Others Have for Us

To the extent that one has a close and positive relationship with a significant other, one may be more likely to be aware of and influenced by the goals this individual has for him or her, both consciously and automatically. Aron, Aron, Tudor, and Nelson (1991), for example, illustrated the cognitive significance of being in a close relationship in terms of how our representations of these individuals may be strongly associated (and even overlap) with our own sense of self. Such overlap may signify stronger self–other associations that extend to the goals these others have for us. Thus such overlap may facilitate the cognitive activation of goals through our representations of others (see also Brewer & Gardner, 1996; Read & Miller, 1989).

Shah (2003a) examined whether priming participants' representation of their father would increase their commitment to a task goal, especially when they perceived their father as wanting them to do well on the task. Participants were told that they would be completing a measure of analytic reasoning—

specifically, an anagram task that required them to unscramble letter strings to form as many words as possible using all of the presented letters. They were then given a questionnaire battery and, in the midst of a number of filler questions, were asked to rate how close they were to their father and how much their father would want them to pursue the task goal. Participants were then primed with words representing their father or with control words. Following this priming manipulation, participants were asked to assess how committed they were to pursuing the upcoming task goal. The dependent variable was the amount of commitment they reported having toward the task goal. As predicted, a Value to Father × Prime Condition interaction was revealed among participants close to their fathers. Specifically, commitment to the task goal significantly varied as a function of whether participants were primed with father-related words and whether they perceived their father as wanting them to pursue the goal.

The Goals That Significant Others Have for Themselves: Goal Contagion

The nature and strength of our relationship to significant others may also increase the degree to which we recognize and nonconsciously adopt the goals that our significant others are themselves actively pursuing. Indeed, we may automatically "catch" these goals—as we may often "catch" moods and mannerisms—via contagion effects (Chartrand & Bargh, 1999; Neumann & Strack, 2000). Aarts, Gollwitzer, and Hassin (2004), for instance, have found considerable evidence that individuals may generally adopt and pursue a goal that is implied through another's behavior, assuming that he or she views the goal as "appropriate." Participants exposed to a story suggesting that an individual had the goal to earn money were subsequently more eager to complete a task that could potentially earn them money than participants not exposed to such a goal prime.

The Goals That Significant Others Embody

Finally, a third possibility is that significant others may themselves come to embody or personify a goal, whether one want to "be like Mike" (as in the case of role models) or to "be with Mike" (as in the case of romantic attachments). Indeed, recent work by Lockwood and Kunda (2000) has convincingly demonstrated the direct motivational impact of role models and the degree to which this impact may vary as a function of the role model's personal relevance. Moreover, work by Andersen and her colleagues on the process of transference has found that the specific interpersonal goals individuals may have to be closer to a significant other may often be transferred to new individuals who resemble this significant other (see Andersen & Berk, 1998; Andersen et al., 1996). This possibility awaits, and warrants, more direct study.

Moderating Conditions: The Self, the Significant Other, and the Relationship

Of course not all of our representations of others have quite the same impact on our motivations and goal pursuits. Different individuals may bring to mind different types of goals and may do so with differing levels of effectiveness. Thus, although some mothers may generally invoke goals relating to our careers or family, other mothers may not invoke such goals so readily. The present analysis also assumes that aspects of the individual, of the significant other, and of the relationship between them may all potentially moderate the degree to which significant others automatically invoke goals (see Andersen et al., 1997, for a similar perspective).

First, specific qualities of one's significant other may boost or diminish his or her implicit motivational impact. One may be more likely to be influenced, for instance, by a relatively powerful or attractive significant other or one that clearly (and unambiguously) conveys what he or she wants you to pursue. Indeed, parents certainly differ in the range of goals they have for their child. While a greater number of goals may suggest a wider range of parental influence, such breadth may actually limit the degree to which a parent invokes any particular goal very strongly. Such a possibility is reminiscent of the classic "fan effect" (Anderson & Berk, 1998) in which the greater the number of specific facts linked to a general mental construct (i.e., the greater the general construct's "fan size"), the less likely any particular fact will be retrieved or recalled. Moreover, even when parents strongly invoke multiple goals in their child, these goals may end up competing with each other for regulatory resources, limiting the degree to which any would be acted upon. Thus, whether through response competition or through spreading activation, the motivational "ambiguity" of our significant other representations may limit the degree to which they invoke any particular goal, all other factors being equal.

With this in mind, Shah (2003a) examined whether the effect of priming participants' significant other on task goal accessibility and task goal commitment were dependent on the number of other goals participants' significant other also had for them. Participants in this study were told that they would complete an anagram task (this time described as "a measure of verbal fluency") and asked to provide the name of a significant other who would want them to do well on the task. Participants were also asked to indicate all the other goals this significant other had for them. Participants then completed the lexical decision task described earlier and were either primed with the name of a significant other or with a control prime. Finally, they were asked to indicate how committed they were to doing well on the upcoming anagram task. As illustrated in the plot of the predicted values presented in Figure 19.2, priming participants' significant other was more likely to affect the accessibility of the task goal and participants' commitment to it when the primed significant other had relatively few other goals for the participant (rather than numerous other goals).

The degree to which one is influenced by significant others may also depend on characteristics of the person and the situation. For example, just as work by Chartrand and Bargh (1999) indicates that empathic individuals are more likely to imitate the social actions of others, so too might empathic individuals be more likely to take on others' goals. Moreover, a strong social pressure to conform (e.g., like that seen in many Asian cultures; see Markus & Kitayama, 1991) may increase the degree to which significant others automatically activate goals. Similarly, various individual differences such as empathy, authoritarianism, and one's interdependent sense of self may all moderate the implicit effect of others. Indeed, van Baaren, Maddux, Chartrand, de Bouter, and van Knippenberg (2003) recently found that differences in self-construals affected nonconscious social behavior more generally. Specifically, individuals primed with words meant to activate their interdependent sense of self were

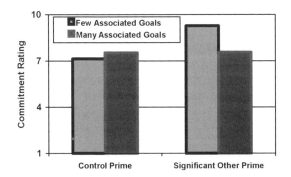

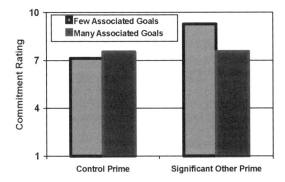

FIGURE 19.2. Goal commitment and accessibility as a function of significant other goal priming and the number of other goals associated with the significant other.

more likely to nonconsciously mimic an interaction partner than individuals primed with words representing their independent self. Such moderation may extend to the nonconscious mimicking of significant others' goals.

Finally, as suggested above, goal priming through significant others may be distinct from other forms of goal priming in being dependent on the often complex relationship we have to our significant others. Shah (2003a), for instance, found that the degree to which significant others primed goals depended on the participants' closeness to their significant other. Indeed, when individuals are not close to their significant other, priming this close other may actually inhibit the goals he or she has for an individual. Similarly, Chartrand, Dalton, and Fitzsimons (2005) recently found that reactant relationships to significant others may lead individuals to adopt the *opposite* goal than that primed by a significant other in an achievement setting. Moreover, individuals' general level of reactance was also found to moderate the effect of significant other goal priming. Whereas individuals with low reactance assimilated to the goal primed by significant others, individuals with high general reactance pursued a goal opposite to that primed by their significant others.

Considering the Conscious Consequences of Significant Other Goal Priming

Significant other representations may do more than simply activate or deactivate goals and goal commitment. Indeed, these representations may have more complex and "conscious" effects on the process of goal pursuit by implicitly affecting how goals are perceived and appraised. There is already a body of literature suggesting that the way we view ourselves and others can be affected by nonconscious mental processes (Bargh, 1990). The large literature on the process of stereotyping, for instance, has recently documented ways in which the activation and application of our stereotypes are influenced by automatic mental processes (Devine, 1989; Kawakami, Dion, & Dovidio, 1998; Lepore & Brown, 1997; Moskowitz, Gollwitzer, & Schaal, 1999).

Goal-Related Appraisals

If priming stereotypes can affect how we see others, priming significant others may certainly affect how we see ourselves, and perhaps our own goals and intentions. Specifically, our representations of significant others may not only activate goal representations and influence goal commitment generally, but might further affect the very nature of our goal representations by implicitly influencing how we appraise these goals. The degree to which we perceive a goal to be difficult or enjoyable, for example, may be implicitly influenced by our thoughts of whether a significant other thinks it will be difficult (or boring) for us to pursue.

Shah (2003b) asked participants to complete an anagram task, which consisted of a set of eight anagram puzzles and was described as "a measure of verbal fluency." Before completing this task, participants were asked to provide the name of a significant other who would most likely appraise the value of the task for them. Participants were also asked to estimate how valuable their significant other would perceive the task goal to be for them. Participants were then either primed with the name of this significant other or with a control nonword. This priming manipulation was followed by an assessment of participants' actual goal pursuit, as measured by how long they persisted on the anagram task and how many solutions they found. As seen in the predicted values presented in Figure 19.3, priming the participants' significant other increased anagram persistence and performance relative to the control prime condition when this significant other perceived the task goal to be valuable for the participant. In contrast, priming the participants' significant other decreased anagram persistence and performance relative to the control prime

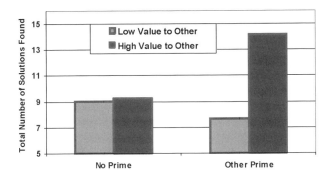

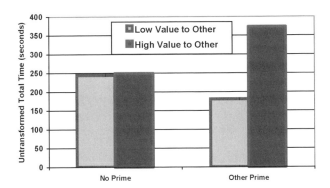

FIGURE 19.3. Anagram performance and persistence as a function of significant other priming and the degree to which the task goal was important to the significant other.

condition when this significant other perceived the task goal to be of little value for the participant.

Shah (2003b) also examined whether priming participants' representation of a significant other would affect their estimations of the difficulty of a presented task goal and their subsequent pursuit of the goal. While completing an anagram task, participants were subliminally primed with either a control word or with the name of a significant other who had an expectation about the task difficulty in order to examine how this priming might influence their estimations of the difficulty of the task. The expectations of a significant other (as perceived by the participants) was found to more strongly influence participants' own appraisals of goal difficulty when the name of this significant other was subliminally primed during the task.

Goal-Related Affective Experiences

Whether we realize it or not, significant other goal priming may also come to affect how we experience goal-related successes and failures. Indeed, the growing body of evidence on "mystery moods" has documented the various ways in which our mood can be mysteriously (i.e., nonconsciously) influenced by processes that occur outside of our awareness, intent, and sometimes control (Chartrand, 2003; Chartrand, van Baaren, & Bargh, in press). That is, an automatic mental process ensues, and as a result we are in a good or bad mood without knowing why. We cannot identify the source or origin of the mood, and we cannot articulate why we feel the way we do.

Can the presence of significant others activate nonconscious self-regulatory processes that ultimately result in mystery moods? Significant other priming has been shown to influence how generally positive or negative one feels about goal attainment and goal failure. Shah (2003b) gave participants an anagram task and primed them with the name of a significant other or a control word. After completing the task, participants were either given feedback that they had attained the task goal of finding 80% of all the possible solutions, feedback that they had not attained this goal, or no feedback. Finally, participants' general satisfaction with their performance was assessed. As can be seen in Figure 19.4, the extent of participants' general reaction to positive and negative feedback varied as a function of whether their significant other had been primed and whether participants' significant other placed a high value on their attainment of the task goal.

Significant others may not only affect the extent of one's general emotional reaction to successful and unsuccessful goal pursuit, but the quality of this emotional reaction. Indeed, Shah (2003b) found evidence suggesting that significant others may alter the way in which goals are perceived to relate to fundamental needs for promotion and prevention, as detailed by regulatory focus theory (Higgins, 1997). This theory has linked the pursuit of promotion-

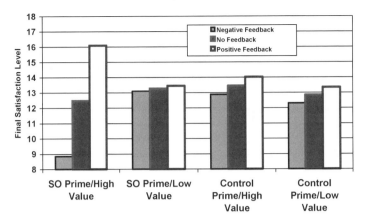

FIGURE 19.4. Final satisfaction rating as a function of significant other priming, the value that the significant other places in the task goal, and performance feedback.

related goals (ideals) to cheerfulness- and dejection-related emotions and the pursuit of prevention-related goals (oughts) to quiescence- and agitation-related emotions (see also Higgins, Shah, & Friedman, 1997). With this theory in mind, Shah examined whether priming participants' representation of their father would influence their regulatory focus with regards to a task goal commensurate with (1) the degree to which participants believed their father wanted them to pursue this goal (thus encouraging a promotion focus with respect to the task goal) and (2) the degree to which they believed their father would view it as their duty or obligation to pursue the goal (thus encouraging a prevention focus with respect to the task goal). Participants again completed an anagram task that was described as "an important measure of analytic reasoning." While they completed this task, they were subliminally primed either with words representing the concept "father" or with control words. This allowed Shah to examine the effect of this priming on participants' emotional reaction to manipulated performance feedback in terms of relaxation- and agitation-related emotions (i.e., emotions pertaining to a prevention focus with respect to the task goal) and cheerfulness- and dejection-related emotions (i.e., emotions pertaining to a promotion focus). The results indicated that priming participants' representation of their father increased participants' emotional reaction to the feedback in terms of cheerfulness- and dejection-related emotions when the participants had perceived that their father would ideally want them to perform well on the task. The results also indicated that priming participants' representation of their father increased participants' emotional reaction to the feedback in terms of relaxation- and agitation-related emotions when the participants had perceived that their father thought that they had a duty or responsibility to perform well on the task.

These results are illustrated in Figure 19.5, which plots the predicted values for participants' emotion scores (with higher scores indicating greater cheerfulness or relaxation).

In summary, then, individuals' relationship to significant others may influence the degree to which they associate a given significant other with goals that the significant other wants them to pursue, is pursuing him- or herself, or that the significant other embodies his- or herself. This interpersonal route to goal priming may be unique in its dependence on the often complex relationship individuals have with their significant others, and may have implications not only for the automatic ignition or extinction of goal pursuit but for the conscious ways in which we appraise and experience goals.

As suggested above, however, this route represents only "half the story" with respect to how and why goals may be associated with significant others. The manner in which our relationship (commitment) to goals may ultimately link them to significant others is considered in some detail below.

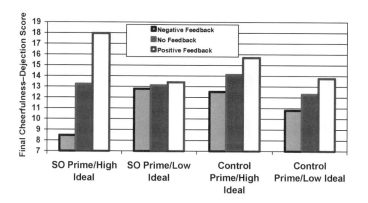

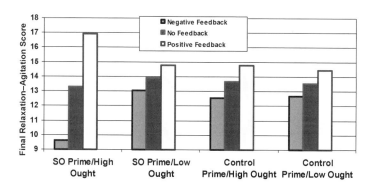

FIGURE 19.5. Final emotion ratings as a function of significant other priming, the regulatory focus that the significant other places in the task goal, and performance feedback.

WHEN GOALS ARE LINKED TO SIGNIFICANT OTHERS

Just as psychology has long noted the social influence on goal pursuit, there is almost an equally long history of examining how people's personal concerns influence their social appraisals. Kelly (1955), for instance, discussed how personal constructs such as "gentleness versus aggressiveness" act as a personal scanning pattern projected on the world that pick up blips of meaning. New Look psychologists have examined how individuals' chronic states (e.g., religious beliefs or economic status) and current concerns (e.g., hunger and thirst) influence how they perceive and appraise relevant objects in the environment (for reviews, see Allport, 1955; Bruner, 1957; Jones & Gerard, 1967).

More recently, Bargh, Gollwitzer, Lee-Chai, Barndollar, and Trötschel (2001) have examined how goal priming may influence social behavior. For example, in an experimentally derived situation in which their teammate (actually a confederate) had performed poorly on a team task, participants primed with the goal to be sociable performed down to the level of their teammate so as not to humiliate him or her. In contrast, participants primed with the goal to achieve strove to excel on the task, regardless of the potential humiliation to their teammate.

The present analysis focuses on another route through which goal activation (either via priming or conscious commitment) may come to have social implications: individuals may come to associate goals with those significant others who would aid their attainment. Such significant others may actively help one attain goals or may simply constitute social mirrors that reflect one's various desired attributes, serving as comparison standards to assess, and possibly facilitate, progress. Indeed, Shah and Kruglanski (2003) have recently found evidence suggesting that goals may be primed by attainment means in a bottom-up fashion, whether these means constitute situations, behaviors, or other individuals. Implicitly associating goals to facilitative significant others may not only have implications for goal progress (because these significant others may actually aid goal attainment), but may also affect how one comes to perceive and act toward a significant other. When actively focused on a goal pursuit, for instance, individuals may implicitly draw psychologically and physically closer to those individuals whom they believe will help them attain the goal.

With this in mind, Fitzsimons and Shah (2005) asked participants to provide the name of a friend who would most help them to achieve academically as well as a friend who would least help them achieve in this domain. After listing a number of other friends and completing a series of filler tasks, participants were either primed with achievement-related words or control words through the use of the scrambled sentence task (see Bargh & Chartrand, 2000). Finally, participants completed a rating of the general importance of these significant others. As illustrated in Figure 19.6, participants were signifi-

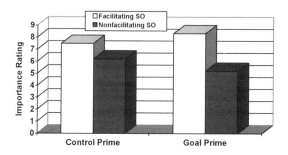

FIGURE 19.6. The effect of goal priming on the importance rating of significant others who are facilitating and nonfacilitating of goal attainment.

cantly more likely to report their "facilitating" friend as important in comparison to their nonfacilitating friend when first primed with the goal to achieve.

Fitzsimons and Shah (2005) also had participants complete a questionnaire after the priming procedure that asked them to indicate how close they felt to their friends, using the Subjective Closeness Index and the Inclusion of Other in Self Scale, and how much time they planned to spend with these friends in the upcoming week. In comparison to the control condition, participants primed with an achievement goal were significantly more likely to report being closer to their friend who facilitated achievement than to their nonfacilitating friend. These participants were also more likely to report the intention to spend more time with their "facilitating" friend than with their "nonfacilitating" friend (see Figure 19.7).

The above analysis can be extended further if one considers the different reasons one may commit to goals. Regulatory focus theory (Higgins, 1997, 1998), for instance, suggests that individuals may adopt goals to fulfill needs for achievement and gain (promotion) or for safety and security (prevention), and that these different reasons may specify how goals are pursued in terms of approach and avoidance behaviors.

Although such a possibility has yet to be examined with respect to individuals' long-standing significant others, Shah, Brazy, and Higgins (2004) have examined how individuals' chronic focus on promotion and prevention may impact behavior toward "situationally defined" significant others—in this case, teammates and competitors in a experimentally defined team competition. In this study, Shah and colleagues measured participants' chronic regulatory focus toward promotion and prevention and then presented them with a "team goal" in which they would be competing with a teammate against two competitors. Based on past research (see Crowe & Higgins, 1997; Shah, Higgins, & Friedman, 1998), it was assumed that participants with a chronic promotion focus (i.e., focus on gain or achievement) would perceive the given

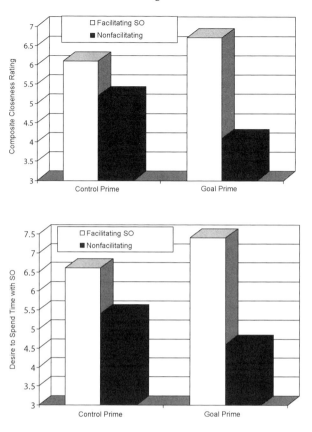

FIGURE 19.7. The effect of goal priming on subjective closeness to significant others who are facilitating or nonfacilitating of goal attainment.

team goal as an "ideal," or an opportunity for advancement, and tend to pursue this goal with approach behavior. Participants with a chronic prevention focus (i.e., focus on security from threat) would perceive the presented goal as an obligation against threat and tend to pursue it using avoidance behavior. It was predicted that such behavioral inclinations would be evident in how participants interacted with teammates and competitors during the team game. Modifying the procedure employed by Macrae, Bodenhausen, Milne, and Jetten (1994), the researchers asked participants to take a seat in a waiting room to await the team game. They were led to believe that one of the seats in this room was already "taken" (as indicated by a bag) by either their teammate or one of their competitors. As indicated in Table 19.1, participants' chronic promotion focus (which presumably caused them to value the task goal as an ideal) positively predicted how close participants sat to the chair they believed

TABLE 19.1. Approach and Avoidance of Teammate versus Competitor as a Function of Regulatory Focus

	Type of interpersonal behavior	
Regulatory focus strength	Teammate approach	Competitor distancing
Ideal strength (promotion)	.31*	−.13
Ought strength (prevention)	−.14	.28*

Note. N = 141.
*p < .05.

belonged to their teammate since this individual would presumably aid goal attainment. Alternatively, participants' prevention focus (which presumably caused them to value the task goal as an obligation) predicted how far participants sat from a competitor, since this individual could presumably hinder goal attainment.

FUTURE DIRECTIONS

Just as the analysis can be expanded to consider different types of "relationships" an individual might have with goals (e.g., promotion- vs. prevention-focused), so might it also be expanded to consider a wider range of social consequences. Future studies, for example, could profitably explore how associating goals with significant others may come to affect the various ways in which we perceive and interact with these individuals.

Goal focus, for instance, may not only affect our approach and avoidance of significant others, and the manner in which we appraise these individuals overall, it may also affect the way in which we appraise our significant others. We may, for instance, be more likely to appraise individuals along an evaluative dimension that is particularly relevant to a current goal pursuit. Shah and Higgins (2001), for instance, found that individuals were quicker to appraise common attitude objects along emotional dimensions that were distinctly relevant to their current regulatory focus. Thus individuals with a relatively strong promotion focus were quicker to appraise these objects in terms of how cheerful and dejected they made them feel, whereas individuals with a relatively strong prevention focus were relatively quicker to appraise objects in terms of how relaxed and agitated they made them feel. The same type of distinct appraisals might also be applied to significant others.

Individuals' goal focus may also affect how individuals perceive the relation between their various significant others. Two significant others may be seen as more similar to each other, or even more substitutable, if both happen to facilitate the attainment of a currently active goal pursuit. Such relational appraisals may have significant implications for friendship patterns and social group interaction and await future study.

AN INTERACTIVE TRIANGLE

Finally, although the above analysis suggests two distinct routes though which significant others may become associated with goals, the "triangular" model of associations detailed in Figure 19.1 also allows one to consider how the two routes detailed above may, in fact, interact with each other. It suggests the possibility, for instance, that the ease by which a significant other may bring to mind a particular goal may be moderated by one's a priori "relationship" or commitment to that goal. Indeed, Bargh (1990) has asserted that a priori acceptance of a goal would be a prerequisite for goal priming generally and increased levels of goal commitment may correspondingly increase one's susceptibility to the corresponding motivational associations of a significant other.

Alternatively, the degree to which a goal may bring to mind a particular significant other may depend not only on the degree to which that significant other helps one to attain the goal but also on one's a priori relation to the significant other. An individual may turn first to close significant others because he or she has a more complete understanding of how these people can help him or her attain a goal or because he or she assumes that a close significant other would be more likely to provide direct assistance.

Such possibilities await more direct examination and only highlight the complex interdependency of our self, goal, and significant other representations and the triangle of associations among them. Clearly, the examination of how these representations influence each other has just begun. The aim of the present chapter is to provide at least an initial framework for continuing this exploration as well as a sense of its importance for a complete understanding of self-regulation and social relations.

REFERENCES

Aarts, H., Gollwitzer, P. M., & Hassin, R. R. (2004). Goal contagion: Perceiving is for pursuing. *Journal of Personality and Social Psychology, 87,* 23–37.

Allport, F. H. (1955). *Theories of perception and the concept of structure.* New York: Wiley.

Andersen, S. M., & Berk, M. S. (1998). Transference in everyday experience: Implications of experimental research for relevant clinical phenomena. *Review of General Psychology, 2,* 81–120.

Andersen, S. M., & Glassman, N. S. (1996). Responding to significant others when they are not there: Effects of interpersonal inference, motivation, and affect. In

R. M. Sorrentino & E. T. Higgins (Eds.), *Handbook of motivation and cognition: Vol. 3. The interpersonal context* (Vol. 3, pp. 262–321). New York: Guilford Press.

Andersen, S. M., Reznik, I., & Chen, S. (1997). The self in relation to others: Motivational and cognitive underpinnings. *Annals of the New York Academy of Sciences, 818,* 233–275.

Andersen, S. M., Reznik, I., & Manzella, L. M. (1996). Eliciting transient affect, motivation, and expectancies in transference: Significant-other representations and the self in social relations. *Journal of Personality and Social Psychology, 71,* 1108–1129.

Aron, A., Aron, E. N., Tudor, M., & Nelson, G. (1991). Close relationships as including other in the self. *Journal of Personality and Social Psychology, 60,* 241–253.

Baldwin, M. W. (1992). Relational schemas and the processing of social information. *Psychological Bulletin, 112,* 461–484.

Baldwin, M. W. (1994). Primed relational schemas as a source of self-evaluative reactions. *Journal of Social and Clinical Psychology, 13,* 380–403.

Baldwin, M. W., Carrell, S. E., & Lopez, D. F. (1990). Priming relationship schemas: My advisor and the pope are watching me from the back of my mind. *Journal of Experimental Social Psychology, 26,* 435–454.

Bargh, J. A. (1990). Auto-motives: Preconscious determinants of social interacting. In E. T. Higgins & R. M. Sorrentino (Eds.), *Handbook of motivation and cognition: Vol. 2. Foundations of social behavior* (pp. 93–130). New York: Guilford Press.

Bargh, J. A., & Chartrand, T. (2000). Studying the mind in the middle: A practical guide to priming and automaticity research. In H. Reis & C. Judd (Eds.), *Handbook of research methods in social psychology* (pp. 253–285). New York: Cambridge University Press.

Bargh, J. A., Gollwitzer, P. M., Lee-Chai, A., Barndollar, K., & Trötschel, R. (2001). The automated will: Nonconscious activation and pursuit of behavioral goals. *Journal of Personality and Social Psychology, 81,* 1014–1027.

Bowlby, J. (1969). *Attachment and loss: Vol. 1. Attachment.* New York: Basic Books.

Brewer, M. B., & Gardner, W. (1996). Who is this "we"?: Levels of collective identity and self representations. *Journal of Personality and Social Psychology, 71,* 83–93.

Bruner, J. S. (1957). On perceptual readiness. *Psychological Review, 64,* 123–152.

Chartrand, T. L. (2003). *Mystery moods and perplexing performance: Consequences of succeeding and failing at a nonconscious goal.* Manuscript under review.

Chartrand, T. L., & Bargh, J. A. (1999). The chameleon effect: The perception–behavior link and social interaction. *Journal of Personality and Social Psychology, 76,* 893–910.

Chartrand, T. L., van Baaren, R., & Bargh, J. A. (in press). Linking automatic evaluation to mood and information processing style: Consequences for experienced affect, information processing, and stereotyping. *Journal of Experimental Psychology: General.*

Chartrand, T. L., Dalton, A., & Fitzsimons, G. J. (2005). *Automatic reactance to significant others.* Work in progress, Department of Psychology, Duke University, Durham, NC.

Cooley, C. H. (1964). *Human nature and the social order.* New York: Schocken Books. (Original work published 1902)

Crowe, E., & Higgins, E. T. (1997). Regulatory focus and strategic inclinations: Promotion and prevention in decision-making. *Organizational Behavior and Human Decision Processes, 69,* 117–132.

Deci, E. L., & Ryan, R. M. (2000). The "what" and "why" of goal pursuits: Human needs and the self-determination of behavior. *Psychological Inquiry, 11,* 227–268.

Devine, P. G. (1989). Stereotypes and prejudice: Their automatic and controlled components. *Journal of Personality and Social Psychology, 56,* 5–18.

Fitzsimons, G. M., & Shah, J. Y. (2005). *Instrumentally yours: How goal pursuits automatically affect social relations.* Manuscript in preparation.

Freud, S. (1958). The dynamics of transference. In J. Strachey (Ed. & Trans.), *The standard edition of the complete psychological works of Sigmund Freud* (Vol. 12, pp. 97–108). London: Hogarth Press. (Original work published 1912)

Glassman, N. S., & Andersen, S. M. (1999). Activating transference without consciousness: Using significant-other representations to go beyond what is subliminally given. *Journal of Personality and Social Psychology, 77,* 1146–1162.

Higgins, E. T. (1997). Beyond pleasure and pain. *American Psychologist, 52,* 1280–1300.

Higgins, E. T. (1998). Promotion and prevention: Regulatory focus as a motivational principle. In M. P. Zanna (Ed.), *Advances in experimental social psychology* (Vol. 30, pp. 1–46). New York: Academic Press.

Higgins, E. T. (1999). Self-discrepancy: A theory relating self and affect. In R. F. Baumeister (Ed.), *The self in social psychology* (pp. 150–181). Philadelphia: Psychology Press.

Hinkley, K., & Andersen, S. M. (1996). The working self-concept in transference: Significant-other activation and self change. *Journal of Personality and Social Psychology, 71,* 1279–1295.

Horney, K. (1946). *Our inner conflicts: A constructive theory of neurosis.* London: Routledge & Kegan Paul.

Jones, E. E., & Gerard, H. B. (1967). *Foundations of social psychology.* New York: Wiley.

Kawakami, K., Dion, K. L., & Dovidio, J. F. (1998). Racial prejudice and stereotype activation. *Personality and Social Psychology Bulletin, 24,* 407–416.

Kelley, H. H. (1952). Two functions of reference groups. In G. E. Swanson, T. M. Newcomb, & E. L. Hartley (Eds.), *Readings in social psychology* (2nd ed., pp. 410–420). New York: Holt, Rinehart & Winston.

Kelly, G. A. (1955). *A theory of personality: The psychology of personal constructs.* New York: Norton.

Kruglanski, A. W. (1996). Goals as knowledge structures. In P. M. Gollwitzer & J. A. Bargh (Eds.), *The psychology of action: Linking cognition and motivation to behavior* (pp. 599–618). New York: Guilford Press.

Lepore, L., & Brown, R. (1997). Category and stereotype activation: Is prejudice inevitable? *Journal of Personality and Social Psychology, 72,* 275–287.

Lockwood, P., & Kunda, Z. (2000). Outstanding role models: Do they inspire or demoralize us? In A. Tesser & R. B. Felson (Eds.), *Psychological perspectives on self and identity* (pp. 147–171). Washington, DC : American Psychological Association.

Macrae, C. N., Bodenhausen, G. V., Milne, A. B., & Jetten, J. (1994). Out of mind but back in sight: Stereotypes on the rebound. *Journal of Personality and Social Psychology, 67,* 808–817.

Markus, H. R., & Kitayama, S. (1991). Culture and the self: Implications for cognition, emotion, and motivation. *Psychological Review, 98*, 224–253.

Mead, G. H. (1934). *Mind, self, and society.* Chicago: University of Chicago Press.

Moretti, M. M., & Higgins, E. T. (1999a). Internal representations of others in self-regulation: A new look at a classic issue. *Social Cognition, 17*, 186–208.

Moretti, M. M., & Higgins, E. T. (1999b). Own versus other standpoints in self-regulation: Developmental antecedents and functional consequences. *Review of General Psychology, 3*, 188–223.

Moskowitz, G. B., Gollwitzer, P. M., Wasel, W., & Schaal, B. (1999). Preconscious control of stereotype activation through chronic egalitarian goals. *Journal of Personality and Social Psychology, 77*, 167–184.

Neumann, R., & Strack, F. (2000). "Mood contagion": The automatic transfer of mood between persons. *Journal of Personality and Social Psychology, 79*, 211–223.

Read, S. J., & Miller, L. C. (1989). Inter-personalism: Toward a goal-based theory of persons in relationships. In L. A. Pervin (Ed.), *Goal concepts in personality and social psychology* (pp. 413–472). Hillsdale, NJ: Erlbaum.

Ryan, R. M., & Deci, E. L. (2000). Intrinsic and extrinsic motivations: Classic definitions and new directions. *Contemporary Educational Psychology, 25*, 54–67.

Schaffer, R. (1968). *Aspects of internalization.* New York: International Universities Press.

Shah, J. Y. (2003a). Automatic for the people: How representations of others implicitly affect goal pursuit. *Journal of Personality and Social Psychology, 84*, 661–681.

Shah, J. Y. (2003b). The motivational looking glass: How significant others implicitly affect goal appraisals. *Journal of Personality and Social Psychology, 85*(3), 424–439.

Shah, J. Y., Brazy, P. B., & Higgins, E. T. (2004). Promoting us or preventing them: Regulatory focus and the nature of ingroup bias. *Personality and Social Psychology Bulletin, 30*, 433–446.

Shah, J. Y., & Higgins, E. T. (2001). Regulatory concerns and appraisal efficiency: The general impact of promotion and prevention. *Journal of Personality and Social Psychology, 80*, 693–705.

Shah, J. Y., Higgins, E. T., & Friedman, R. F. (1998). Performance incentives and means: How regulatory focus influences goal attainment. *Journal of Personality and Social Psychology, 74*, 285–293.

Shah, J. Y., & Kruglanski, A. W. (2003). When opportunity knocks: Bottom-up priming of goals by means and its effects on self-regulation. *Journal of Personality and Social Psychology, 84*, 1109–1122.

Sherif, M. (1948). *An outline of psychology.* New York: Harper.

Sullivan, H. S. (1940). *Conceptions of modern psychiatry.* New York: Norton.

Sullivan, H. S. (1953). *The interpersonal theory of psychiatry.* New York: Norton.

Triplett, N. (1898). Dynamogenic factors in pacemaking and competition. *American Journal of Psychology, 9*, 507–533.

van Baaren, R., Maddux, W. W., Chartrand, T.L., de Bouter, C., & van Knippenberg, A. (2003). It takes two to mimic: Behavioral consequences of self-construals. *Journal of Personality and Social Psychology, 84*, 1093–1102.

CHAPTER 20

Succeeding at Self-Control through a Focus on Others

The Roles of Social Practice and Accountability in Self-Regulation

ELIZABETH A. SEELEY
WENDI L. GARDNER

Whenever I am tempted I think of my kids and it helps
me make better decisions.
—Posted May 29, 2004, on the 3FC
Healthy Community Weight Loss Board

Hundreds of comments like the one above, recently volunteered by a member of a weight loss support website, are posted across a variety of bulletin boards that share the common goal of helping people to maintain self-control. Whether an individual is quitting smoking, losing weight, or combating an alcohol, drug, sex, or even shopping addiction, the sentiments expressed in the quote above are omnipresent: thoughts of loved ones are believed to provide an effective shield against temptation. It is, upon reflection, a somewhat odd notion. *Self*-control is, by definition, an individual process, often cast as an internal battle in which the executive (or ego) attempts to restrain the dangerous desires of the id (Freud, 1923/1961). Yet, when that drink, cigarette, or hot fudge sundae seems irresistibly enticing, individuals seem to recruit thoughts of others to assist them in their struggle to achieve a desired goal.

The current chapter, like the others in this volume, examines the inter-play between interpersonal relationships and intrapersonal processes. Spe-cifically, we are interested in the manner in which external social relationships often pervade the seemingly internal process of self-control. What role do close others play in prompting and maintaining self-regulatory endeavors? In this chapter we discuss just a few of the potential functions social relationships may serve in the self-regulation process. First, we discuss the social underpin-nings of self-regulation in general. Second, we review research examining individual differences in social sensitivity, and argue that maintaining harmo-nious social relations serves to strengthen self-regulatory "muscles." Third, we discuss how disclosing goals to close others may spur self-regulatory success through enhancing accountability, removing the burden of choice from the self-control process.

THE SOCIAL ROOTS OF SELF-REGULATION

Why would humans engage in self-regulation at all? At first glance the abil-ity to refuse fattening foods or attractive potential mates would not necessar-ily seem a skill that evolutionary forces would favor. Indeed, the media often argue that it is the ancestral appeal of some of these temptations that makes them so difficult to resist, that their allure is woven into our very DNA (see, e.g., "How We Grew So Big"; Lemonick, 2004). What these views may have overlooked, however, is the equally primal and powerful pull of belonging needs (e.g., Baumeister & Leary, 1995; Caporael, 1997; Gardner, Pickett, & Brewer, 2000; Heatherton & Vohs, 1998; Williams, 2001).

According to Heatherton and Vohs (1998), self-control is a fundamentally social process, shaped through cultural forces and driven by our basic need to be socially accepted. Their argument rests on an evolutionary perspective. They argue that those individuals who were able to control their behavior to meet group requirements would have avoided being expelled from social groups and would have derived numerous benefits (e.g., shared resources and workloads). Help from others would have increased chances of survival and reproduction, thereby perpetuating the need to belong and the accompanying self-regulatory skills. Although the requirements of our social groups may change over time (e.g., share the day's catch vs. don't smoke in public spaces), the need to override one's impulses in order to satisfy the group is still the same today.

Complementing the evolutionary perspective on the social roots of self-regulation are perspectives that emphasize the modern importance of a desire to fit in and get along with close others (e.g., Jackson, Mackenzie, & Hobfoll, 2000; Vohs & Ciarocco, 2004). For example, Jackson and colleagues (2000) focus on more contemporary times, but still emphasize the role of close others in our attempts to self-regulate. They argue that individuals often look toward others within their social network for behavioral guidance, for confirmation of appropriate display of actions or emotions, and as a source for modeling appropriate behavior. Thus, whether the need to belong is embraced as a part of our ancestral heritage or presented as a more current concern, the perspective shared by all of these theorists represents self-regulation as a fundamentally interpersonal endeavor.

SOCIAL SENSITIVITY AND REGULATORY STRENGTH

The limited strength model of self-regulation, developed in recent years, provides a possible mechanism through which social pressures could enhance self-regulatory success (e.g., Baumeister, 2000; Baumeister & Heatherton, 1996; Baumeister, Heatherton, & Tice, 1994; Baumeister, Muraven, & Tice, 2000; Muraven & Baumeister, 2000). This model proposes that the human ability to self-regulate is a limited resource, a type of energy or strength that can be spent and exhausted. The expenditure of this limited resource is analogous to the use of physical energy and the exhaustion of muscles after exertion. When the resource is spent, a person is considered "depleted." Just as a person's arms may tire after carrying a series of heavy moving cartons up the stairs, making each successive burden heavier, a person's regulatory strength may be depleted after engaging in a series of self-control tasks, making subsequent self-control increasingly difficult. In a state of depletion a person is no longer able to effectively regulate him- or herself, and may lose inhibition or succumb to temptation.

Working from the assumption that self-regulatory failure is often the result of self-regulatory depletion, recent work has focused on understanding the nature of depletion. In this effort, researchers have manipulated self-regulatory exertion and examined the consequences of our intentional efforts to self-control. Findings indicate that being in a depleted state may lead people to react more negatively to their close relationship partners, responding to interpersonal conflict with less constructive, less accommodating behaviors (Finkel & Campbell, 2001). Likewise, depletion may lead to the greater use of stereotyping in our evaluations of others (Gordijn, Hindriks, Koomen, Dijksterhuis, & Van Knippenberg, 2004). Repeatedly, research has demonstrated that people are less persistent in pursuing their goals when they are depleted (e.g., Baumeister, Bratsklavsky, Muraven, & Tice, 1998; Muraven, Tice, & Baumeister, 1998; Vohs & Schmeichel, 2003). In short, findings suggest that the intentional exertion of self-control will rapidly lead to depletion of this resource and that depletion will lead to far-ranging negative consequences.

Importantly, one aspect of the limited strength model of self-regulation allows for a gradual increase in the strength of self-regulation; over time, engaging in self-regulation may ultimately improve our ability to self-control. Specifically, researchers have found that individuals who *practice* at self-control are able to improve their abilities (Muraven, Baumeister, & Tice, 1999). Rather than becoming depleted after each brief attempt to engage in self-control, people who have frequently and consistently engaged in self-regulation efforts may become less prone to depletion. In one study, participants who spent 2 weeks practicing a self-control exercise showed significant improvement in their general self-regulatory performance. In this experiment, participants' self-regulatory stamina was tested by asking them to squeeze a handgrip exerciser for as long as they could persist, a task primarily requiring self-regulatory exertion (e.g., Hejak, 1989; Rethlingshafer, 1942; Thornton, 1939). They were then asked to engage in 5 minutes of thought suppression, a task also shown to require self-regulatory exertion (e.g., Wegner, Schneider, Carter, & White, 1987), followed by another attempt to persist at the handgrip task. The difference in the time participants spent squeezing the handgrip at attempts 1 and 2 served as an initial measure of self-regulatory depletion. If the thought suppression task had significantly tapped their self-regulatory resources, participants would not have been able to persist at the increasingly irritating, painful handgrip task. To examine the effects of practice at self-regulation, participants then worked for 2 weeks to either constantly try to improve their posture or to keep a careful diary of all the food they had eaten. In a control condition, participants did not practice any self-regulatory exercises. At the end of this practice period, participants returned to the lab where their self-regulatory stamina was tested again. When their postpractice results were compared to their prepractice baseline results, researchers found that participants who had practiced at self-control did not show the customary decrease in the amount of time they could squeeze the handgrip. Only participants who had practiced self-control appeared to retain their self-regulatory stamina and avoided showing signs of self-regulatory depletion. Muraven and colleagues (1999) concluded that just as a series of exercises may ultimately build physical strength, repeated acts of self-control seem successful in building self-regulatory strength.

The strengthening of self-control through practice provides one pathway through which interpersonal relationships may influence self-regulation. One natural opportunity to "practice" self-control is in our daily interactions with others. As previously noted, self-control is thought to be a central component of successful social functioning (e.g., Heatherton & Vohs, 1998; Jackson et al., 2000). The research by Finkel and Campbell (2001) demonstrating the impact of regulatory depletion on responses to relationship partners illustrates just one way harmonious social relationships are maintained through self-control.

The fact that Finkel and Campbell's (2001) participants showed diminished constructive relationship behavior when depleted speaks to the natural engagement of self-control mechanisms in our social interactions. Of course, there are presumably individual differences in the engagement of socially motivated self-control efforts. Although, as Finkel and Campbell showed, most individuals would attempt to control their more selfish instincts in a conflict with a romantic partner, fewer may be apt to engage in such control for less important social relationships (e.g., with neighbors, coworkers, or acquaintances). Thus individual differences in social sensitivity, or the motivation to maintain harmonious social interactions, may be one important factor contributing to individual differences in the day-to-day exertion of self-control. After all, if one important impetus for self-regulation is social pressure, then individuals who are most sensitive to this pressure should engage in the most frequent self-regulation.

Sensitivity to social pressure may take a variety of forms. Although everyone is impacted by the approval and disapproval of others (Leary, Gallagher, & Fors, 2003), it is possible that some individuals may take greater notice of others' expectations, or be trained to respond to these expectations with greater accommodation. The desire to control oneself in order to respond appropriately to social cues may stem, among other things, from personality characteristics, cultural forces, recent social experiences, or even attachment style (e.g., Gaines et al., 1997; Markus & Kitayama, 1991; Pickett & Gardner, 2005; Singelis, 1994; Snyder, 1974). We recently explored two potential factors that may lead to socially induced practice at self-regulation: the collectivist worldview and the self-monitoring personality trait (Seeley & Gardner, 2003).

In comparison to more individualistic cultures, collectivist cultures place great emphasis on social harmony and concern for the welfare of the group (e.g., Markus & Kitayama, 1991). In order to maintain this harmony, it is important for individual members of society to know their role and to fulfill the obligations of that role. Children are taught about their place in relation to society and of the obligations they have to others (e.g., Wang & Leichtman, 2000; Yue & Ng, 1999). Likewise, collectivist cultures are more likely to promote the notion of obedience to parents, teachers, employers, and other authority figures (e.g., Buck, Newton, & Muramatsu, 1984; Hwang, 1977; Kashiwagi, 1986; Munroe & Munroe, 1975). In order to meet these various standards, we argued that members of collectivist cultures would need to engage in self-regulation far more often than members of individualistic cultures, where being "true to oneself" and "following one's own path" are highly valued characteristics (e.g., Markus & Kitayama, 1991). Indeed, self-control is considered fundamental to the development of the self in collectivist cultures (Sinha & Tripathi, 1996) and is a skill emphasized in parenting and early schooling (e.g., Julian, McKenry, & McKelvey, 1994; Kashiwagi, 1986). In collectivist cultures, learning to suppress personal desires is considered a sign of maturity (e.g., Markus & Kitayama, 1991).

Further evidence that practice at self-control may be more frequent in collectivist cultures is a meta-analytic review by Bond and Smith (1996). This meta-analysis established that collectivist cultures tend to show higher levels of conformity than individualistic cultures. In fact, the cultural difference was the largest found in their meta-analysis of conformity. In order to conform to cultural norms and standards, members of more collectivist cultures must, by definition, work to control their own behavior (see Kashiwagi, 1986). Over time, this repeated effort at self-control should lead to enhanced self-regulatory ability.

To more directly test this hypothesis, we recently compared undergraduates who had been raised in individualistic (the United States) and collectivist (various East Asian countries) cultures in their self-control abilities following a regulatory depletion task (Seeley & Gardner, 2003). In the depletion condition, participants performed a thought suppression task similar to that employed by Muraven and colleagues (1999). They were told to speak out loud into a tape recorder for 5 minutes about anything they wanted, but to suppress any thoughts they had of white bears. In the control condition, participants were provided the same instructions, but they were not encouraged to suppress thoughts of white bears. After the task, all participants were asked to squeeze a handgrip exerciser for as long as they could.

Results revealed the predicted pattern of self-regulatory performance for Asian and American students. The two groups held the handgrip for a similar number of seconds in the control condition. However, when the handgrip task was performed after suppressing thoughts of a white bear, Asian students performed significantly better than U. S. students. Additionally, in keeping with the pattern repeatedly found by Baumeister and colleagues (e.g., Baumeister, Muraven, & Tice, 1998), the U.S. students performed marginally worse in the suppression than in the control condition. The Asian students, who were expected to have had a greater history of practice at self-control, did not differ in the two conditions. In short, the suppression task appeared to cause self-regulatory depletion for the U.S. students, but not for the students raised in Asian cultures.

To further explore the impact of social sensitivity on self-regulatory performance, we examined participants' endorsement of collectivist values, as measured by the Singelis Self-Construal Scale (Singelis, 1994). We hoped to exploit differences in independent and interdependent self-construals, which have been shown to differ not only *across* cultures but also *within* cultures (e.g., Gardner, Gabriel, & Lee, 1999; Singelis, 1994; Triandis, 1996). Importantly, the Singelis Self-Construal Scale measures differences in self-construal that can be theoretically linked to the frequent conformity, obedience to authority, and accommodation to others that has been predicted to lead to greater self-regulatory ability. For example, items such as "I will sacrifice my self-interest for the benefit of the group I am in," "It is important for me to maintain harmony within my group," "I act the same way no matter who I am with" (reversed), and "I will stay in a group if they need me, even when I'm not happy with the group" are reflective of an interdependent self-construal, and of a highly controlled person. Not surprisingly, results revealed that regardless of the participant's culture of origin, those with more interdependent self-construals had an advantage when it came to self-regulatory stamina. Participants who endorsed items related to the frequent exercise of self-regulation performed better than participants with low endorsement of these items. Those low in interdependence performed significantly worse in the suppression condition than they did in the control condition. In contrast, participants high in collectivist orientation repeated the pattern suggested by the comparison of Asian and U.S. students. Highly interdependent participants' performance was unimpaired after the thought suppression task. In sum, we theorized that growing up in a collectivist culture or ascribing to the values of that culture would lead to more habitual efforts at self-control. In turn, we expected that over time these frequent efforts at self-control would lead to greater self-regulatory stamina. These predictions were supported by our preliminary work.

To provide further evidence that sensitivity to the concerns of others may play a defining role in the frequency with which we self-regulate, we sought a different measure of "social sensitivity." We reasoned that any social orientation that prompts chronic self-regulatory "practice" should produce the same pattern of results. Thus in a second study we selected another measure of social sensitivity, one devoid of cultural implications (Seeley & Gardner, 2003; Study 2). A desire to *directly* measure people's motivation to control their own behavior in social settings led us to the Other-Directedness component of Snyder's (1974) Self-Monitoring Scale (Briggs, Cheek, & Buss, 1980).[1] This component of the Self-Monitoring Scale assesses the extent to which people pay attention to their social environment. Moreover, the items directly measure the extent to which people are chronically motivated to control their behavior in order to get along with others and to behave in a socially appropriate fashion. Items from the Other-Directedness component of the Self-Monitoring Scale include "When I am uncertain how to act in social situations, I look to the behavior of others for cues" and "In order to get along and be liked, I tend to be what people expect me to be rather than anything else." If people are able to accurately reflect on their socially motivated efforts at self-regulation, then we should see greater self-regulatory stamina by those who report high levels of other-directed self-monitoring.

Indeed, to the extent that participants reported above-average concern with adapting their behavior to please others, we found greater self-regulatory stamina. Once again, we replicated the self-regulatory depletion effect of

Muraven and colleagues (1998) for individuals who were not socially moti-vated to self-regulate on a consistent basis. Utilizing the same method used in the cultural comparison study, we found that low other-directed individuals held the handgrip for less time in the suppression condition than in the con-trol condition. In contrast, the high other-directed individuals held the grip for roughly the same time in the control and in the suppression conditions. Thus participants who acknowledged regulating their behavior in response to the social cues around them did not show signs of self-regulatory depletion. These participants were able to complete two self-regulatory tasks without showing diminished ability to self-control. On the other hand, participants who reported a lesser likelihood of self-regulating in response to the concerns of others showed a sizable impairment when they were asked to exert self-control on two consecutive tasks. These participants showed adequate self-regulatory performance when they were rested, but when asked to exert self-control they quickly showed signs of depletion.

Although our original work was limited to the two mechanisms of social sensitivity mentioned above, these were only selected to serve as examples. One can imagine additional factors that should lead to the same results. Any mechanism that spurs frequent self-regulation in the pursuit of positive inter-personal relations should result in greater self-regulatory ability. For example, an extensive research literature suggests that people with relatively little power are more inclined to adapt to the perceived wishes of the powerful than vice versa. In one such study, Copeland (1994) randomly assigned participants to a high- or a low-power role and indicated that the high-power party would have the opportunity to select a partner for a potentially rewarding game. In introductory conversations between the two parties, the high-power partici-pants were more concerned with learning about their partners than the low-power participants, who were generally more concerned with facilitating favorable interactions. In this study, the low-power party's outcomes were contingent on the decisions of the more powerful party, leading the low-power party to be highly motivated to please the other person. In their recent review of the literature, Keltner, Gruenfeld, and Anderson (2003) identified this as a typical reaction for those whose outcomes will be determined by someone else. These authors provided an extensive review suggesting that the behavior of people in positions of low power is highly constrained. They asserted that those low in power are likely to attend to possible threats or pun-ishments in the environment, are likely to engage in controlled informa-tion processing, and are likely to inhibit their social behavior. Specifically, they note that low-power individuals inhibit their speech (Holtgraves & Lasky, 1999; Hosman, 1989), inhibit their emotional displays (Keltner, Young, Heerey, Oemig, & Monarch, 1998), curtail the expression of their opinions in public debate (e.g., Noelle-Neumann, 1991), and are less likely to behave in accordance with their self-reported internal states (Hecht & LaFrance, 1998).

In short, their review points to the conclusion that people who do not control their own outcomes tend to inhibit their automatic reactions and replace them with reactions deemed more suitable. We believe that this repeated effort at self-regulation should also, over time, lead to greater self-regulatory ability.

There are others who may be relatively practiced at self-control. As another example of interpersonally motivated efforts at self-control, we might consider those with secure attachment styles (see Hazan & Shaver, 1987). Individuals with a secure attachment style are those who are comfortable depending on others and who do not often worry about being abandoned or about others getting too close. In a study of close relationships, Gaines and colleagues (1997) established that individuals with secure attachment styles often respond to conflict in their relationships with self-regulation. Although all romantic relationship partners behave badly at times (see Finkel & Campbell, 2001), there is evidence that the response of the nonoffending partner plays a major role in the ultimate health of the relationship (e.g., Gottman, 1998). Whereas people's automatic and immediate response to the destructive behavior of a close relationship partner is likely the reciprocation of negative behavior (Yovetich & Rusbult, 1994), this response can be inhibited. Rather than responding to destructive behavior in kind, securely attached individuals are more likely than those with insecure attachment styles to "accommodate"—that is, to inhibit this negative response and replace it with a more constructive response. Although those with an anxious–ambivalent attachment style are highly relationship-oriented, perhaps to the point of being obsessed with their relationships, they are focused less on their relationship partner and his or her needs than on themselves. They may fixate on their fear of abandonment or their desire to feel love and closeness, rather than on their partner (e.g., Gaines et al., 1997). It is not surprising, then, that they are less likely than securely attached individuals to accommodate to their partners. Over time, the desire to maintain a healthy romantic relationship may lead to frequent self-regulation. This practice at self-control should translate into enhanced self-regulatory ability.

Based on the assertion that self-regulation is fundamentally driven by our desire for social approval (e.g., Heatherton & Vohs, 1998), we have outlined a number of possible mechanisms through which self-regulation may be practiced and enhanced. Ultimately, this "social sensitivity" is more than a mere acknowledgment of the judgment of others: It is a desire (or a need) to control oneself to better achieve interpersonal goals. The examples we have provided are only for illustration. It is easy to imagine others. Chronic dieters may become practiced at self-regulation in an effort to appear more attractive to others (Kahan, Polivy, & Herman, 2003) and regimented athletes may become practiced at self-regulation in an effort to outperform the competition. In theory, any endeavor that drives a person to control his or her own behavior on a chronic basis should result in an increasing ability to self-regulate.

ACCOUNTABILITY TO OTHERS:
A STRATEGY FOR SUCCESSFUL SELF-REGULATION

We have argued that self-regulation may have evolved as an interpersonal process; the desire to please others and to be accepted by important groups may be the catalyst for a majority of our attempts to self-regulate (see Heatherton & Vohs, 1998). We have demonstrated that those who are more sensitive to this social pressure will engage in greater daily efforts at self-control, and that this practice will lead to better self-regulatory ability (see Seeley & Gardner, 2003). Finally, we would argue that there are often situations in which an individual is able to exploit the experience of social pressure to achieve his or her own self-regulatory aims.

A few years ago one of us (W. L. G.) decided to quit smoking. She immediately told her spouse, family, friends, and coworkers of the decision she had made and the "quit date" she had selected. Indeed, she even mentioned her quitting smoking to the neighbors she was friendly with in her building, the acquaintances she frequently chatted with at the gym, and the staff she saw daily at the neighborhood coffee shop. The end result of all of this disclosure was an invisible but powerful network of public accountability. Short of traveling to a distant locale (which was considered, longingly, on more than one occasion), there was now nowhere she might "sneak" a cigarette without being seen by someone who knew of her goal to quit.

Utilizing self-disclosure in this way may be a strategy for some people to improve their self-regulatory stamina. It is highly taxing to attempt to thwart our habitual impulses and replace them with carefully selected alternatives (e.g., replacing cigarettes with gum, cookies with carrots, or hours on the sofa with miles on a treadmill). As we have reviewed, even brief exertions of self-control may leave many people depleted (e.g., Baumeister & Heatherton, 1996). Although we have established that "socially sensitive" individuals may have stronger self-regulatory stamina, their resources are not limitless. Presumably, they should show the same patterns of self-regulatory depletion when their resources are spent. To avoid this depletion, it is possible that socially oriented individuals may make themselves accountable to close others. This accountability may enhance assistance with the goal, motivation for achieving the goal, and even enhance self-regulatory resources through removing the perception of choice.

Confiding one's self-regulatory goals to another person increases the likelihood of assistance in future situations requiring self-regulation. In the most straightforward context, a person might tell a close other, "I am on a diet. Please don't let me have any of those cookies," thereby initiating a direct relationship of accountability. If the person later appears ready to give in to the temptation of the plate of cookies, the confidant is expected to respond. Thus, when close others are informed of our goals, they may at times make self-regulation easier through the physical removal of temptation (e.g., removing the cookies) or through a verbal reminder of the goal.

However, even when a person has not explicitly asked for his or her confidant's direct assistance in self-regulating, we believe that simply disclosing the goal provides psychological assistance through the feeling of accountability. Failing to self-regulate in front of important others may engender feelings of embarrassment or even shame about disappointing one's audience. Indeed, disclosure of a self-regulatory goal may institute a type of "psychological contract." A *psychological contract* is an individual's belief about the terms and conditions of an agreement with another person, a belief that some form of promise has been made and that the terms are accepted by both parties. By confiding self-regulatory goals to friends, family, or coworkers, a person may feel as if he or she has made a promise to another person and may feel a greater sense of obligation to meet those goals. Thus people who have shared their self-regulatory goals with others should feel more pressure to succeed at those goals.

Feeling accountable to others may thus increase a person's motivation to succeed at his or her self-regulatory goals. This motivation may be strongest for people who are socially sensitive. People who are particularly attuned to the expectations of others and who work hardest to meet those expectations should be highly motivated to self-regulate when they are feeling accountable. Research supports this assertion. First, the belief that one may be required to justify actions to others often results in aligning actions with the expectations of others (e.g., Tetlock, 1983; Tetlock, Skitka, & Boettger, 1989). In particular, when a person feels accountable to an audience whose views are known, the most likely response is a shift in attitudes or behaviors in the direction of that audience (see Lerner & Tetlock, 1999). Importantly, Quinn and Schlenker (2002) established that it is the goal of getting along with others that leads people to conform to audiences with known views. When people do not have this goal, they do not conform. When people are particularly socially sensitive, this pressure may be acute. For instance, people who score high in self-monitoring (Snyder, 1974) score low in individuation (Maslach, Stapp, & Santee, 1985), and those who score high in social anxiety show a greater tendency to conform to the expectations and views of a prospective audience than do their less socially oriented counterparts (e.g., Brockner, Rubin, & Lang, 1981; Chen, Shecter, & Chaiken, 1996; Maslach, Santee, & Wade, 1987; Turner, 1977). The common tendency for people to conform when they are feeling accountable thus appears to be heightened in individuals who are socially oriented.

Confiding in close others should help a potential self-regulator manage the expectations of his or her presumed audience. For instance, a wife's announcement that she is going to join her husband at the gym each morning will create that expectation in her spouse. What was once only her personal self-regulatory goal becomes a tacit interpersonal agreement that the couple will exercise together each morning. The social pressure to meet her husband's expectation is, by her own doing, added pressure to achieve her own self-regulatory goals. By adding a layer of accountability, however, this socially sensitive wife should feel more motivated to accomplish her fitness goals. The strategy of confiding our goals to others when we are experiencing a moment of conviction should help us sustain our motivation when we experience moments of weakness. In summary, we expect that confiding in close others will lead to feelings of accountability, which will only heighten the pressure that socially sensitive individuals may already feel. Whereas they are already more motivated to self-regulate in order to meet others' expectations, accountability should serve to enhance this motivation.

Of course, as a strategy for successful self-regulation, increasing one's motivation may be an excellent approach. To the extent that socially oriented individuals are aware of this fact on some level, they may use self-disclosure as a strategy for increasing their adherence to self-regulatory goals. By increasing his or her motivation, a person should have greater success at self-regulation. Recent research demonstrates that individuals with greater motivation to complete a task are better able to avoid the effects of self-regulatory depletion. For example, Muraven and Slessareva (2003) induced a state of self-regulatory depletion in half of their participants. Those participants who had been motivated by the experimenter (e.g., they were told that the research was important) performed as well on the subsequent task as participants who had not been depleted. Thus motivation appears to be a crucial component of effective self-regulation. Maintaining sufficient levels of motivation should be a primary goal in any self-regulatory regimen. In sum, if self-disclosure increases accountability, then accountability should increase the motivation to succeed at self-regulatory goals, particularly for those who are socially sensitive. Motivation has been directly linked to success at self-regulation.

Over time, the benefits of making oneself accountable may accrue. The repeated pairing of a close relationship partner and a specific self-regulatory goal may create a link between the constructs. Eventually, the mere psychological presence of the relationship partner may trigger interpersonal goals that are then pursued nonconsciously (Fitzsimons & Bargh, 2003). In several studies, Fitzsimons and Bargh (2003) demonstrated that priming participants with thoughts of close others produced goal-directed behavior in line with the goals associated with those relationships. In short, thoughts of relationship partners should increase our motivation to pursue our self-regulatory goals without requiring conscious intention or control.

Enhanced motivation alone may allow people to persist at self-regulation when they might otherwise desist. However, confiding in others may have an additional benefit for self-regulators. Confiding a self-regulatory goal to a friend, family member, or colleague may change the regulatory focus of that goal. Regulatory focus theory outlines the fundamental differences that may exist between different types of goals (Higgins, 1997). Whereas a *promotion-focused goal* is driven by a desire for accomplishment or growth, and is focused on hopes, ideals, and aspirations, a *prevention-focused goal* is driven by a desire for safety and security. Prevention-focused goals are driven by a sense of duty, obligation, and "ought," and are generally viewed as necessities whose attainment is immediately required. In contrast, promotion-focused goals are often viewed as less pressing (Freitas, Liberman, Salovey, & Higgins, 2002; Shah, Friedman, & Kruglanski, 2002; Shah & Higgins, 1997). Confiding one's self-regulatory goal to close others may shift the nature of that goal from something one would ideally like to accomplish to something that one feels obligated to accomplish. In other words, accountability may shift a goal from a promotion focus to a prevention focus, increasing the sense that that goal is a necessity and its attainment required.

Framing one's goals as prevention-focused may help stave off self-regulatory depletion. In a fascinating series of studies, Shah, Friedman, and Kruglanski (2002) demonstrated that focusing on an important goal tends to inhibit the accessibility of competing goals. Their "goal-shielding theory" posits that we have overlearned this strategy to the point that is it automatically applied without conscious awareness. Thus, if a person's focal goal is to finish writing a paper, any goals that might diminish the chances of accomplishing that goal (by competing for time, attention, or self-regulatory resources) will be inhibited. Notably, these researchers found that regulatory focus is an important moderator of this effect. The more that goals were seen as duties or obligations (i.e., prevention-focused), the more they inhibited their alternatives. In contrast, the more that goals were seen as aspirations or ideals (i.e., promotion-focused), the less they inhibited their alternatives. Likewise, greater inhibition of competing goals was related to better performance at participants' focal goals. When participants were freed from the distraction of their competing goals, they were better able to persist at their focal goals and to succeed at those goals.

Inhibiting alternative goals allows a person to attend more closely to his or her focal goal. If confiding one's goals to another person increases the extent to which a goal is viewed in a prevention-focused frame, it should increase the extent to which the focus on that goal inhibits its alternatives. A prevention-focused frame may assist the self-regulatory effort in that fewer self-regulatory resources may be required by this approach. Although the inhibition of alternative goals is done automatically and nonconsciously (requiring few regulatory resources), the distraction of competing goals may require significant resources to overcome. Avoiding those goals that have not been successfully inhibited should require greater self-regulatory effort. Thus, to the extent that alternative goals have been automatically inhibited, self-regulators should have more resources to commit to their focal self-regulatory project. Viewing his or her goals in a prevention-focused frame should improve a person's self-regulatory stamina. When fewer resources are expended in a self-regulatory attempt, less depletion should result.

Finally, whether breaking an old habit or creating a new one, self-regulatory goals consist of a series of daily choices (e.g., cookie or carrot, TV or treadmill). However, because feelings of accountability to others may make people feel more constrained in their behavior, it may remove the perception of choice. If a person is truly concerned about the repercussions his or her actions may have on his or her relationships or social standing, he or she may feel that he or she has less choice about whether to persist at his or her focal self-regulatory goal. Instead, he or she may feel obligated to follow through. In essence, the die is cast; the person curtailed his or her ability to choose when he or she opted to share his or her self-regulatory goal with someone else. With his or her actions relatively predetermined, this person will need to expend less energy deciding how to behave.

The benefit of feeling such behavioral constraint is that making choices is in itself depleting. When a person works to make a decision, he or she uses self-regulatory energy (e.g., Baumeister et al., 1998; Kahan et al., 2003; Vohs et al., 2005). Researchers have repeatedly found that people asked to make a series of choices show subsequent declines in self-regulatory performance—the same as those seen after other types of self-regulatory exertion. Because making choices is depleting, feeling the pressures of accountability may help a person to avoid these depleting effects. People feeling accountable may engage in less rigorous decision making, simply acceding to the presumed wishes of their audience. For example, in a decision-making context, people who are accountable to an audience with known views tend to think in less self-critical and less integratively complex ways (Tetlock, 1983; Tetlock et al., 1989). Importantly, they also consider fewer perspectives on the issue under consideration and make fewer attempts to try to anticipate the objections that others might raise to positions that they might take (Tetlock, 1983; Tetlock et al., 1989). When people know what others expect of them, they appear to engage in less rigorous contemplation of issues. This less intensive decision-making process should lead to less self-regulatory depletion. In essence, facing a refrigerator stocked with both cookies and carrots when a dieter is alone may require a difficult and depleting choice, but when in the presence of an audience (even a private audience; see Baldwin & Holmes, 1987) who knows the dieter's goals, there may be no perception of a choice at all—one simply takes the carrot.

CONCLUSION

The current chapter has discussed several means through which interpersonal relationships both permeate and moderate the intrapersonal process of self-control and the likelihood of success of self-regulatory endeavors. Much of the work reviewed here presents initial explorations of the impact of social relationships upon self-regulatory processes. Despite its early stages, we believe research at the intersection of these two areas has the potential to illuminate how people typically engage in self-regulatory pursuits. The folk wisdom of thinking of your family to resist temptation, expressed on the dieting website at the opening of this chapter, appears to be supported on both theoretical and empirical grounds. At least for some individuals, a focus on others heightens self-regulatory success.

NOTE

1. The remaining two subscales of the Self-Monitoring Scale measure, Acting (e.g., "I would probably make a good actor") and Extraversion (e.g., "In a group of people I am rarely the center of attention" [reversed]), did not address our theoretical interest in socially motivated attempts at self-control.

REFERENCES

Baldwin, M. W., & Holmes, J. G. (1987). Salient private audiences and awareness of the self. *Journal of Personality and Social Psychology, 52,* 1087–1098.

Baumeister, R. F. (1998). The self. In D. T. Gilbert & S. T. Fiske (Eds.), *The handbook of social psychology* (Vol. 1, pp. 680–740). Boston: McGraw-Hill.

Baumeister, R. F. (2000). Ego depletion and the self's executive function. In A. Tesser & R. B. Felson (Eds.), *Psychological perspectives on self and identity* (pp. 9–33). Washington, DC: American Psychological Association.

Baumeister, R. F., Bratslavsky, E., Muraven, M., & Tice, D. M. (1998). Ego depletion: Is the active self a limited resource? *Journal of Personality and Social Psychology, 74,* 1252–1265.

Baumeister, R. F., & Heatherton, T. F. (1996). Self-regulation failure: An overview. *Psychological Inquiry, 7,* 1–15.

Baumeister, R. F., Heatherton, T. F., & Tice, D. M. (1994). *Losing control: How and why people fail at self-regulation.* San Diego, CA: Academic Press.

Baumeister, R. F., & Leary, M. R. (1995). The need to belong: Desire for interpersonal attachments as a fundamental human motivation. *Psychological Bulletin, 117,* 497–529.

Baumeister, R. F., Muraven, M., & Tice, D. M. (2000). Ego depletion: A resource model of volition, self-regulation, and controlled processing. *Social Cognition, 18,* 130–150.

Bond, R., & Smith, P. B. (1996). Culture and conformity: A meta-analysis of studies using Asch's (1952b, 1956) line judgment task. *Psychological Bulletin, 119,* 111–137.

Briggs, S. R., Cheek, J. M., & Buss, A. H. (1980). An analysis of the Self-Monitoring Scale. *Journal of Personality and Social Psychology, 38,* 679–686.

Brockner, J., Rubin, J. Z., & Lang, E. (1981). Face-saving and entrapment. *Journal of Experimental Social Psychology, 17,* 68–79.

Buck, E. B., Newton, B. J., & Muramatsu, Y. (1984). Independence and obedience in the U.S. and Japan. *International Journal of Intercultural Relations, 8,* 279–300.

Caporael, L. R. (1997). The evolution of truly social cognition: The core configurations model. *Personality and Social Psychology Review, 1,* 276–298.

Chen, S., Shecter, D., & Chaiken, S. (1996). Getting at the truth or getting along: Accuracy- versus impression-motivated heuristic and systematic processing. *Journal of Personality and Social Psychology, 71,* 262–275.

Copeland, J. T. (1994). Prophecies of power: Motivational implications of social power for behavioral confirmation. *Journal of Personality and Social Psychology, 67,* 264–277.

Finkel, E. J., & Campbell, W. K. (2001). Self-control and accommodation in close relationships: An interdependence analysis. *Journal of Personality and Social Psychology, 81,* 263–277.

Fitzsimons, G. M., & Bargh, J. A. (2003). Thinking of you: Nonconscious pursuit of interpersonal goals associated with relationship partners. *Journal of Personality and Social Psychology, 84,* 148–163.

Freitas, A. L., Liberman, N., Salovey, P., & Higgins, E. T. (2002). When to begin?: Regulatory focus and initiating goal pursuit. *Personality and Social Psychology Bulletin, 28,* 121–130.

Freud, S. (1961). The ego and the id. In J. Strachey (Ed. & Trans.), *The standard edition of the complete works of Sigmund Freud* (Vol. 19, pp. 3–66). London: Hogarth Press. (Original work published 1923)

Gaines, S. O. Jr., Reis, H. T., Summers, S., Rusbult, C. E., Cox, C. L., Wexler, M. O., et al. (1997). Impact of attachment style on reactions to accommodative dilemmas in close relationships. *Personal Relationships, 4,* 93–113.

Gardner, W. L., Gabriel, S., & Lee, A. Y. (1999). "I" value freedom, but "we" value relationships: Self-construal priming mirrors cultural differences in judgment. *Psychological Science, 10,* 321–326.

Gardner, W. L., Pickett, C. L., & Brewer, M. B. (2000). Social exclusion and selective memory: How the need to belong influences memory for social events. *Personality and Social Psychology Bulletin, 26,* 486–496.

Gordijn, E. H., Hindriks, I., Koomen, W., Dijksterhuis, A., & Van Knippenberg, A. (2004). Consequences of stereotype suppression and internal suppression motivation. *Personality and Social Psychology Bulletin, 30,* 212–224.

Gottman, J. M. (1998). Psychology and the study of marital processes. *Annual Review of Psychology, 49,* 169–197.

Hazan, C., & Shaver, P. (1987). Romantic love conceptualized as an attachment process. *Journal of Personality and Social Psychology, 52,* 511–524.

Heatherton, T. F., & Vohs, K. D. (1998). Why is it so difficult to inhibit behavior? *Psychological Inquiry, 9,* 212–216.

Hecht, M., & LaFrance, M. (1998). License or obligation to smile: The effect of power and sex on amount and type of smiling. *Personality and Social Psychology Bulletin, 24,* 1332–1342.

Hejak, P. (1989). Breath holding and success in stopping smoking: What does breath holding measure? *International Journal of the Addictions, 24,* 633–639.

Higgins, E. T. (1997). Beyond pleasure and pain. *American Psychologist, 52,* 1280–1300.

Holtgraves, T., & Lasky, B. (1999). Linguistic power and persuasion. *Journal of Language and Social Psychology, 18,* 196–205.

Hosman, L. A. (1989). The evaluative consequences of hedges, hesitations, and intensifiers: Powerful and powerless speech styles. *Human Communication Research, 15,* 383–406.

Hwang, C.-H. (1977). Filial piety from the psychological point of view. *Bulletin of Educational Psychology, 10,* 11–20.

Jackson, T., Mackenzie, J., & Hobfoll, S. E. (2000). Communal aspects of self-regulation. In M. Boekaerts & P. R. Pintrich (Eds.), *Handbook of self-regulation* (pp. 275–300). San Diego, CA: Academic Press.

Julian, T. W., McKenry, P. C., & McKelvey, M. W. (1994). Cultural variations in parenting: Perceptions of Caucasian, African-American, Hispanic, and Asian-American parents. *Family Relations: Interdisciplinary Journal of Applied Family Studies, 43,* 30–37.

Kahan, D., Polivy, J., & Herman, C. P. (2003). Conformity and dietary disinhibition: A test of the ego-strength model of self-regulation. *International Journal of Eating Disorders, 33,* 165–171.

Kashiwagi, K. (1986). Development of self-regulations. *Japanese Psychological Review, 29,* 3–24.

Keltner, D., Gruenfeld, D. H., & Anderson, C. (2003). Power, approach, and inhibition. *Psychological Review, 110,* 265–284.

Keltner, D., Young, R. C., Heerey, E. A., Oemig, C., & Monarch, N. D. (1998). Teasing in hierarchical and intimate relations. *Journal of Personality and Social Psychology, 75,* 1231–1247.

Leary, M. R., Gallagher, B., & Fors, E. (2003). The invalidity of disclaimers about the effects of social feedback on self-esteem. *Personality and Social Psychology Bulletin, 29,* 623–636.

Lemonick, M. D. (2004, June 7). How we grew so big. *Time,* pp. 58–64.

Lerner, J. S., & Tetlock, P. E. (1999). Accounting for the effects of accountability. *Psychological Bulletin, 125,* 255–275.

Markus, H. R., & Kitayama, S. (1991). Culture and the self: Implications for cognition, emotion, and motivation. *Psychological Review, 98,* 224–253.

Maslach, C., Santee, R. T., & Wade, C. (1987). Individuation, gender role, and dissent: Personality mediators of situational forces. *Journal of Personality and Social Psychology, 53,* 1088–1093.

Maslach, C., Stapp, J., & Santee, R. T. (1985). Individuation: Conceptual analysis and assessment. *Journal of Personality and Social Psychology, 49,* 729–738.

Munroe, R. L., & Munroe, R. H. (1975). Levels of obedience among U.S. and East African children on an experimental task. *Journal of Cross-Cultural Psychology, 6,* 498–503.

Muraven, M., & Baumeister, R. F. (2000). Self-regulation and depletion of limited resources: Does self-control resemble a muscle? *Psychological Bulletin, 126,* 247–259.

Muraven, M., Baumeister, R. F., & Tice, D. M. (1999). Longitudinal improvement in self-regulation through practice: Building self-control strength through repeated exercise. *Journal of Social Psychology, 139,* 446–457.

Muraven, M., & Slessareva, E. (2003). Mechanisms of self-control failure: Motivation and limited resources. *Personality and Social Psychology Bulletin, 29,* 894–906.

Muraven, M., Tice, D. M., & Baumeister, R. F. (1998). Self-control as a limited resource: Regulatory depletion patterns. *Journal of Personality and Social Psychology, 74,* 774–789.

Noelle-Neumann, E. (1991). The theory of public opinion: The concept of the spiral of silence. In J. A. Anderson (Ed.), *Communication yearbook* (pp. 256–308). Thousand Oaks, CA: Sage.

Pickett, C. L., & Gardner, W. L. (in press). The social monitoring system: Enhanced sensitivity to social cues and information as an adaptive response to social exclusion and belonging need. In K. Williams, J. Forgas, & W. von Hippel (Eds.) *The social outcast: Ostracism, rejection, social exclusion and bullying.* New York: Psychology Press.

Quinn, A., & Schlenker, B. R. (2002). Can accountability produce independence?: Goals as determinants of the impact of accountability on conformity. *Personality and Social Psychology Bulletin, 28,* 472–483.

Rethlingshafer, D. (1942). Relationship of tests of persistence to other measures of continuance of activities. *Journal of Abnormal Social Psychology, 37,* 71–82.

Seeley, E. A., & Gardner, W. L. (2003). The "selfless" and self-regulation: The role of chronic other-orientation in averting self-regulatory depletion. *Self and Identity, 2,* 103–117.

Shah, J. Y., Friedman, R., & Kruglanski, A. W. (2002). Forgetting all else: On the antecedents and consequences of goal shielding. *Journal of Personality and Social Psychology, 83,* 1261–1280.

Shah, J., & Higgins, E. T. (1997). Expectancy × value effects: Regulatory focus as determinant of magnitude and direction. *Journal of Personality and Social Psychology, 73,* 447–458.

Singelis, T. M. (1994). The measurement of independent and interdependent self-construals. *Personality and Social Psychology Bulletin, 20,* 580–591.

Sinha, D., & Tripathi, R. C. (1996). Individualism in a collectivist culture: A case of coexistence of opposites. In K. Uichol & H. C. Triandis (Eds.), *Individualism and collectivism: Theory, method and applications. Cross-cultural research and methodology series* (pp. 123–136). Thousand Oaks, CA: Sage.

Snyder, M. (1974). Self-monitoring of expressive behavior. *Journal of Personality and Social Psychology, 30,* 526–537.

Tetlock, P. E. (1983). Accountability and complexity of thought. *Journal of Personality and Social Psychology, 45,* 74–83.

Tetlock, P. E., Skitka, L., & Boettger, R. (1989). Social and cognitive strategies for coping with accountability: Conformity, complexity, and bolstering. *Journal of Personality and Social Psychology, 57,* 632–640.

Thornton, G. R. (1939). A factor analysis of tests designed to measure persistence. *Psychological Monographs, 51,* 1–42.

Triandis, H. C. (1996). Theoretical and methodological approaches to the study of collectivism and individualism. In U. Kim, H. C. Triandis, C. Kagitcibasi, S.-C. Choi, & G. Yoon (Eds.), *Individualism and collectivism: Theory, method, and applications* (pp. 41–51). Thousand Oaks, CA: Sage.

Turner, R. G. (1977). Self-consciousness and anticipatory belief change. *Personality and Social Psychology Bulletin, 3,* 438–441.

Vohs, K. D., Baumeister, R. F., Twenge, J. M., Schmeichel, B. J., Tice, D. M., & Crocker, J. (2005). *Decision fatigue exhausts self-regulatory resources—But so does accommodating to unchosen alternatives.* Unpublished manuscript, University of Minnesota.

Vohs, K. D., & Ciarocco, N. J. (2004). Interpersonal functioning requires self-regulation. In R. F. Baumeister & K. D. Vohs (Eds.), *Handbook of self-regulation* (pp. 392–407). New York: Guilford Press.

Vohs, K. D., & Schmeichel, B. J. (2003). Self-regulation and the extended now: Controlling the self alters the subjective experience of time. *Journal of Personality and Social Psychology, 85,* 217–230.

Wang, Q., & Leichtman, M. D. (2000). Same beginnings, different stories: A comparison of American and Chinese children's narratives. *Child Development, 71,* 1329–1346.

Wegner, D. M., Schneider, D., Carter, S. R., & White, T. L. (1987). Paradoxical effects of thought suppression. *Journal of Personality and Social Psychology, 55,* 5–13.

Williams, K. D. (2001). *Ostracism: The power of silence.* New York: Guilford Press.

Yovetich, N. A., & Rusbult, C. E. (1994). Accommodative behavior in close relationships: Exploring transformation of motivation. *Journal of Experimental Social Psychology, 30,* 138–164.

Yue, X., & Ng, S. H. (1999). Filial obligations and expectations in China: Current views from young and old people in Beijing. *Asian Journal of Social Psychology, 2,* 215–226.

Index